CELL PROLIFERATION, CANCER, AND CANCER THERAPY

A CONFERENCE IN HONOR OF
ANNA GOLDFEDER

ANNALS OF THE NEW YORK ACADEMY OF SCIENCES

Volume 397

CELL PROLIFERATION, CANCER, AND CANCER THERAPY
A CONFERENCE IN HONOR OF ANNA GOLDFEDER

Edited by Renato Baserga

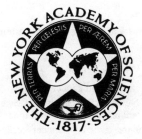

The New York Academy of Sciences
New York, New York
1982

Library of Congress Cataloging in Publication Data

Main entry under title:

Cell proliferation, cancer, and cancer therapy.
  (Annals of the New York Academy of Sciences; v. 397)
  Includes bibliographical references and index.
    1. Cancer—Congresses. 2. Cancer cells—Congresses.
3. Cell proliferation—Congresses. I. Goldfeder, Anna. II.
Baserga, Renato. III. Series. [DNLM: 1. Cell division
—Congresses. 2. Medical oncology—Congresses. 3.
Neoplasms—Therapy—Congresses. W1 AN626YL v. 397
/ QZ 266 C393 1982]

Q11.N5 vol. 397 [RC261]   500s [616.99'4]   82-19073
ISBN 0-89766-184-2
ISBN 0-89766-185-0 (pbk.)

PCP
Printed in the United States of America
ISBN 0-89766-184-2 (cloth)
ISBN 0-89766-185-0 (paper)

ANNALS OF THE NEW YORK ACADEMY OF SCIENCES

VOLUME 397

December 10, 1982

CELL PROLIFERATION, CANCER, AND CANCER THERAPY: A CONFERENCE IN HONOR OF ANNA GOLDFEDER *

Editor
RENATO BASERGA

———◆———

CONTENTS

* This volume is the result of a conference entitled Cell Proliferation, Cancer, and Cancer Therapy, held on February 17–19, 1982 by The New York Academy of Sciences.

Financial assistance was received from:

- AMERICAN CANCER SOCIETY (GRANT NO. RD-132)
- BURROUGHS WELLCOME CO.
- DOW CHEMICAL CO.
- E. I. DU PONT DE NEMOURS & COMPANY
- HOFFMANN-LA ROCHE, INC.
- LEDERLE LABORATORIES
- MC NEIL PHARMACEUTICAL
- NATIONAL CANCER INSTITUTE, NATIONAL INSTITUTES OF HEALTH
- NEWPORT PHARMACEUTICALS INTERNATIONAL, INC.
- SCHERING CORPORATION
- SMITH KLINE & FRENCH LABORATORIES
- THE UPJOHN COMPANY
- WARNER-LAMBERT COMPANY
- WYETH LABORATORIES

A TRIBUTE TO ANNA GOLDFEDER

Sol   Spiegelman

*Comprehensive Cancer Center and
Institute of Cancer Research
Columbia University
New York, New York 10032*

The truly extraordinary story of Anna Goldfeder started at a most unlikely time and in an even more improbable place. Over 80 years ago a child was born to Jewish parents in the Polish town of Lublin. This infant was destined to become the internationally renowned cancer researcher whom we know today as Dr. Anna Goldfeder. The religious, political and antifeminist barriers that had to be surmounted in those days to achieve this goal staggers the imagination, and yet the goal was attained.

After finishing the Gymnasium she matriculated in 1918 at two of the major universities of Europe, Charles University and the German University in Prague. Anna received her D.Sc. Degree in the natural sciences in 1923. At that time she was offered and accepted a position in the newly organized Masaryk University, in Brno, Czechoslovakia, where she worked in the Department of Pathology and the Institute of Physiology. She also pursued the preclinical medical courses for which she received the MUC (Medicine Universal Candidate) degree.

Anna was introduced to and became attracted to the cancer problem as a result of a stay at the University of Vienna in the Department of Pathology, headed by Dr. Carl Sternberg. From that time on, understanding the cancer problem became and remained the principal goal of her professional efforts. In making this early decision, Anna Goldfeder illustrated the fearless courage that was uniquely characteristic of this woman's life and work. She was warned by Professor Sternberg that cancer research has ruined many more reputations than it has ever made. The reasons for this are inherent in the very nature of the scientific enterprise. Most recognized advances are made by those who succeed in isolating and reducing a problem of nature to the status of a puzzle. Compared with a problem, a puzzle has two useful features. One is the guaranteed existence of a unique solution. The second is that a mechanism is usually available for arriving at the required answer. Thus, when the solution is found, the achievement is readily apparent to all. Under the circumstances, it is not surprising that talented investigators often avoid problems and focus on puzzles. There are, however, problems of such obvious importance to mankind that one cannot wait until they are converted into puzzles. Cancer is one of these problems, where solutions in a unique sense may not even exist, but where partial advances can improve diagnosis or treatment long before a full understanding is achieved. Such gains are difficult to identify and are rarely recognized. It takes the courage of an Anna Goldfeder to make an early commitment to this kind of research.

As a result of her interest and work on the cancer problem, she received an invitation in 1931 to continue her cancer research in the United States, where she remained. She continued to expand her technical expertise in

ix

various laboratory disciplines such as tissue culture, the application of radioactive isotopes, electron microscopy and immunogenetics.

I should like to note briefly just a few of her contributions to provide at least a slight indication of her originality and foresight. (1) Anna Goldfeder was one of the first to succeed in establishing tissue culture with human epithelial cells—an achievement made even more monumental by the fact that it was accomplished prior to the introduction of antibiotics. (2) She was one of the first to identify the importance of ensuring isogenicity of the host in attempting to obtain useful therapeutic and biological information from tumor transplants. (3) Anna established the therapeutic value of fractionated and localized radiation in treating tumors and showed that cures could in fact be obtained using animal models. These results had a significant impact on the design of protocols for clinical radiotherapy. (4) She developed the famous XgF strain of mice, which were highly resistant to spontaneous as well as to induced tumors. These mice became a useful experimental tool for the analysis of questions related to both the cure and cause of cancer.

In 1940, during the reign of Mayor Fiorello H. LaGuardia, Dr. Goldfeder was appointed to a newly created civil service position in the Department of Hospitals of the City of New York, as a principal research scientist in cancer research, and Director of the Cancer and Radiobiology Research Laboratory. This laboratory was established at the newly built Frances Delafield Hospital, a cancer hospital affiliated with the Columbia-Presbyterian Medical Center. Subsequently, a wing of this hospital was added to house the Institute for Cancer Research of the Columbia College of Physicians & Surgeons.

I made my first personal contact with Dr. Goldfeder when I assumed the directorship of the Institute of Cancer Research in 1969. Soon after my arrival, an incident occurred that I kept quiet about then and that I believe I never communicated to Dr. Goldfeder. I received a letter from the then Commissioner of Public Health of New York City saying essentially the following:

Dear Dr. Spiegelman—I would like your advice on a matter of some concern to me. It has come to my attention that a Dr. Anna Goldfeder is on our payroll and doing cancer research supported by funds from the City. The problem is that she is well beyond mandatory retirement. I would deeply appreciate it if you would let me know if her work is of such importance as to warrant retaining her on the payroll despite the fact that this is clearly illegal.

When I received this letter, two facts were clear to me. One was that at all costs I must avoid any kind of dialogue with this individual on whether or not Dr. Goldfeder's work was of such importance as to warrant breaking the law. This was an argument that I was not likely to win with a public official. The second thing I was sure of was that the survival time of Dr. Goldfeder was quite a bit longer than that of a Commissioner of Public Health in New York City. Consequently, I decided that the simplest and safest thing for me to do was to ignore the letter and allow the Commissioner to disappear, which is precisely what happened. Within a year he was gone and the whole issue vanished along with any threats to Dr. Goldfeder's continued activity. Of course this was not a permanent solution, for the crisis reappeared several years later when the city decided to close Delafield Hospital. This meant of course that we had to relocate the Institute, a problem solved by the construction of the Hammer Health Sciences Building. We could, and did, help Dr. Goldfeder in the care and housing of her mouse colony, but the resolution of the question of her laboratory space was more difficult. She was negotiating to move her laboratory to New York University. However, this took some time. In the interval, she had to hang on to the physical facilities in the defunct Delafield Hospital, even though it was closed for at least two years. Ultimately she managed to solve the problem.

In this connection, I would like to quote an illuminating account that appeared in the "About New York" column of *The New York Times* in early 1977, written by Francis X. Clines, a perceptive and compassionate reporter. The subtitle of the article was "Waiting for a Benefactor," and Mr. Clines describes a visit to Dr. Goldfeder's laboratory in the empty Delafield Hospital:

> There is harmonica music from the watchman's radio sounding through the empty building that was once-busy Delafield Hospital, and downstairs 80-year-old Dr. Anna Goldfeder will not give up her five decades with the mice and mysteries of cancer research.
>
> She bought space heaters to keep her mice alive through the empty winter of the deserted hospital. And even after the city cut off her budget, she managed enough of a Federal grant to keep a lab staff of three going through the routine of her various cancer research experiments.
>
> This unseen effort in the tomblike hospital gets at the essence of all problems, survival. Survival on the physical level of studying the floridly living death of carcinoma, and on the spirit level of the woman's fight to keep her long life of special intelligence moving forward.
>
> Moving away from the harmonica music, very proud in her white smock and very precise in her accented discourse, the small woman seems like a finely wrought antimacassar glinting in the dimness of a shuttered mansion. Her heels click in the corridors. In a walk with a stranger to her lab, views of the Hudson cut brilliantly into the corridor dimness of the waterfront building at 164th Street and Fort Washington Avenue.
>
> "I'm waiting for a benefactor," she says and the remark is not as hopelessly Pinteresque as it sounds. For while Delafield has been turned into a warehouse in the two years since it closed, Dr. Goldfeder will not be stored away. She has a promise of space from New York University, but needs renovation money, about $60,000, to set up all the cages, microscopes and radiation equipment. "I need money—I would put an appropriate memorial plaque on my new office, of course."
>
> Downstairs, the remaining mice look healthy except for the ones with tiny carefully measured cancers about them. A man washes test tubes. A student peers through a microscope. Everyone is quiet. The X-ray machine looks worn and tired from years of silently burning out life pieces.
>
> The doctor tracks everything. An autobiographical essay she published last year in Cancer Research had 64 footnotes of documentation of the various phases of her career in a field of diabolical frustrations. "Unfortunately, in cancer research the tendency is to reach a point where you think you have something but then find you can't go forward."
>
> So 50 years can amount to valuable threads in an unfinished fabric. Her latest thread seems particularly cherished because it takes Dr. Goldfeder full cycle from her undergraduate, magna cum laude days in Prague, where her devotion to science was first spun from curiosity about the basic growth, structure and metabolism of the cell.
>
> "This is the mystery of life itself," Dr. Goldfeder says in outlining her current isotope research into the kinetics of cellular growth.

Money seems only slightly less a mystery and life force for a cancer scientist. She recalls the richer days of former Mayor Fiorello H. LaGuardia when any self-respecting branch of government wanted its own separate cancer-research institute, and she became a principal in the city's own. While she no longer has the city budget line, she still has the title of director of the city's Cancer and Radiobiological Research Laboratory, this forgotten outpost at Delafield. For years, the city post gave her Civil Service protection and a salary. That plus helpful grants from the National Cancer Institute helped her get this far, to the point of fighting to go farther.

"You can't throw living animals in the Hudson," she says of her loss of city financing. "So I stand up and say you can't throw me out." But the city seems to be simply passing her by silently, in its own metabolic ague.

In her resistance, among the first to be protected were thousands of creatures designated X/Gf mice. This is an albino strain the doctor developed for research that are exceptionally free of spontaneous cancers and so provide a reliable test subject for certain needs. She found a home for this research stock at Columbia University, but only a temporary home, she emphasizes, until that benefactor cuts through the gloom at Delafield.

Dr. Goldfeder stays scientific when she discusses herself, offering facts the way she holds the mice—briefly by the tail, between thumb and index finger while she quickly sweeps the underbelly for salient information. As a girl she was proud when the teacher offered several problems to solve and she chose the most difficult. As an old woman, she regrets giving up the violin and her weekly ticket to the opera, but she had to cut back and lives alone directly across from the hospital.

Friends die and it is sad, and she feels "humiliated" moreover, when cancer is the cause and she cannot help them. She goes to the lab mostly seven days a week and the watchman sees her safely across the street. Clearly it is everything. "I am grateful to nature," she says. But more life, if you please. "I always felt life was like a big wave. You either keep swimming or sink to the bottom."

On the way out, there is rock music on the watchman's radio, and the doctor brushes off questions about how many more decades of cancer research will be needed. She repeats that she is willing to put up a plaque for that benefactor. [© 1977 by The New York Times Company. Reprinted by permission.]

I would like to supplement Francis Clines' moving description with some verse I wrote in tribute to Anna and to others like her who live lives that sing praises to the wonder of our universe and thus add honor to the human condition:

THE GENTLE GIANTS

There are the gentle giants
Who walk softly through our lives.

No shrill demand for early recognition
Commands our attentive admiration.

No blinding glare of brilliance
Announces their presence amongst us.

They are the quietly courageous ones
Who plant for future generations.

They are the creators and searchers
Who teach and celebrate the truth.

THE REGULATION OF CELL PROLIFERATION BY SERUM GROWTH FACTORS

W. J. Pledger, P. H. Howe, and E. B. Leof

*Department of Pharmacology and the Cancer Research Center
University of North Carolina School of Medicine
Chapel Hill, North Carolina 27514*

Platelet-derived growth factor (PDGF) is the mitogenic activity in serum that stimulates the cellular proliferation of density-arrested fibroblast cultures.[1, 2] It has been purified to homogeneity.[3, 4] PDGF is a cationic polypeptide that is stored in the α-granules of platelets.[5] When blood clots, PDGF is released into the serum. Pure PDGF has been shown to bind to fibroblast cells, apparently to a specific PDGF receptor.[6] PDGF induces the initial event in the growth response of density-arrested BALB/c-3T3 fibroblast cells by rendering them competent to respond to a second set of growth factors derived from platelet-poor plasma.[7, 8] The second set of factors is required for competent cells to undergo progression through the cell cycle.

The growth of normal fibroblast cell populations at sparse cell density is dependent on PDGF.[9] Nontransformed fibroblasts grow in serum-supplemented medium, but not in medium supplemented with platelet-poor plasma. Addition of PDGF to plasma-supplemented medium allows normal growth parameters. Transformed cells (spontaneous, viral, or chemical transformants) grow in medium supplemented with platelet-poor plasma. Not only did transformation alter the cellular requirement for PDGF, but infection with SV40 also was demonstrated to alter the plasma requirements necessary for progression.[10]

The G_0/G_1 portion of the cell cycle contains important biochemical regulatory events necessary for proper control of cellular growth. PDGF-treated competent cells in plasma-supplemented medium have a minimum G_1 lag time of 12 hours before the initiation of DNA synthesis.[7] Two plasma-dependent arrest points have been described within this portion of the cell cycle.[8] Other reports of sequential control events in G_0/G_1 have been published that demonstrate multiple serum factors acting at different times affecting the regulation of cell cycle traverse.[11] Clearly, the growth control mechanisms regulated by serum growth factors should be delineated in order to understand normal growth control and how transformation arises.

Little is understood about the mechanism of action of PDGF. Smith and Stiles have demonstrated that the competence state can be transferred from a PDGF-treated donor cell to an untreated recipient cell.[12] This transfer was apparently dependent on a cytoplastic factor(s). The acquisition of competence was temperature-dependent, but was not dependent on nutrients.[7, 13]

The treatment of density-arrested BALB/c-3T3 cells with PDGF rapidly stimulated the preferential synthesis of several cytoplasmic proteins (molecular weights 29,000 to 70,000).[14] The induction of one of these proteins (molecular weight 29,000), termed pI, was shown to be dependent on the concentration of PDGF. The synthesis of pI was shown to be induced by pure PDGF and fibroblast growth factor (FGF), but the synthesis of pI was not induced by platelet-poor plasma, insulin, or epidermal growth factor (EGF). The increase in the amount of pI synthesized in response to PDGF was related to the percent

1

0077–8923/82/0397–0001 $1.75/0

of the cell population rendered competent. We have now investigated the induction of the synthesis of pI by PDGF in density-arrested BALB/c-3T3 cells in relationship to unique phases of the cell cycle. The synthesis of pI is apparently a G_0 specific event: only cells in G_0 could be induced to synthesize pI by PDGF.

The delineation of the mechanism whereby a cell is rendered competent is important; however, the mechanisms by which plasma-derived factors control progression through G_1 and entry into S phase are equally important. In order to investigate how growth factors regulate the progression of competent cells and bring about commitment of DNA synthesis, the necessary plasma-derived factors and their sites of action in progression must be elucidated. These types of studies will provide a distinct advantage compared to similar types of studies that employed serum to obtain traverse of the cell cycle. We have shown that epidermal growth factor (EGF) and somatomedin C can be employed as a substitute for plasma to regulate progression of unique areas of G_0/G_1.[15] The growth factor requirements for distinct portions of the G_0/G_1 phase have now been determined.

PDGF-INDUCED PREFERENTIAL PROTEIN SYNTHESIS

Since PDGF initiates the proliferation of density-inhibited BALB/c-3T3 cells and plasma does not, we have developed a strategy to investigate biochemical events specific for the initiation of the cell cycle. Biochemical processes induced by PDGF but not by plasma may be unique, necessary prerequisites for the stimulation of growth. This allows the study of events induced by the serum growth mitogen, PDGF, while employing the other nonmitogenic serum component, platelet-poor plasma, as a control. Specific plasma factors such as EGF, insulin, and somatomedin C can also be used to compare with cellular responses to PDGF. This experimental approach was used to determine that PDGF induced the synthesis of unique proteins that may be involved in competence formation and the initiation of cell proliferation.

Density-inhibited BALB/c-3T3 cells were transferred to prewarmed (37° C) Dulbecco's modified Eagle's medium containing 2.5% of the standard methionine concentrations. Some cultures contained highly purified PDGF, while other cultures received medium supplemented with 5% plasma and no PDGF. The highly purified PDGF was obtained from heat-treated platelet extracts that had been chromatographed on CM Sephadex® and Bio-Gel® P150.[3] The cultures were incubated for various times and then given 30–50 μCi of [35S] methionine (Amersham) per ml. Incubation continued for 20 minutes, at which time the cells were collected, washed, and suspended in reticulocyte saline buffer (0.01 M NaCL, 0.01 M Tris HCl, 0.015 M MgCl$_2$, pH 7.4) containing 1% Nonidet P-40. The nuclei were removed by centrifugation. Samples were heated at 100° C with 1% sodium dodecyl sulfate and α-mercaptoethanol. Equal amounts of incorporated counts were applied to 6–18% exponential gradients of polyacrylamide, electrophoresed,[16] and processed for fluorography.[17] The exposure of cells to PDGF brought about the preferential synthesis of at least five proteins whose synthesis was not stimulated by plasma (FIG. 1).

As seen in FIGURE 1, at the earliest time tested, 1.5 hours, a 29 K protein (pI) was preferentially induced by PDGF. The synthesis of pI was induced by pure PDGF and FGF, but not plasma or EGF.[14] Two-dimensional polyacrylamide gel electrophoresis confirmed the PDGF induction of the preferential synthesis of pI.[14]

Our studies suggested that the pI was the first preferentially synthesized protein that we could observe following exposure of density-arrested BALB/c-3T3 cells to PDGF. In order to further investigate the time required for PDGF to bring about the synthesis of pI, cultures of quiescent cells were incubated with [35S] methionine following 20, 40, and 60 minutes of exposure to PDGF. After incubation with the radiolabeled methionine, cells were processed and

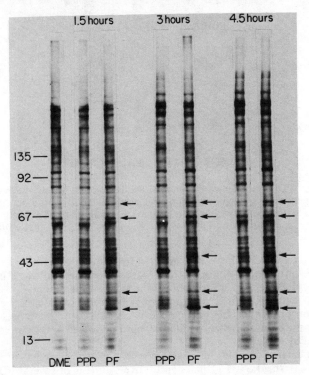

FIGURE 1. PDGF stimulates selective synthesis of five cytoplasmic proteins.[14] Density-inhibited BALB/c-3T3 cells were transferred to incorporation medium alone (DME) or medium supplemented with either dialyzed PPP at 5% or partially purified PDGF (PF) at 25 μg/ml. At the indicated times, [35S]methionine was added, and 20 min later the cultures were harvested for gel electrophoresis. The arrows indicate proteins that were preferentially synthesized in response to PDGF. The positions of molecular weight markers ($M_r \times 10^3$) are shown.

electrophoretic profiles were obtained on 15% polyacrylamide gels. The pI protein was visible after only 40 minutes' exposure of the density-arrested cells to PDGF (FIG. 2).

When RNA synthesis was inhibited, PDGF did not induce the pI protein. Cultures of density-arrested cells were treated with actinomycin D (5 μg/ml) for 30 minutes to inhibit greater than 95% of the RNA synthesis. These cultures were then transferred to medium containing PDGF. Some cultures, not

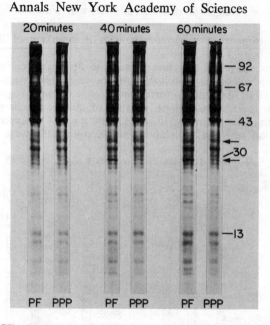

FIGURE 2. PDGF stimulates preferential synthesis of pI within 40 min.[14] Density-arrested cells were treated with partially purified PDGF (PF) at 25 μg/ml or 5% PPP for the indicated times prior to the addition of [^{35}S] methionine. Ten minutes later the cultures were harvested. The arrow indicates the position of pI.

receiving actinomycin D, were transferred to medium containing either plasma or PDGF. At various times the cells were incubated with [^{35}S]methionine. Cells were processed for electrophoresis on 15% polyacrylamide gels. FIGURE 3 shows that cultures treated with actinomycin D did not synthesize detectable amounts of pI. Other inhibitors of RNA synthesis, camptothecin and 5,6-dichloro-β-D-ribofuranosylbenzimidazole, also inhibited induction of the synthesis of pI by PDGF.

It is of interest to point out that a spontaneous transformant of the BALB/c-3T3 cells (termed ST3T3) had constitutive synthesis of several PDGF-modulated proteins, including pI.[14] The ST3T3 cells were shown to have lost the growth requirement for PDGF. ST3T3 cells grew in medium containing only plasma. It is important to point out that these transformed cells had lost the PDGF requirement, normal growth control, and they synthesized pI in a constitutive manner (in plasma- or PDGF-supplemented medium and in unsupplemented medium).

PDGF-INDUCED pI SYNTHESIS DURING EARLY G$_1$

The induction of the synthesis of pI was of particular interest because pI was the first protein that we could detect preferentially synthesized after the exposure of quiescent cell populations to PDGF. The period of time was studied in which pI was synthesized after density-arrested cells were stimulated to initiate DNA synthesis with fresh medium containing PDGF and plasma.

Density-arrested cells were changed to medium containing a low methionine concentration with 10 μg/ml PDGF and 10% plasma. At various times cultures were incubated with [^{35}S] methionine for 20 minutes. The cells were collected and processed for polyacrylamide gel electrophoresis. In these experiments we estimated the approximate amount of label in the pI band by estimating densities of autoradiograms using densitometer tracings. TABLE 1 shows that pI was maximally synthesized for approximately 4 hours after the cells were stimulated in the medium containing PDGF and plasma. Cells incubated in this medium for more than 6 hours did not preferentially synthesize pI as compared to cultures treated with plasma-supplemented medium. During the course of this experiment, plasma did not induce the synthesis of pI. These results were not a result of an inadequate supply of PDGF because addition of more PDGF at 6 hours after stimulation did not bring about further synthesis of the pI protein.

The G_0/G_1 minimum lag time has been shown to be 12 hours in plasma-supplemented medium. Pledger *et al.*[8] had described two plasma-dependent arrest points within the G_0/G_1 phase. One of these arrest points, termed the "V" point, preceded DNA synthesis by 6 hours. Stiles *et al.*[13] demonstrated a nutrient arrest point, brought about by stimulating density-inhibited cells in medium deficient in amino acids, that also arrested progression 6 hours prior to the S phase. In addition to showing growth arrest in medium deficient in

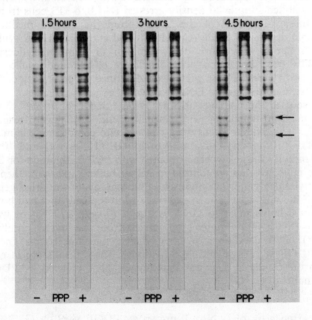

FIGURE 3. Actinomycin D inhibits PDGF-stimulated pI and pII synthesis.[14] Density-inhibited cells were treated with 25 μg/ml of partially purified PDGF (+ and −) or 5% PPP for the indicated times prior to addition of [^{35}S]methionine. The cultures were harvested 20 min later. Some PDGF-treated cultures (+) were incubated with actinomycin D at 5 μg/ml for 30 min prior to growth factor addition, whereas other PDGF-treated cultures (−) received no actinomycin D. Plasma-treated cultures received no actinomycin D. The arrows indicate pI (*below*) and pII (*above*).

TABLE 1

PREFERENTIAL SYNTHESIS OF pI AFTER STIMULATION OF QUIESCENT
BALB/c-3T3 CELLS WITH PDGF AND PLASMA

Culture Condition	Time after Stimulation (hr)				
	2	4	6	8	10
PPP	1.0	0.9	1.1	1.2	0.8
PDGF + PPP	7.5	7.9	2.1	0.9	1.1

NOTE: Density-inhibited Balb/c-3T3 cells were transferred to medium with low methionine and 10 μg/ml PDGF with 10% plasma (PPP). Other cultures received medium with only 10% plasma. At the indicated times, cells were incubated with [^{35}S] methionine for 20 min and were then processed for polyacrylamide electrophoresis. Data are given as fold increase of pI compared to pI at 2 hours in plasma-supplemented medium.

amino acids, recently Leof et al.[18] have also shown that elevated intracellular cyclic AMP levels produced by cholera toxin and isobutylmethylxanthine (IBMX) inhibited stimulated density-arrested BALB/c-3T3 cells from initiating DNA synthesis. Removal of the IBMX from the culture medium brought about a rapid decline in cyclic AMP levels and entry into DNA synthesis after a lag of 6 hours. Therefore, the inhibition of stimulated density-arrested BALB/c-3T3 cells by amino acid deficiency or elevated cyclic AMP may produce growth arrest at the previously described V point, a location in mid G_0/G_1 phase, 6 hours prior to DNA synthesis.

We have used the methods of Stiles et al.[13] and Leof et al.[18] to arrest cells due to amino acid deficiency and elevated cyclic AMP levels, respectively, at mid G_0/G_1. The inhibited cells were released into complete medium containing either PDGF (10 μg/ml), 10% PPP or PDGF (10 μg/ml) and 10% plasma. After 120 minutes the cells were incubated with [^{35}S] methionine for 20 minutes. Cells were collected and solubilized in NP40 buffer, and were then processed for polyacrylamide gel electrophoresis. Fluorograms of the dried gels indicated that PDGF did not induce the synthesis of pI in the cells that had been arrested at the point 6 hours prior to DNA synthesis (TABLE 2). No pI was induced at 30, 120, 180 or 600 minutes after release from the mid G_1 inhibition (data not shown). Both conditions of arrest yielded the same results: no induction of pI by PDGF in cells at mid G_0/G_1 phase. These results are in good agreement with the results in TABLE 1 that suggest pI is induced by PDGF during the first 6 hours of G_0/G_1.

SYNTHESIS OF pI IS NOT INDUCED BY PDGF IN S OR G_2 PHASE

Density-inhibited BALB/c-3T3 cells stimulated to initiate proliferation by exposure to PDGF and then transferred to medium containing plasma and 100 nM methotrexate were "growth-arrested" in early S phase.[19] Once these inhibited cells were removed from the medium containing methotrexate and placed in medium containing plasma, 106 nM hypoxanthine and 10 nM thymidine, they continued through the cell cycle. Scher et al.[19] have shown that such cells do not initiate another cycle of proliferation after they undergo cell division. However, treatment of the S phase or G_2 phase cells with a transient exposure to PDGF stimulates the cells to enter another cycle of cell proliferation. Therefore, these investigators concluded that PDGF produced a memory effect on the premitotic cells that the postmitotic daughter cells remembered and to which they responded by reinitiating the cell cycle.

Density-inhibited quiescent BALB/c-3T3 cells were stimulated for 18 hours with PDGF and PPP in medium containing methotrexate. These cells were released from the methotrexate inhibition into medium containing hypoxanthine, thymidine, and a low concentration of methionine. Some culture received medium that contained either PDGF or plasma, or PDGF and plasma. At various times after release from the methotrexate inhibition the cells were incubated with [^{35}S] methionine for 20 minutes. Cells were processed for polyacrylamide gel electrophoresis. TABLE 3 shows that no new synthesis of pI was observed in any of the conditions for as long as 20 hours after release from early S phase inhibition. The addition of fresh PDGF to cells incubated in plasma-containing medium at the times indicated in TABLE 3 also did not bring about the appearance of pI synthesis.

Our data suggest that pI was induced after response to PDGF within the first 6 hours of the G_0/G_1 phase. Apparently this synthesis occurs only in quiescent cells that require a 12-hour G_0/G_1 lag time before DNA synthesis. Scher *et al.*[19] have also shown that cells that undergo cell division in plasma-supplemented medium and receive PDGF within 8 hours have a minimum G_1 lag time of only 6 hours. This 6-hour G_1 time is in agreement with the time for G_1 traverse in growing cells. If PDGF is added after 8 hours post cell division a 12-hour G_0/G_1 lag is obtained before DNA synthesis begins. Cells that had undergone division, but apparently were not arrested in G_0 such that a required 12-hour G_0/G_1 lag time was required, did not synthesize pI in response to PDGF. Our preliminary data suggested that once pI was synthesized and the cells were placed in plasma-supplemented medium to allow progression,

TABLE 2

pI Is Not Induced at Mid G_1

Condition of Arrest	(Hours prior to S phase)	Increase in pI Synthesis		
		Plasma	PDGF	PDGF & Plasma
Density inhibition	12	1.0	6.7	6.2
Amino acid deficiency	6	0.9	1.0	1.0
Elevated cyclic AMP (cholera toxin and IBMX)	6	1.0	1.1	1.0

NOTE: PDGF-rendered competent density-arrested Balb/c-3T3 cells were arrested during the progression of G_0/G_1 by the methods of Stiles[13] and Leof.[18] The cells were released from arrest as described and placed into medium containing low methionine and supplemented as indicated. After incubation for 120 min, the cells were then incubated with [^{35}S] methionine. Data are expressed as fold increase in pI synthesis as in TABLE 1.

TABLE 3

SYNTHESIS OF pI IS NOT INDUCED IN S PHASE OR G$_2$

Culture Conditions after MTX Removal	Time after MTX Removal (hr)						
	1	3	5	8	10	15	20
PPP	1.0	0.9	1.1	0.8	1.2	0.9	1.0
PDGF	1.0	0.8	1.2	0.9	1.1	1.0	0.9
PDGF and plasma	0.9	1.0	1.1	0.6	1.0	0.9	0.0
PDGF added to cells in PPP at indicated times	0.9	0.0	0.9	1.0	1.2	0.9	1.1

NOTE: Density-inhibited Balb/c-3T3 cells were stimulated with PDGF (15 μg/ml) and 10% plasma in medium containing 100 nM methotrexate. After incubation for 16–20 hours, cells were washed and placed in medium containing 106 nM hypoxanthine, 16 nM thymidine, and 10% plasma or 10% PPP with PDGF (20 μg/ml). Other cultures received only PDGF. Some cultures transferred to medium containing plasma received 30 μg/ml PDGF at the indicated times with an additional 1.5 hours' incubation. At the indicated times, the cultures received [^{35}S] methionine and were processed for electrophoresis. Control values for density-inhibited cells that were placed in medium with either plasma or PDGF for a 2-hour incubation before labeling gave values of 1.0 (plasma) and 8.5 (PDGF). Data are given as fold increase when compared to cells in plasma medium for 2 hours as in TABLE 1.

the pI remains in the cell for 10–12 hours. After competent cells begin progression and as long as the cells are continuously cycling with PDGF present, the synthesis of pI may not be required. One possible explanation is that other proteins (pII–pV) or other cellular components made in response to PDGF can be synthesized once pI has been synthesized. The continued synthesis of one or more secondary PDGF-induced proteins may be required for continuous cell cycling and may also be involved in the inhibition of the synthesis of pI. Therefore, the pI protein would only be synthesized in cells that are quiescent and in G$_0$, with a 12-hour lag before DNA synthesis.

PLASMA FACTOR REQUIREMENTS FOR THE PROGRESSION OF COMPETENT CELLS

The stimulation of density-arrested BALB/c-3T3 cells to initiate DNA synthesis is controlled by two different sets of serum factors. Cells are first rendered competent by exposure to PDGF, a serum component derived from platelets. The progression of competent cells through the G$_0$/G$_1$ phase is controlled by serum factors derived from platelet-poor plasma. The 12-hour plasma-controlled progression of G$_0$/G$_1$ has two plasma-controlled arrest points. One of these points, V, bisects the midpoint of G$_0$/G$_1$ and precedes the S phase by 6 hours. The other point, W, immediately precedes S phase and is thought to be the point at which commitment to DNA synthesis occurs.

Recently, Leof *et al.* have shown that epidermal growth factor (EGF) and somatomedin C (SmC) can replace plasma in allowing competent cells to enter

DNA synthesis. Leof *et al.*[15] have also reported that only somatomedin C was required for the progression of the last 6 hours of G_0/G_1 and commitment to DNA synthesis. We have used temporal exposures of various combinations of EGF and Sm C to PDGF-rendered competent cells to determine how far into G_0/G_1 the various factors allowed progression to continue. Temporal location in the cell cycle was determined by the entry time into S phase after addition of 5% plasma to the competent cells that were incubated in medium supplemented with limiting variations of EGF and SmC.

When density-inhibited BALB/c-3T3 cells were made competent by a transient exposure to PDGF and then incubated in an optimal concentration of EGF (5–20 ng/ml) for 12 hours, these cells had not progressed into G_0/G. When plasma was added to the cells in the EGF-containing medium, the cells required 12 hours before the population began to enter S phase. However, the addition of optimal EGF (5–20 ng/ml) with suboptimal somatomedin C (0.25–0.75 ng/ml) to the competent cells allowed partial progression through G_0/G_1. Even though this condition did not allow entry into S phase, when plasma was added only a 6-hour lag was observed before entry into S phase began. The suboptimal concentration of SmC also did not allow competent cells to progress into G_0/G_1. Using these data we have constructed a schematic diagram to illustrate the time in G_0/G_1 required for the various progression factors to be present in culture medium (FIG. 4). The specific G_0/G_1 period for specific factor requirements agreed with previously described plasma-controlled G_0/G_1 divisions.

CONCLUSIONS

Platelet-derived growth factor induced a unique state—termed competence—in density-arrested fibroblasts. The competent state may be the result of unique proteins whose synthesis was induced by PDGF. One of these proteins, induced by PDGF, had a molecular weight of 29,000. The synthesis of this protein, pI, required RNA synthesis and appeared within 40 minutes after density-arrested cells were placed in PDGF-containing medium. The pI appeared in fact to be a protein whose synthesis was unique to cells that are quiescent in the G_0 state. Therefore, the synthesis of this protein may be required for G_0 cells to become competent and enter the cell cycle.

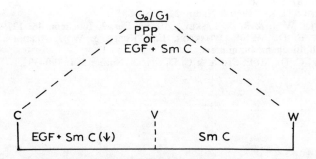

FIGURE 4. Schematic illustration of the EGF and somatomedin C requirements for the progression of competent cells during portions of G_0/G_1.

We have also shown that EGF and somatomedin C can substitute for plasma in allowing competent cells to enter DNA synthesis. EGF was required only during the first 6 hours of the G_0/G_1 phase. This is not to say that the biological effect of EGF was not required for the entire G_0/G_1 phase. While suboptimal concentrations of SmC were required during the first 6 hours of G_0/G_1, only SmC (at optimal concentrations of 5–20 ng/ml) was required during the last 6 hours of G_0/G_1 and commitment to DNA synthesis.

REFERENCES

1. Ross, R., B. Glomset, B. Karuja & L. Harker. 1974. Proc. Natl. Acad. Sci. USA **71:** 1207–1210.
2. Kohler, N. & A. Lipton. 1974. Exp. Cell Res. **87:** 297–301.
3. Antoniades, H. N., C. D. Scher & C. D. Stiles. 1979. Proc. Natl. Acad. Sci. USA **76:** 1809–1813.
4. Heldin, C. H., B. Westermark & A. Wasteson. 1970. Proc. Natl. Acad. Sci. USA 00: 3722–3726.
5. Kaplan, D. R., F. C. Chao, C. D. Stiles, H. N. Antoniades & C. D. Scher. 1979. Blood
6. Heldin, C. H., B. Westermark & A. Wasteson. 1981. Proc. Natl. Acad. Sci. USA **78:** 3664–3668.
7. Pledger, W. J., C. D. Stiles, H. N. Antoniades & C. D. Scher. 1977. Proc. Natl. Acad. Sci. USA **74:** 4481–4484.
8. Pledger, W. J., C. D. Stiles, H. N. Antoniades & C. D. Scher. 1978. Proc. Natl. Acad. Sci. USA **75:** 2839–2843.
9. Scher, C. D., W. J. Pledger, P. Martin, H. N. Antoniades & C. D. Stiles. 1978. J. Cell. Physiol. **97:** 371–380.
10. Stiles, C. D., G. T. Capone, C. D. Scher, H. N. Antoniades, J. J. Van Wyk & W. J. Pledger. 1979. Proc. Natl. Acad. Sci. USA **76:** 1279–1283.
11. Jimenez de Asua, L. 1980. *In* Control Mechanisms in Animal Cells. L. Jimenez de Asua, R. Levi-Montalcini, R. Shields & S. Iacobelle, Eds.: 173–198. Raven Press. New York, NY.
12. Smith, J. C. & C. D. Stiles. 1981. Proc. Natl. Acad. Sci. USA **78:** 4363–4367.
13. Stiles, C. D., R. R. Isberg, W. J. Pledger, H. N. Antoniades & C. D. Scher. 1979. J. Cell. Physiol. **99:** 395–406.
14. Pledger, W. J., C. A. Hart, K. L. Locatell & C. D. Scher. 1981. Proc. Natl. Acad. Sci. USA **78:** 4358–4362.
15. Leof, E. B., W. Wharton, J. J. Van Wyk & W. J. Pledger. 1980. J. Cell. Biol. **87:** 5 (abstract).
16. Laemmli, U. K. 1970. Nature **227:** 680–685.
17. Bonner, W. J. & R. A. Laskey. 1974. Eur. J. Biochem. **46:** 1279–1283.
18. Leof, E. D., W. W. Wharton, E. O'Keefe & W. J. Pledger. 1982. J. Cell. Biochem. 19: in press.
19. Scher, C. D., M. E. Stone & C. D. Stiles. Nature **281:** 390–392.

EPIDERMAL GROWTH FACTOR *

Graham Carpenter, Christa M. Stoscheck, and
Ann Mangelsdorf Soderquist

Department of Biochemistry
Vanderbilt University School of Medicine
Nashville, Tennessee 37232

Epidermal growth factor (EGF) is a small polypeptide (molecular weight 6000) that stimulates the proliferation of the epidermis and several internal epithelial tissues *in vivo*.[1] Also, the growth factor enhances the carcinogenic potential of methylcholanthrene on animal skin.[2] In cell culture systems EGF stimulates the growth of a variety of different cell types.[1] The EGF-mediated growth stimulation of cultured human fibroblasts is accompanied by decreased sensitivity to density-dependent inhibition of growth[3] and a decreased dependence on extracellular serum[4] and calcium[5] concentrations. Although these changes are reminiscent of the behavior of transformed cells in culture, EGF does not appear to induce the transformed phenotype, particularly since anchorage-dependent growth is not abrogated by the growth factor.

Recent studies of EGF have centered on its mechanism of action and have begun to yield biochemical details of the mechanisms by which growth-regulating characteristics may be altered by an extracellular mitogenic signal.

INTERACTION OF EGF WITH INTACT CELLS

Studies with ^{125}I-labeled EGF established the presence of specific, high-affinity receptor molecules on the surface of responsive cell types.[1] The formation of hormone:receptor complexes at the cell surface is followed by the internalization of these complexes and the degradation of ^{125}I-EGF. This pathway is illustrated in FIGURE 1. There are sufficient experimental data to support steps 1 through 10, which depict: step 1, the binding of EGF to surface receptors[6]; steps 2 and 3, the clustering of EGF:receptor complexes on the surface[7]; steps 4 and 5, the internalization of the complexes in endocytotic vesicles[7,8]; steps 6 to 8, the fusion of these vesicles with multivesicular bodies, presumably lysosomes[7,8]; and step 9, the extensive degradation of EGF within the lysosome[6-8]. When the fate of cell-bound ^{125}I-EGF is determined, the only degradation product to be found is ^{125}I-labeled monoiodotyrosine, which rapidly appears in the media (step 10).[6] Because the iodine tracer may selectively label a particular portion of the polypeptide molecule, we cannot be sure that all of the growth factor is degraded to the level of free amino acids. It is possible that small fragments that do not contain iodinated tyrosine residues are generated in this process and somehow pass into the cytoplasm. Also, it is not

* The authors were supported by research Grants CA24071 from the National Cancer Institute (G.C.) and BC–294A from the American Cancer Society (G.C.) and by Fellowships HD–07043 (C.S.) and CA09313 (A.M.S.) from the United States Public Health Service. G.C. is the recipient of an Established Investigator Award from the American Heart Association.

11

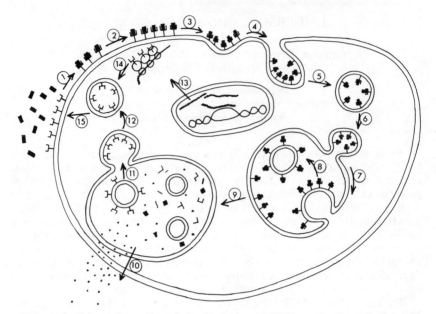

FIGURE 1. Schematic outline of the formation of EGF:receptor complexes on the surface of intact cells and the intracellular metabolism of the cell-bound complexes.

clear whether the internalization and/or degradation steps have a significant or critical role in the mechanism by which EGF produces a mitogenic response.

In regard to the fate of internalized EGF receptors, as shown in FIGURE 1, there is no direct information to date to substantiate the possible recycling of internalized receptor molecules (steps 12 and 15). Nor is there a good understanding of whether the receptors are degraded as is the growth factor. The data of Das and Fox,[9] however, indicate that at least a small percentage (approximately 2%) of the internalized receptors are degraded to products of 37,000 to 62,000 daltons.

Little is known of the mechanism of receptor biosynthesis (steps 13 to 15) or what role receptor biosynthesis may play in the mitogenic process if, in fact, internalized receptors are degraded and not recycled.

Binding of EGF to its surface receptors is required for the stimulation of DNA synthesis in quiescent cells, and several studies [3, 10] have shown that the interaction between free EGF in the media and cell surface receptors must take place for a relatively long period of time, greater than 6 hours, before a significant number of cells are committed to enter the S phase of the cell cycle. This time period is considerably longer than the time (1 hour) required to achieve maximal binding. In view of the lengthy requirement of persistent EGF: receptor interactions at the cell surface, it seems reasonable to investigate plasma-membrane-localized biochemical responses to the formation of EGF: receptor complexes, which may be of significance in elucidating the mechanism by which a mitogenic response is produced by EGF.

BIOCHEMISTRY OF CELL PROLIFERATION

Understanding the primary biochemical changes elicited by EGF binding to membrane receptors is a task that requires a system amenable to biochemical analysis. The intact cell is a poor system with which to attempt this sort of analysis, and therefore a suitable subcellular system was sought. The cell-free system has many advantages from a biochemical point of view, but does have the disadvantage that it is not always possible to extrapolate the biochemical response measured *in vitro* to the biological response *in vivo*. An additional difficulty to be expected in a hormonal system is that regulatory reactions may be difficult to detect because of the relatively small number of hormone:receptor complexes formed, the high association constants involved, and the rapidity with which responses may occur.

The discovery by Fabricant *et al.*[11] that a human epidermoid carcinoma cell line, designated A-431, bound large quantities of ^{125}I-EGF was an important step in finding a responsive system to study EGF action *in vitro*. These cells contain approximately 2×10^6 receptors for EGF per cell—nearly 20-fold more than other cell lines such as 3T3 or human fibroblasts.[12] Carpenter *et al.*[13] prepared membranes from these cells and found that the membrane preparations retained the capacity to bind high quantities of ^{125}I-EGF—approximately 16 picomoles of growth factor were bound per milligram of membrane protein. The binding was specific for EGF and rapid, with binding equilibrium attained after 5 minutes at 0° or 25° (FIGURE 2).

Since protein phosphorylation is known to occur in membranes and since some hormonal mechanisms are known to involve protein phosphorylation systems (mostly of the cyclic-nucleotide-dependent variety), the A-431 subcellular membrane preparations were assayed for protein kinase activity in the presence and absence of EGF. The data shown in FIGURE 3 demonstrate that when the membranes were preincubated for 10 minutes with EGF and then [γ-^{32}P]ATP was added, there was a three-fold increase in the transfer of labeled phosphate to endogenous membrane proteins compared to membranes not preincubated with EGF. Since phosphatase activity is selectively decreased at

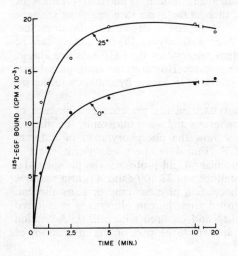

FIGURE 2. Time course of ^{125}I-EGF binding to A-431 membranes. (From Carpenter *et al.*[13] Reprinted by permission.)

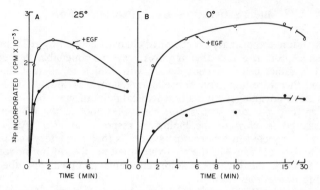

FIGURE 3. Effect of temperature on phosphorylation of A-431 membranes. EGF stimulated the incorporation of [³²P]phosphate from [³²P]ATP into A-431 cell membranes. (From Carpenter *et al.*[13] Reprinted by permission.)

low temperatures, the effect of EGF was most evident at 0°. Further analysis demonstrated that this EGF-sensitive protein phosphorylation was independent of cyclic nucleotides, calcium, or calmodulin.[13] The activation by EGF is very rapid; when binding and phosphorylation are started simultaneously, the growth factor is able to increase phosphorylation within 30 seconds at 0°.[14]

Exogenous proteins such as histones or tubulin can be utilized as substrates,[13, 15] although this does not necessarily identify these proteins as substrates *in vivo*. Interestingly, the phosphate acceptors on endogenous and exogenous protein substrates were shown to be tyrosine residues,[16] even though protein kinases nearly always phosphorylate either serine or threonine residues. The only tyrosine-specific kinases are (1) coupled to hormone receptors, such as EGF, platelet-derived growth factor,[17] and insulin[18]; and (2) products of the transforming gene of retroviruses, such as the avian sarcoma virus *src* gene product.[19] Two independent studies[20, 21] suggest a degree of relatedness between these two groups of kinases since antibody to the *src* kinase can be recognized and used as a phosphorylation substrate by the EGF-sensitive kinase, whereas control antibody is not phosphorylated. However, the antigenic relatedness is not sufficient for precipitation of the EGF kinase by antibody to the *src* kinase.

If A-431 membranes are phosphorylated in the presence and absence of EGF and analyzed by SDS gel electrophoresis and autoradiography, densitometer scans of the autoradiograms show how the phosphorylation of different classes of proteins is affected by EGF (FIG. 4). The predominant effect is observed on 170,000 and 150,000 molecular weight proteins. The phosphorylation of membrane proteins of 80,000 daltons and 22,500 daltons is also sensitive to EGF.[22] The EGF-sensitive phosphorylation of membrane proteins also can be demonstrated with membranes derived from human placenta,[22, 23] cultured human fibroblasts,[17, 22] rat kidney cells,[8] and cultured glial cells.[17] Activation of protein kinase activity, therefore, appears to be part of the mechanism of EGF action in all cells.

Purification and Characterization of the Receptor/Kinase

Membranes from A-431 cells have been solubilized in Triton X-100 and subjected to affinity chromatography on EGF–agarose.[14, 15] After adsorption and washing, the bound material can be eluted with either EGF or 5 mM ethanolamine at pH 9.0. Depending on the initial procedure used to prepare the membranes from intact cells, the predominant (90% of the Coomassie blue staining material) protein species eluted from the affinity gel have apparent molecular weights of 170,000 or 150,000.[15] Available data strongly indicate that 170,000 daltons is the size of the native EGF receptor and that the 150,000-dalton species is a fragment of the receptor produced by proteolysis during certain membrane preparation procedures.[15] Both the 170,000- and 150,000-dalton species bind ^{125}I-EGF with similar affinities and are each immunoprecipitated with antisera prepared against the 170,000-dalton species.[15]

Interestingly, the EGF-sensitive protein kinase copurifies with the receptor on the EGF affinity column.[14] Addition of [γ-^{32}P]ATP to the purified material results in EGF-sensitive phosphorylation of both the 170,000 and the 150,000 band. Data from several laboratories indicate (1) that the molecular weight of covalently linked EGF–receptor complexes is about 170,000 daltons[25]; (2) that there is an ATP binding site in the 170,000-dalton species[26]; and (3) that antibodies to the purified 170,000-dalton material can immunoprecipitate EGF-sensitive protein kinase activity and ^{125}I-EGF binding activity[27]. These data suggest that the 170,000-dalton protein is both an EGF receptor and a protein kinase. A direct response to EGF binding, at least *in vitro*, is activation of the protein kinase activity, which potentiates autophosphorylation of the receptor–kinase molecules, phosphorylation of other membrane proteins whose functions are not known, and possible phosphorylation of cytoplasmic proteins. The last conclusion requires that the kinase activity be localized on the cytoplasmic side of the membrane, which has not yet been demonstrated.

Treatment of intact cells with EGF increases the phosphorylation of cytoplasmic proteins, some of which also are phosphorylated by activation of the sarcoma virus *src* protein kinase.[28] It is not clear, however, whether these

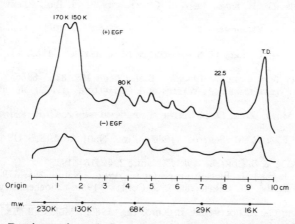

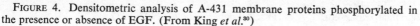

FIGURE 4. Densitometric analysis of A-431 membrane proteins phosphorylated in the presence or absence of EGF. (From King *et al.*[30])

cytoplasmic proteins, which may be second messenger candidates for EGF, are phosphorylated by the 170,000-dalton membrane-localized receptor–kinase or by another unidentified kinase whose activity is regulated by the EGF kinase.

The receptor has been purified to near homogeneity by affinity chromatography, but further information on the biochemical characteristics is delayed by the fact that relatively small amounts of material can be purified. Antibodies to the affinity-purified 170,000-dalton material isolated on an SDS gel have been produced.[27] Immunoprecipitation of extracts of cells prelabeled with ^{3}H-glucosamine or ^{35}S-methionine have established the glycoprotein nature of the 170,000-dalton receptor.[29] Similar immunoprecipitations performed after labeling cells with ^{35}S-methionine in the presence of tunicamycin (to prevent N-linked glycosylation) indicate that the protein portion of the receptor is approximately 130,000 daltons.

REFERENCES

1. CARPENTER, G. & S. COHEN. 1979. Annu. Rev. Biochem. **48:** 193–216.
2. ROSE, S. P., R. STAHN, D. S. PASSOVOY & H. HERSCHMAN. 1976. Experientia **32:** 913–915.
3. CARPENTER, G. & S. COHEN. 1976. J. Cell. Physiol. **88:** 227–237.
4. CARPENTER, G. & S. COHEN. 1978. *In* Molecular Control of Proliferation and Differentiation. J. Papaconstantinou & W. J. Rutter, Eds.: 13–31. Academic Press. New York, NY.
5. McKEEHAN, W. L. & K. A. McKEEHAN. 1979. Exp. Cell Res. **123:** 397–400.
6. CARPENTER, G. & S. COHEN. 1976. J. Cell Biol. **71:** 159–171.
7. HAIGLER, H., J. A. McKANNA & C. COHEN. 1979. J. Cell Biol. **81:** 382–395.
8. McKANNA, J. A., H. HAIGLER & S. COHEN. 1979. Proc. Natl. Acad. Sci. USA **76:** 5689–5693.
9. DAS, M. & C. F. FOX. 1978. Proc. Natl. Acad. Sci. USA **75:** 2644–2648.
10. HAIGLER, H. & G. CARPENTER. 1980. Biochim. Biophys. Acta **598:** 314–325.
11. FABRICANT, R. N., J. E. DeLARCO & G. J. TODARO. 1977. Proc. Natl. Acad. Sci. USA **74:** 565–569.
12. HAIGLER, H., J. F. ASH, S. J. SINGER & S. COHEN. 1978. Proc. Natl. Acad. Sci. USA **75:** 3317–3321.
13. CARPENTER, G., L. KING, JR. & S. COHEN. 1979. J. Biol. Chem. **254:** 4884–4891.
14. COHEN, S., G. CARPENTER & L. KING, JR. 1980. J. Biol. Chem. **255:** 4834–4842.
15. COHEN, S., H. USHIRO, C. STOSCHECK & M. CHINKERS. 1982. J. Biol. Chem. **257:** 1523–1531.
16. USHIRO, H. & S. COHEN. 1980. J. Biol. Chem. **255:** 8363–8365.
17. EK, B., B. WESTERMARK, A. WASTESON & C. HELDIN. 1982. Nature **295:** 419–420.
18. KASUGA, M., Y. ZICK, D. L. BLITHE, F. A. KARLSSON & C. R. KAHN. Submitted for publication.
19. HUNTER, T. & B. M. SEFTON. 1980. Proc. Natl. Acad. Sci. USA **77:** 1311–1315.
20. CHINKERS, M. & S. COHEN. 1981. Nature **290:** 516–519.
21. KUDLOW, J. E., J. E. BUSS & G. N. GILL. 1981. Nature **290:** 519–521.
22. KING, L. E., JR., G. CARPENTER & S. COHEN. 1980. Biochemistry **19:** 1524–1528.
23. CARPENTER, G., L. POLINER & L. KING, JR. 1980. Mol. Cell. Endocrinol. **18:** 189–199.
24. FERNANDEZ-POL, J. A. 1981. Biochemistry **20:** 3907–3912.

25. DAS, M., T. MIYAKAWA, C. F. FOX, R. M. PRUSS, A. AHARONOV & H. R. HERSCH-MAN. 1977. Proc. Natl. Acad. Sci USA **74:** 2790–2794.
26. BUHROW, S. A., S. COHEN & J. V. STAROS. 1982. J. Biol. Chem. **257:** 4019–4022.
27. STOSCHECK, C., S. COHEN & G. CARPENTER. Manuscript in preparation.
28. HUNTER, T. & J. A. COOPER. 1981. Cell **24:** 741–752.
29. SODERQUIST, A. M. & G. CARPENTER. Manuscript in preparation.
30. KING, L., G. CARPENTER & S. COHEN. Unpublished data.

GROWTH FACTORS FROM PLATELETS, MONOCYTES, AND ENDOTHELIUM: THEIR ROLE IN CELL PROLIFERATION *

Russell Ross, Elaine Raines, and Daniel Bowen-Pope

Departments of Pathology and Biochemistry
School of Medicine
University of Washington
Seattle, Washington 98195

INTRODUCTION

During the past decade a number of polypeptide hormones, or growth factors, have been discovered that are capable of stimulating cells to proliferate in culture. Several of these have been purified to homogeneity, and their mode of action upon cells is under intensive study.

There are a number of ways in which these factors can be classified; however, from a biological point of view, we suggest that they be considered in four possible categories. These are:

a. Growth factors that may be associated with embryogenesis, and normal growth and development. Such factors include epidermal growth factor,[1] fibroblast growth factor,[2] the somatomedins,[3] and nerve growth factor.[4]

b. Growth factors associated with those populations of cells in the adult that have continual or intermittent turnover, such as epithelial cells lining body cavities and the different hematopoietic cells. These growth factors include colony-stimulating factor[5] and erythropoietin[6] as modulators of hematopoiesis, and possibly epidermal growth factor as one of the factors controlling turnover of epithelial cells in the epidermis, gut, or urogenital tract.

c. Growth factors associated with the proliferative response to injury, as may occur in wound repair, in chronic inflammatory responses, and potentially in atherosclerosis. Such factors include platelet-derived growth factor (PDGF),[7] monocyte/macrophage-derived growth factor (MDGF),[8] and possibly the endothelial-cell-derived growth factor (EDGF).[9]

d. Growth factors formed by some populations of tumor cells, including some virally transformed cells, which may act as self-mitogens. These factors, termed tumor growth factors,[10] can elicit a transformed phenotype when applied to nontransformed cells, but do not permanently alter the phenotype of the cells.

We have been particularly interested in the growth factors of category (c) that may play important roles in a number of tissue responses to injury. These factors include the platelet-derived growth factor (PDGF), monocyte/macro-

* This work was supported in part by Grants AM 13970 and HL 18645 from the United States Public Health Service.

phage-derived growth factor (MDGF), and the endothelial-derived growth factor (EDGF).

PLATELET-DERIVED GROWTH FACTOR

Platelet-derived growth factor was discovered in 1974 [7, 11] and was found to be one of the principal mitogens present in whole blood serum and missing from plasma-derived serum. Platelets were demonstrated to be the source of this factor, since material derived from frozen-thawed platelets or platelets exposed to purified thrombin could replace all of the mitogenic activity lacking in cell-free plasma and plasma-derived serum (PDS) and present in whole blood serum (WBS).[7] This factor was mitogenic for smooth muscle cells,[7] fibroblasts,[12] 3T3 cells,[11] and glial cells,[13] but was not mitogenic for arterial endothelial cells.

Several laboratories have purified this factor close to homogeneity [15-18] and have established that it is a protein with a molecular weight of approximately 30,000, consisting of two chains of approximately 17,000 and 14,000 molecular weight joined by disulfide bonds. Retention of the disulfide bonds in the native configuration is necessary for activity. In its pure form, 6 ng per ml (2×10^{-10} M) of PDGF stimulates DNA synthesis in 3T3 cells, smooth muscle cells, and fibroblasts to a level equivalent to that produced by 5% whole blood serum. As is the case for many mitogens, the exposure of PDGF to cells leads to an increased rate of incorporation of thymidine into DNA beginning 12–16 hours after exposure, and reaching a maximum rate 24–32 hours after exposure to the mitogen. PDGF stimulates many activities in cells that occur much earlier than increased thymidine incorporation. These include an increased rate of endocytosis of tracer molecules such as ^{14}C-sucrose within an hour after exposure [14]; increased cholesterol synthesis [18]; increased binding of low-density lipoprotein (LDL) to the specific high-affinity receptor for this lipoprotein [18]; increased turnover of phospholipids [20]; and it has been shown to be chemotactic for cells such as fibroblasts and smooth muscle [21]. The latter response could be important in attracting cells such as fibroblasts into wound sites or into areas where injury and blood coagulation have occurred. This response could also be important during the development of intimal smooth muscle lesions of atherosclerosis. If PDGF was deposited at sites of endothelial injury in the artery wall, it could help to attract smooth muscle cells into the intima from the media.

Platelet-derived growth factor has been purified by several laboratories.[15-18] Most of the strategies for purification of this mitogen have used similar approaches. The starting material is either platelets purified from fresh platelet-rich plasma, or more commonly, outdated human platelet-rich plasma.[15] In the latter instance, approximately 90% of the PDGF is released into the plasma during the outdating process and therefore both plasma and platelets must be processed to purify the PDGF.[17, 18] The purification schemes have employed various combinations of ion exchange chromatography, gel filtration, and hydrophobic chromatography. The approach that is used in our laboratory is shown in TABLE 1 and demonstrates a purification of greater than 500,000-fold with an overall yield of 21%.[15] Material purified in this manner consists of four components of molecular weights of 27,000, 28,500, 29,000 and 31,000 when examined by silver-stained SDS polyacrylamide gel electrophoresis under

TABLE 1

PURIFICATION OF PLATELET-DERIVED GROWTH FACTOR FROM OUTDATED
PLATELET-RICH PLASMA

	Specific Activity (μg/ml media)	Growth-Promoting Activity (units/mg)	Percentage of Recovery of Activity from Starting Material
5% Calf Serum Standard Conditions	2350	1.0	
Human platelet-rich plasma, frozen-thawed, defibrinogenated	1075	3.0	100
CM-Sephadex, fraction III	2.0	1625	40
Sephacryl S-200	0.5	6500	28
Heparin-Sepharose CL-6B	0.087	37,356	23
Phenyl-Sepharose CL-6B	0.0064	507,808	21

nonreducing conditions. All four components are biologically active, as determined on the basis of elution from SDS gels and analysis of cell-bound ^{125}I-PDGF. Reduction with 2-mercaptoethanol converts PDGF to three inactive chains of molecular weights of 14,400, 16,000, and 17,500. These chains cannot be reassociated to produce an active molecule. The heterogeneity noted above was further investigated by analyzing proteinase-K digests of each individual band (reduced or nonreduced) followed by two-dimensional peptide map analysis. These studies demonstrated that the four nonreduced species were closely related. Of the reduced species, the 16,000- and 17,500-dalton peptides were very similar, whereas the 14,400-dalton species showed many differences and thus appeared to be different. These data are consistent with a model in which the small chain is disulfide-crosslinked to one of the two larger chains.[19]

Purified PDGF has been radioiodinated with full retention of biological activity using an iodine monochloride method.[22] ^{125}I-PDGF binds with high affinity to Swiss 3T3 cells, arterial smooth muscle cells, and human fibroblasts in a saturable and specific fashion. The binding of this molecule is highly competed for by whole blood serum, by purified unlabeled PDGF, and by material obtained after each stage of purification of PDGF.[22] Other mitogens, including epidermal growth factor, fibroblast growth factor, and insulin, show no competition for binding to the PDGF receptor. For all of the cells that have demonstrated high-affinity receptors, PDGF shows an apparent dissociation constant (K_d) of about 10^{-11} M, comparable to the range in which it is mitogenic. In those cells that have been studied, the apparent number of receptors per cell for PDGF ranges from 600,000 to 0 (TABLE 2.) Binding of ^{125}I-PDGF to monolayer cultures of different cells was examined at 4° C. Under these conditions, equilibrium binding at low concentrations of the molecule requires more than 7 hours, unless the binding medium is continuously agitated and mixed during this period of time. The binding does not require calcium or magnesium ion, but is reduced if both monovalent and divalent cations are missing from the binding mixture and replaced with isotonic sucrose. Binding of ^{125}I-PDGF is more rapid at 37° C than at 4° C; however, at 37° C the cell-associated material declines after approximately 60 minutes of incubation, reflecting a degradation in previously bound ^{125}I-PDGF and a reduction in the number of PDGF receptors.[22]

The PDGF receptor itself was further studied using affinity labeling techniques developed by Massaque *et al.*[23] in which bifunctional crosslinking reagents are used to covalently link radiolabeled polypeptide hormones to cell surface receptors. In our studies, we have found that a cell surface component with most of the characteristics expected of a PDGF receptor can be identified in autoradiographs of polyacrylamide gels after crosslinking ^{125}I-PDGF to cell surface components.[24] The labeled complex has a molecular weight of 194,000, implying a cell surface component of 164,000. The formation of this complex was reduced by preincubation with unlabeled PDGF, but not with insulin, FGF, EGF, LDL, or acetylated LDL. The amount of complex formed was greatly reduced by treatments that reduce the binding capacity of the cells for PDGF, including trypsin treatment and preincubation with PDGF at 37° C to permit downregulation to occur. The complex was not seen on cell types that do not demonstrate specific binding of PDGF.[24]

MACROPHAGE-DERIVED GROWTH FACTOR

A second cell, the peripheral blood monocyte, is the source of a growth factor that may be as important biologically as the growth factor derived from the platelet. This may be particularly true in association with the type of fibroproliferative response that is commonly found in chronic inflammatory responses and possibly in atherosclerosis as well. If macrophage activity is inhibited in healing wounds by local administration of antimacrophage sera in a monocytopenic animal, the rate of healing is reduced, as are fibroblast proliferation and connective tissue formation.[25]

Culture medium, using plasma-derived serum and lacking platelet-derived growth factor, was shown to be suitable to culture peritoneal macrophages. Upon stimulation, such macrophages released a potent growth factor into the culture medium.[8] Similar observations have been made by Greenburg and Hunt[26] and by Martin *et al.*[27] Recently, we[28] studied the capacity of human peripheral blood monocytes to produce such a growth factor. Utilizing techniques of counterflow centrifugation (elutriation), it was possible to obtain 95% pure preparations of monocytes in suspension. Lysates of these freshly

TABLE 2

PDGF RECEPTORS ON DIFFERENT CELL STRAINS

	Number of PDGF Receptors per Cell
3T3 (mouse cell line)	1.3×10^5
High-binding 3T3	6.2×10^5
Monkey smooth muscle	7.9×10^4
Human foreskin fibroblasts	4.5×10^4
Human smooth muscle	3.8×10^4
A-431 human carcinoma	—0—
3T3 variant clone PF 2	2.5×10^3

isolated monocytes failed to demonstrate any growth factor activity, suggesting that the cells either contained no prepackaged growth factor, or, if they did, that the factor was present in an inactive form. The latter does not appear to be the case since once these cells were stimulated to form growth factor, approximately 4 hours were required before any sizable amount of factor is produced; further experiments will be required to determine whether this is the case.[28]

When cultures of purified peripheral blood monocytes were stimulated with endotoxin, concanavalin A, or zymosan, they began to release a potent growth factor into the culture medium within 4 hours, and continued to release this material for up to 22 hours. After 22 hours, there did not appear to be any increase in release upon continued stimulation. The cells appeared to release more factor when they were grown in culture medium containing autologous plasma rather than homologous plasma, and the density of the monocytes in the culture affected the amount of growth factor formed.[28]

On the basis of several observations it can be seen that the monocyte/macrophage-derived growth factor appears to be different from PDGF. MDGF does not compete for binding to the PDGF receptor, and the activity of MDGF is not inhibited by antiserum directed against PDGF (unpublished observations). The purification of this molecule and further studies of its biological properties should provide both interesting and important data to assist in our understanding of inflammation and its associated fibroproliferative response.

Endothelial-Cell-Derived Growth Factor

Arterial endothelial cells also synthesize and release a growth factor in culture.[9] It is made by endothelial cells in culture in serum-free medium as well as in medium containing plasma-derived serum. Partial purification of this factor suggests that it has a molecular weight of approximately 20,000. It appears to be different from PDGF in terms of its chromatographic characteristics and the fact that antiserum against PDGF has no effect upon its activity (unpublished observations). Antiserum directed against epidermal growth factor also has no effect upon EDGF, suggesting that these two molecules are different (unpublished observations). Since multiplication of endothelial cells of many types is associated with a number of proliferative phenomena, further study of this growth factor and its role in biology should yield important data.

Summary

Of the various biological roles assigned to growth factors at the beginning of this article, the factors described here are largely associated with the response to injury. These represent a special type of factor since two of them, PDGF and MDGF, are carried in the circulation by the platelet and the monocyte respectively, and can therefore be delivered to sites where a proliferative response would be an important event in the restitution of tissue continuity. The role of the endothelial-derived growth factor in these phenomena is not clear at present.

Atherosclerosis has been suggested to represent a protective proliferative response that has gone awry and become disease.[29, 30] In this instance both PDGF and MDGF could play important roles, since platelets have been associated with the early injury phenomenon and macrophages appear to be present in virtually all phases of the development of the lesions of atherosclerosis from the fatty streak to the fibrous plaque and the complicated lesion. In each of these circumstances the macrophage may be important in lesion progression and possibly in lesion initiation. PDGF may also be important in initiation of some lesions, and in some instances would undoubtedly participate in the fibroproliferative response that occurs during organization of a thrombus.

REFERENCES

1. COHEN, S. 1962. Isolation of a mouse submaxillary gland protein accelerating incisor eruption and eyelid opening in the newborn animal. J. Biol. Chem. **237:** 1555–1562.
2. GOSPODAROWICZ, D. 1975. Purification of a fibroblast growth factor from bovine pituitary. J. Biol. Chem. **250:** 2515–2520.
3. VAN WYK, J. J., L. E. UNDERWOOD, J. B. BASEMAN, R. L. HINTZ, D. R. CLEMMONS & R. N. MARSHALL. 1975. Explorations of the insulinlike and growth-promoting properties of somatomedin by membrane receptor assays. Adv. Metab. Disord. **8:** 127–150.
4. LEVI-MONTALCINI, R. & P. U. ANGELETTI. 1968. Nerve growth factor. Physiol. Rev. **48:** 534–569.
5. BURGESS, A. W., D. METCALF, H. M. RUSSELL & N. A. NICOLA. Granulocyte/macrophage-, megakaryocyte-, eosinophil- and erythroid-colony-stimulating factors by mouse spleen cells. J. Biol. Chem. **185:** 301–314.
6. MIYAKE, T., C. K.-H. KUNG, & E. GOLDWASSER. 1977. Purification of human erythropoietin. J. Biol. Chem. **252:** 5558–5564.
7. ROSS, R., J. GLOMSET, B. KARIYA & L. A. HARKER. 1974. Platelet-dependent serum factor that stimulates the proliferation of arterial smooth muscle cells *in vitro*. Proc. Natl. Acad. Sci. USA **71:** 1207–1210.
8. LEIBOVICH, S. J. & R. ROSS. 1976. A macrophage-dependent factor that stimulates the proliferation of fibroblasts *in vitro*. Am. J. Pathol. **84:** 501–513.
9. GADJUSEK, C., P. DiCORLETO, R. ROSS & S. SCHWARTZ. 1980. An endothelial cell derived growth factor. J. Cell Biol. **85:** 467–472.
10. DELARCO, J. E., R. REYNOLDS, K. CARLBERG, E. ENGLE & G. TODARO. 1980. Sarcoma growth factor from mouse sarcoma virus-transformed cells. J. Biol. Chem. **255:** 3685–3690.
11. KOHLER, N. & A. LIPTON. 1974. Platelets as source of fibroblast growth-promoting activity. Exp. Cell Res. **87:** 297–301.
12. RUTHERFORD, R. B. & R. ROSS. 1976. Platelet factors stimulate fibroblasts and smooth muscle cells quiescent in plasma serum to proliferate. J. Cell Biol. **69:** 196–203.
13. HELDIN, C.-H., B. WESTERMARK & A. WASTESON. 1981. Specific receptors for platelet-derived growth factor on cells derived from connective tissue and glia. Proc. Natl. Acad. Sci. USA **78:** 3664–3668.
14. DAVIES, P. F. & R. ROSS. 1978. Mediation of pinocytosis in cultured arterial smooth muscle and endothelial cells by platelet-derived growth factor. J. Cell Biol. **79:** 663–671.
15. RAINES, E. & R. ROSS. 1982. Platelet-derived growth factor. I. High yield purification and evidence for multiple forms. J. Biol. Chem. **257:** 5154–5160.
16. HELDIN, C.-H., B. WESTERMARK & A. WASTESON. 1981. Structural studies on platelet-derived growth factor isolated by a large-scale purification procedure. Biochem. J. **93:** 907.
17. DEUEL, T. F., J. S. HUANG, R. T. PROFFITT, J. R. BAENZIGER, D. CHANGE & B. B. KENNEDY. 1981. Human platelet-derived growth factor—Purification and resolution into two active protein factors. J. Biol. Chem. **256:** 8896–8899.

18. ANTONIADES, H. N., C. D. SCHER & C. D. STILES. 1979. Purification of human platelet-derived growth factor. Proc. Natl. Acad. Sci USA **76:** 1809–1813.
19. CHAIT, A., R. ROSS, J. ALBERTS & E. BIERMAN. 1980. Platelet-derived growth factor stimulates low density lipoprotein receptor activity. Proc. Natl. Acad. Sci USA **77:** 4084–4088.
20. HABENICHT, A. J. R., J. A. GLOMSET, W. C. KING, C. NIST, C. D. MITCHELL & R. ROSS. 1981. Early changes in phosphatidylinositol and arachidonic acid metabolism in quiescent Swiss 3T3 cells stimulated to divide by platelet-derived growth factor. J. Biol. Chem. **256:** 12329–12335.
21. GROTENDORST, G. R., H. SEPPA, H. K. KLEINMAN & G. R. MARTIN. 1981. Attachment of smooth muscle cells to collagen and their migration toward platelet-derived growth factor. Proc. Natl. Acad. Sci. USA **78:** 3669–3672.
22. BOWEN-POPE, D. & R. ROSS. 1982. Platelet-derived growth factor. II. Specific binding to cultured cells. J. Biol. Chem. **257:** 5161–5171.
23. MASSAQUE, J., B. GUILLETTE & M. CZECH. 1981. Affinity labeling of multiplication stimulating activity receptors in membranes from rat and human tissues. J. Biol. Chem. **256:** 2122–2125.
24. GLENN, K. C., D. BOWDEN-POPE & R. ROSS. 1982. Platelet-derived growth factor. III. Identification of a PDGF receptor by affinity labeling. J. Biol. Chem. **257:** 5172–5176.
25. LEIBOVICH, S. J. & R. ROSS. 1975. The role of the macrophage in wound repair: A study with hydrocortisone and antimacrophage serum. Am. J. Pathol. **78:** 71–92.
26. GREENBURG, G. & T. HUNT. 1978. The proliferative response *in vitro* of vascular endothelial and smooth muscle cells exposed to wound fluids and macrophages. J. Cell. Physiol. **97:** 353–360.
27. MARTIN, B. M., M. A. GIMBRONE, JR., E. R. URANUE & R. S. COTRAN. 1981. Stimulation of non-lymphoid mesenchymal cell proliferation by a macrophage-derived growth factor. J. Immunol. **126:** 1510–1515.
28. GLENN, K. & R. ROSS. 1981. Human monocyte-derived growth factor(s) for mesenchymal cells: Activation of secretion by endotoxin and concanavalin A (Con A). Cell **25:** 603–615.
29. ROSS, R. & J. GLOMSET, JR. 1976. The pathogenesis of atherosclerosis. N. Engl. J. Med. **295:** 369–377, 420–425.
30. ROSS, R. 1981. Atherosclerosis: A problem of the biology of arterial wall cells and their interactions with blood components. Arteriosclerosis **1:** 293–311.

A PLATELET-DERIVED GROWTH FACTOR ANALOG PRODUCED BY A HUMAN CLONAL GLIOMA CELL LINE *

Monica Nistér,† Carl-Henrik Heldin,‡ Åke Wasteson,‡ and
Bengt Westermark †§

† The Wallenberg Laboratory and Department of
Clinical Pathology, and
‡ Institute of Medical and Physiological Chemistry
University of Uppsala
Uppsala, Sweden

More than a decade ago, Holley and Kiernan [1] demonstrated that the saturation density of mouse 3T3 cells depends on the serum concentration in the medium. These authors suggested the presence in serum of specific mitogenic substances which are operational in the regulation of normal mammalian cellular growth. In contrast to normal cells, transformed cells in general multiply more or less independent of the serum concentration, leading to the suggestion that such cells may produce their own growth factors.[2] Therefore, the elucidation of the biochemistry and biology of naturally occurring growth factors may be of vital importance for the understanding of the normal cycle control mechanisms as well as the deficient control of neoplastic cells.

Several studies have shown that platelet-derived growth factor (PDGF) is the major growth-promoting agent of serum for various fibroblastic and glial cells in culture (see Westermark et al.[3] for a recent review). Human PDGF is a ~30 kilodalton protein consisting of two polypeptide chains linked by disulfide bonds.[4, 5] A single class of high-affinity receptors for PDGF has been demonstrated on responsive cells using ^{125}I-labeled ligand.[6-8] The receptor is specific for PDGF in the sense that other growth factors such as epidermal growth factor, fibroblast growth factor, or insulin do not compete with ^{125}I-PDGF for binding.[6] In addition, various unresponsive cells such as those of epithelial origin show no significant specific binding of ^{125}I-PDGF.

We have previously demonstrated a growth-promoting activity in serum-free, conditioned medium of a human osteosarcoma cell line.[9] Application of purification principles similar to those used for PDGF resulted in an about 50% pure preparation of a growth factor, denoted osteosarcoma-derived growth factor (ODGF).[10] The similarities in physicochemical properties of PDGF and ODGF in conjunction with the observation that ^{125}I-ODGF was recognized by an antibody to PDGF and competed with PDGF for binding to glial cells led to the conclusion that PDGF and ODGF are closely related or identical.[10]

The availability of a receptor-binding assay using ^{125}I-PDGF has made it possible to further search for PDGF analogs in conditioned media of cultured

* This work was supported by Grants 689, 786, and 1794 from the Swedish Cancer Society, Grants 4486 and 02X-4 from the Swedish MRC, and by a grant from the O.E. and Edla Johansson Foundation.

§ Address for correspondence: Dr. Bengt Westermark, Department of Tumor Biology, The Wallenberg Laboratory, PO Box 562, S-751 22 Uppsala, Sweden.

0077-8923/82/0397-0025 $01.75/0 © 1982, NYAS

cell lines. The present report demonstrates a growth-promoting activity released by a human clonal glioma cell line; this activity blocks the binding of ^{125}I-PDGF to human fibroblast receptors.

MATERIALS AND METHODS

Cell Culture

A number of human normal and neoplastic cell lines were used (TABLE 1). These were routinely maintained in Eagle's minimum essential medium supplemented with 5% newborn calf serum (GIBCO) and antibiotics. Cells were

TABLE 1

DISPLACEMENT OF ^{125}I-PDGF FROM FIBROBLASTS BY CONDITIONED MEDIA

Cell	Origin	Cell Type	Percentage of Displacement
AG 1523	Foreskin	Fibroblast	4
U-2 OS	Osteosarcoma	Sarcoma cell[17]	29
U-4 SS	Synovial sarcoma	Sarcoma cell[17]	19
U-393 OS	Osteosarcoma	Sarcoma cell *	14
U-787 CG	Brain tissue	Glia-like cell[18]	8
U-1508 CG	Brain tissue	Glia-like cell[18]	1
U-178 MG	Glioma	Glioma cell[19]	−5
U-251 MG	Glioma	Glioma cell[19]	18
U-343 MG	Glioma	Glioma cell[19]	22
U-343 MGa	Glioma	Clonal cell[20]	37
U-1752	Squamous carcinoma	Carcinoma cell †	5
PDGF (10 ng/ml)			30

NOTE: Confluent cultures were grown for 3–4 days in F-10 medium supplemented with fetal calf serum. Media were harvested and analyzed for their ability to displace ^{125}I-PDGF from human fibroblasts, as described in the MATERIALS AND METHODS section in text. The figures represent displacement obtained with undiluted media.
  * Unpublished line of the Wallenberg Laboratory.
  † Kindly provided by Dr. J. Bergh.

grown in 5-cm Nunc petri dishes, and maintained at 37° C in humidified air containing 5% CO_2. For collection of conditioned medium, cells were grown to confluency in 10-cm Nunc petri dishes. The cell number was then determined, and cultures were incubated in F-10 medium, 2 ml per 10^6 cells, supplemented with 1% fetal calf serum. Media were harvested after 3–4 days of incubation and stored at −20° C. The lines AG 1523 and U-343 MGa Cl 2 were also incubated in serum-free F-10 medium. U-343 MGa Cl 2 was maintained under serum-free conditions and medium was harvested every 3–4 days and used for partial purification.

Purification and Radiolabeling of PDGF

PDGF was purified from fresh platelets as described.[4, 5] The final product was >99% pure as estimated from sodium dodecyl sulfate/polyacrylamide gel electrophoresis. PDGF was labeled with ^{125}I according to the method of Hunter and Greenwood [11] as described.[12] The specific activity was 20,000 cpm/ng.

Assay of ^{125}I-PDGF-Displacing Activity

Binding of ^{125}I-PDGF was analyzed using the human foreskin fibroblast cell line AG 1523, provided by the Human Mutant Cell Repository, Institute for Medical Research (Camden, NJ). For binding experiments, cells were seeded in 12-well plates (4.5 cm^2 per well) and grown to confluency. After a wash with binding medium (phosphate-buffered saline, containing human serum albumin at 1 mg/ml, $CaCl_2 \cdot 2H_2O$ at 0.01 mg/ml and $MgSO_4 \cdot 7H_2O$ at 0.01 mg/ml), duplicate wells then received appropriate dilutions of conditioned media (clarified by centrifugation at 10,000 $\times$ g for 20 min), fraction samples, or standard PDGF and were incubated for 2 hr at 4° C. After this period of preincubation, the cultures were washed once with ice-cold binding medium and then received 0.5 ml of binding medium per well together with 5 ng (100,000 cpm) of ^{125}I-PDGF. After binding for 1 hr at 4° C, experiments were terminated by five washes with binding medium containing 1% newborn calf serum rather than albumin. Cell-associated radioactivity was collected by extracting the cells with 0.5 ml of 1% Triton X-100, 20 mM HEPES, pH 7.4, 10% (vol/vol) glycerol containing bovine serum albumin at 0.1 mg/ml. Radioactivity was determined in a gamma spectrometer. ^{125}I-PDGF-displacing activity of test samples was compared with that afforded by unlabeled, pure PDGF (10–100 ng/ml).

PDGF Radioimmunoassay

A PDGF antiserum was raised in a rabbit using pure PDGF [5] as immunogen; 15-μg portions of PDGF were injected subcutaneously at 14-day intervals. After 6–7 injections 40-ml portions of blood were collected each 2 weeks. Serum samples were stored at −20° C.

For the radioimmunologic determination of PDGF, 5 μl of PDGF antiserum diluted 1:300 in RIA-buffer (0.5 M NaCl, 0.01 M phosphate, pH 7.4, 0.5% bovine serum albumin, 0.1% Tween 80) was mixed with a 20-μl test sample appropriately diluted in RIA-buffer. The samples were incubated at room temperature for 16 hr with agitation. Five microliters of ^{125}I-PDGF (30,000 cpm) were then added and samples were again incubated for 2 hr at room temperature with agitation. Twenty-five microliters of a 20 % (w/v) suspension of *Staphylococcus aureus* (Cowan strain) were added and samples were incubated at room temperature for 30 min, again under shaking. One milliliter of RIA-buffer was then added and the bacteria were washed three times by centrifugation (10,000 $\times$ g, 2 min). Radioactivity was determined using a gamma spectrometer. The radioimmunoassay was standardized by the use of pure unlabeled PDGF (2–500 ng/ml).

Assay for Growth-Promoting Activity

Growth-promoting activity was determined using the method of ^{3}H-thymidine incorporation in serum-free cultures of human glial cells described previously.[13] The activity of test samples was compared with that displayed by various concentrations of pure PDGF (0.5–10 ng/ml).

RESULTS

^{125}I-PDGF-Displacing Activity in Conditioned Media of Human Cell Lines

Conditioned media from various human normal and neoplastic cell lines were screened with regard to their ability to displace ^{125}I-PDGF from human fibroblasts. The results are summarized in TABLE 1. A consistently high displacing activity was recovered from the conditioned medium of a clonal human glioma line, U-343 MGa Cl 2. Also, as expected, line U-2 OS was positive; it has previously been demonstrated as an ODGF-producing cell line.[10] Lower amounts of activity were found in the other two sarcoma lines (U-4 SS and U-393 OS) and in some of the glioma lines (U-251 MG and U-343 MG). In contrast, no significant displacing activity was recovered from the normal cell lines, that is, glial and foreskin fibroblast cell lines.

FIGURE 1 shows a typical displacement curve obtained with various dilutions of serum-free conditioned U-343 MGa Cl 2 medium. By a comparison of the displacing activity of the medium with that obtained with various concentrations of unlabeled PDGF it was estimated that undiluted conditioned medium contained an activity equivalent to 10–20 ng of PDGF per milliliter.

Properties of the Clonal Glioma Line U-343 MGa Cl 2

The cell line U-343 MGa is derived from a human glioblastoma multiforme and has all the properties of a human glioma line: aneuploidy, immortality, growth at high cell density, low serum requirement (see Pontén[14]). U-343 MGa Cl 2 is a clonal derivative of this cell line. An astrocytic origin of the clonal line is demonstrated by its high content of the astrocyte-specific marker glial fibrillary acidic protein (GFAP).[15] The intracellular distribution of this antigen is demonstrated by indirect immunofluorescence staining using rabbit antiGFAP serum and fluorescein isothiocyate conjugated antirabbit Ig (FIG. 2).

Partial Purification and Characterization of the ^{125}I-PDGF-Displacing Activity from U-343 MGa Cl 2

In order to further characterize the glioma-derived, ^{125}I-PDGF-displacing activity, 1.5–2 liters of serum-free, conditioned medium was harvested from U-343 MGa Cl 2 cultures. The active component was then adsorbed to a heparin-substituted Sepharose gel, following the protocol for the purification of ODGF from U-2 OS medium.[10] The heparin–Sepharose was eluted with 2 M NaCl, and the eluate precipitated with 70% ammonium sulfate. The precipitate was dissolved in 1 M NaCl, 0.01 M phosphate buffer pH 7.4 and

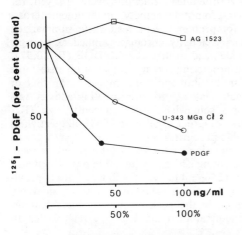

FIGURE 1. ^{125}I-PDGF-displacing activity in serum-free conditioned medium of U-343 MGa Cl 2 glioma cell line. Conditioned media were harvested from the clonal glioma line and the human foreskin fibroblast line AG 1523 was used as a control. Pure PDGF was used as a standard. Note the displacing activity of the glioma-derived medium and the absence of such activity in the fibroblast medium.

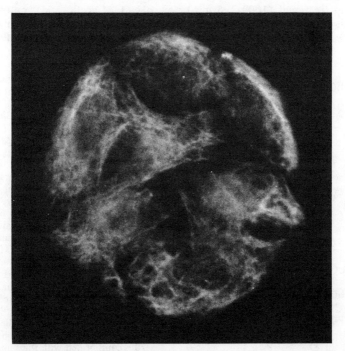

FIGURE 2. Immunofluorescence of glial fibrillary acidic protein (GFAP) of U-343 MGa Cl 2. Cells were grown on a coverslip, fixed in 2% paraformaldehyde (20 minutes at room temperature) and acetone (1 min at −20° C). Indirect immunofluorescence staining was performed at room temperature using rabbit antiGFAP (1:100) in the first layer and fluorescein isothiocyanate conjugated goat antirabbit Ig (1:20) in the second layer. Note the fibrillary distribution of GFAP.

chromatographed on Sephadex G-200; effluent fractions were assayed for ^{125}I-PDGF-displacing activity, growth-promoting activity, immunologic cross-reactivity with human PDGF, and for protein.[16] The results are summarized in FIGURE 3. The ^{125}I-PDGF-displacing activity chromatographed as a single component with an elution position identical to that of ^{125}I-PDGF (K_{av} 0.57). Also, the major portion of the growth-promoting activity and all of the detectable RIA-positive material showed similar distributions, superimposable on that of authentic PDGF. In addition, a small peak of growth-promoting activity was observed with an elution indicating a somewhat larger molecular size (K_{av} 0.27). It was concluded that the three different aspects of PDGF-like activities had essentially similar chromatographic properties, suggesting that they were all confined to the same molecule. Examination of the relative potencies of these activities revealed that the growth-promoting activity (1 μg/ml in peak fractions) and the ^{125}I-PDGF-displacing activity (2 μg/ml in peak fractions) were approximately equivalent, whereas the immunologic crossreactivity was considerably lower, corresponding only to 20 ng/ml in the peak fractions. These findings would seem to indicate a closer functional than immunologic relationship to human PDGF.

Heat treatment (100° C, 5 min), low pH (1 M acetic acid), or treatment with dissociating agents (4 M guanidine hydrochloride, 1% sodium dodecyl sulfate) had little effect on the ^{125}I-PDGF-displacing activity (TABLE 2). In

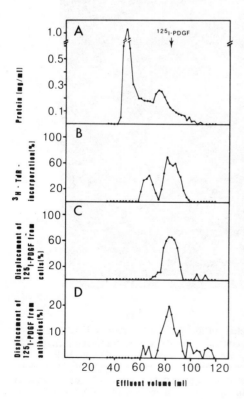

FIGURE 3. Chromatography on Sephadex G-200 of concentrated serum-free glioma conditioned medium. Two liters of serum-free medium from cultures of U-343 MGa Cl 2 were mixed with 100 ml of 1 M acetate buffer, pH 5.0, and pumped through a 2×5 cm column of heparin-Sepharose (25 ml per hr, 4° C). After washing with 100 ml of 0.15 M NaCl, 0.05 acetate buffer, pH 5.0, the column was eluted with 60 ml of 2 M NaCl, 0.01 M phosphate buffer, pH 7.4. Solid ammonium sulfate was added to 70% saturation. After end-over-end mixing for 2 hr at 4° C, the precipitate was collected by centrifugation at 20,000 $\times$ g for 30 min. The precipitate was dissolved in 1.5 ml of 1 M NaCl, 0.01 M phosphate buffer, pH 7.4, and applied to a 150×1 cm column of Sephadex G-200, equilibrated with the same buffer. The column was eluted at a flow rate of 4 ml per hr. Effluent fractions were analyzed for protein (**A**), growth promoting activity (**B**), ^{125}I-PDGF-displacing activity (**C**), and by the PDGF radioimmunoassay (**D**). The elution position of ^{125}I-PDGF is indicated by an arrow.

TABLE 2

SUSCEPTIBILITY OF GLIOMA-DERIVED ^{125}I-PDGF-DISPLACING ACTIVITY AND
GROWTH-PROMOTING ACTIVITY TO DISSOCIATIVE AGENTS AND HEAT

	Remaining Activity (%)	
Treatment	^{125}I-PDGF-Displacing Activity	Growth-Promoting Activity
Control, untreated	100	100
4 *M* guanidine–HCl, 4°, 24 hr	103	37
1%, SDS, 4° C, 24 hr	84	39
1 *M* HAc, 4° C, 24 hr	81	63
100° C, 5 min.	108	44

contrast, the same treatment resulted in a marked reduction in growth-promoting activity (TABLE 2).

DISCUSSION

The present results demonstrate that an astrocyte-derived human clonal cell line releases a factor that inhibits ^{125}I-PDGF binding to its fibroblast receptor. The glioma-derived factor showed a considerable homology to PDGF. In addition to its ^{125}I-PDGF-displacing activity, this factor was mitogenic for serum-deprived glial cells and crossreacted with PDGF in the radioimmunoassay. Moreover, all these activities had the same chromatographic behavior on Sephadex G-200, identical to that of authentic PDGF. However, it seems unlikely that the glioma-derived factor is identical to PDGF since the immunologic crossreactivity was only about 1–2% compared with the ^{125}I-PDGF-displacing activity. Furthermore, the mitogenic activity was markedly reduced by heat treatment, low pH, and denaturing agents, whereas PDGF is more resistant to such treatments.[21] Rather, the glioma-derived factor would seem to represent some variant, such as an immature or modified form of PDGF with certain structural features distinct from those of PDGF. These hypothetical differences would then lead to reduced immunologic crossreactivity and reduced resistance towards denaturation, without affecting the binding capability to the PDGF receptor or the mitogenic property. The reason why heat treatment destroyed the mitogenic activity of the glioma-derived factor but not the ^{125}I-PDGF-displacing activity is not known, but does not necessarily indicate that the two activities are associated with two different molecules. It is interesting to note that, similarly, cyanogen bromide treatment of EGF has a different effect on the same variables, the effect on mitogenicity being more marked than that on the receptor binding activity.[22]

A variety of oncogenically transformed, mainly rodent cells, produce polypeptide growth factors.[23-25] Some of these have been shown to interfere with receptors for known growth factors. Thus, murine sarcoma virus transformed cells release a factor (sarcoma growth factor, SGF) that displaces EGF from its receptor.[23] SGF is, however, antigenically distinct from EGF.[24] An interesting property of SGF and a few other growth factors derived from tumor cells is that they can induce anchorage-independent growth of normal mouse and rat cell lines.[23, 24] Since anchorage independence is correlated with transformation and tumorigenicity,[26] these factors have been denoted transforming growth factors (TGFs). Whether PDGF analogs, like the one described in the present report, can function as transforming factors is the object of current investigation.

ACKNOWLEDGMENTS

We thank S. Hermansson and A. Magnusson for technical assistance, and Dr. D. Dahl for kindly providing antiGFAP serum.

REFERENCES

1. HOLLEY, R. W. & J. A. KIERNAN. 1968. Proc. Natl. Acad. Sci. USA 60: 300–304.
2. TEMIN, H. M., R. W. PIERSON, JR. & N. C. DULAK. 1972. In Growth, Nutrition and Metabolism of Cells in Culture. G. H. Rothblatt and V. J. Cristofalo, Eds.: 50–81. Academic Press, New York, NY.
3. WESTERMARK, B., C.-H. HELDIN, B. EK, A. JOHNSSON, K. MELLSTRÖM, M. NISTÉR & Å. WASTESON. 1982. In Growth and Maturation Factors. G. Guroff, Ed. John Wiley. New York, NY. In press.
4. HELDIN, C.-H., B. WESTERMARK & Å. WASTESON. 1981. Biochem. J. 193: 907–913.
5. JOHNSSON, A., C.-H. HELDIN, B. WESTERMARK & Å. WASTESON. 1982. Biochem. Biophys. Res. Commun. 104: 66–74.
6. HELDIN, C.-H., B. WESTERMARK & Å. WASTESON. 1981. Proc. Natl. Acad. Sci. USA 78: 3664–3668.
7. HELDIN, C.-H., B. WESTERMARK & Å. WASTESON. 1982. J. Biol. Chem. In press.
8. BOWEN-POPE, D. F. & R. ROSS. 1982. J. Biol. Chem. In press.
9. WESTERMARK, B. & Å. WASTESON. 1975. In Advances in Metabolic Disorders. R. Luft and K. Hall, Eds. Vol. 8: 85–100. Academic Press. New York, NY.
10. HELDIN, C.-H., B. WESTERMARK & Å. WASTESON. 1980. J. Cell Physiol. 105: 235–246.
11. HUNTER, W. M. & F. C. GREENWOOD. 1962. Nature 194: 495–496.
12. HELDIN, C.-H., B. WESTERMARK & Å. WASTESON. 1979. Proc. Natl. Acad. Sci. USA 76: 3722–3726.
13. HELDIN, C.-H., Å. WASTESON & B. WESTERMARK. 1977. Exp. Cell Res. 109: 429–437.
14. PONTÉN, J. 1975. In Human Tumor Cells in Vitro. J. Fogh, Ed.: 175–206. Plenum Press. New York, NY.
15. BIGNAMI, A., L. ENG, D. DAHL & C. T. UYEDA. 1972. Brain Res. 43: 429–435.
16. LOWRY, O. H., N. J. ROSEBROUGH, A. L. FARR & R. J. RANDALL. 1951. J. Biol. Chem. 193: 265–275.
17. PONTÉN, J. & E. SAKSELA. 1967. Int. J. Cancer 2: 434–447.
18. PONTÉN, J. & E. MACINTYRE. 1968. Acta Path. Microbiol. Scand. Sec. A. 74: 465–486.
19. WESTERMARK, B., J. PONTÉN & R. HUGOSSON. 1973. Acta Pathol. Microbiol. Scand. Sec. A. 81: 791–805.
20. PONTÉN, J. & B. WESTERMARK. 1978. Med. Biol. 56: 184–193.
21. HELDIN, C.-H., B. WESTERMARK & Å. WASTESON. 1979. In Hormones and Cell Culture. G. Sato and R. Ross, Eds. Vol. 6: 17–31. Cold Spring Harbor Laboratory.

22. SCHREIBER, A. B., Y. YARDEN, & J. SCHLESSINGER. 1981. Biochem. Biophys. Res. Commun. **101:** 517–523.
23. DE LARCO, J. E. & G. J. TODARO. 1978. Proc. Natl. Acad. Sci. USA **75:** 4001–4005.
24. TODARO, G. J. & J. E. DE LARCO. 1980. *In* Control Mechanisms in Animal Cells: Specific Growth Factors. J. de Asua, R. Levi-Montalcini, R. Shields and S. Iacobelli, Eds. Vol. **1:** 223–243. Raven Press. New York, NY.
25. OZANNE, B., R. J. FULTUN & P. L. KAPLAN. 1980. J. Cell. Physiol. **105:** 163–180.
26. SHIN, S.-I., V. H. FREEDMAN, R. RISSER & R. POLLACK. 1975. Proc. Natl. Acad. Sci. USA **72:** 4435–4439.

CELLULAR HETEROGENEITY IN MALIGNANT NEOPLASMS AND THE THERAPY OF METASTASES

George Poste *

Smith Kline and French Laboratories
Philadelphia, Pennsylvania 19101; and
Department of Pathology and Laboratory Medicine
University of Pennsylvania, Medical School
Philadelphia, Pennsylvania 19104

INTRODUCTION

The spread of malignant tumor cells from the primary tumor to form metastases at distant sites is the most feared aspect of cancer and is a major cause of death in cancer patients. Treatment of metastases poses formidable problems. First, metastases are often too small to be detected at the time the primary tumor is treated, and widespread dissemination of malignant tumor cells typically occurs before clinical symptoms of metastatic disease are evident. Second, most patients suffer from multiple metastases. This, together with their dispersed anatomic locations, hinders their surgical removal and limits the effective concentration of anticancer drugs that can be delivered to sites of metastasis. The third, and most formidable, problem concerns the frequent resistance of metastases to conventional therapy and the varied response to therapy of individual metastases in the same patient.

There is an enormous literature of clinical and experimental observations describing the relationship of cytokinetic variables to the response of metastases to therapy.[1-4] Although knowledge of cell cycle and DNA synthesis times, tumor-doubling times, the size of the growth fraction, and the extent of cell loss is valuable in predicting the response of a tumor to therapy and in the staging of treatment protocols, it is now clear that the phenotypic heterogeneity of tumor cells represents the single most important factor responsible for the present general lack of success in treating metastases.

Tumors are not uniform entities populated by cells with similar properties, but are highly heterogeneous and contain multiple subpopulations of cells with different properties, including differences in responsiveness to the various modalities commonly used in cancer therapy.[4-6] Tumor cell heterogeneity and the extensive variation in the susceptibility of different subpopulations of tumor cells to killing by cytotoxic drugs, radiation, and hyperthermia dictate that the successful therapy of neoplastic disease will require modalities which can circumvent this cellular diversity and against which resistance is unlikely to develop. If this challenging goal is to be achieved, we need to understand better the factors responsible for the generation of cellular diversity in malignant tumors and how such diversity is controlled.

This chapter presents a brief survey of current knowledge of how cellular diversity may be generated within tumors and the factors that may influence this process.

* Address for correspondence: Dr. G. Poste, Smith Kline & French Laboratories, 1500 Spring Garden Street, Philadelphia, Pennsylvania 19101.

0077-8923/82/0397-0034 $01.75/0 © 1982, NYAS

CELLULAR HETEROGENEITY IN MALIGNANT NEOPLASMS:
TUMOR CELL SUBPOPULATIONS WITH DIFFERENT METASTATIC
CAPACITIES AND RESPONSES TO THERAPY

The cellular heterogeneity of neoplasms has been known since the last century, when histologic studies first identified morphologic differences among cells within the same tumor. Since then the use of increasingly sophisticated methods to study tumor cells *in vivo* and *in vitro* has revealed significant heterogeneity in the expression of myriad phenotypic properties by tumor cells in both primary and metastatic lesions from the same host. These include differences in karyotype, antigenicity, immunogenicity, biochemical properties, growth behavior, and cellular susceptibility to chemotherapeutic drugs.[4-7] More recently, studies done in several laboratories using animal tumors of diverse histologic origins have revealed significant variation in the metastatic capabilities of subpopulations of cells isolated from the same tumor.

The possibility that cells with differing metastatic capabilities might coexist within the same tumor was first suggested by Koch,[8] who isolated a highly metastatic subline from the Ehrlich carcinoma tumor by serially transplanting lymph node metastases. In 1955, Eva Klein[9] demonstrated that gradual conversion of some solid murine neoplasms into ascites variants was due to the selective overgrowth of a small number of cells which differed from the parental population in their ability to proliferate in the peritoneal cavity and metastasize to the lungs. Since the change was stable and heritable, Klein concluded that the gradual conversion of the solid tumor to the ascites form involved mutation/ selection and not adaptation. Further evidence of heterogeneity in the metastatic potential of tumor cells has come from more recent experiments, in which selective harvesting of cells from metastases during successive passages of tumors cells *in vivo* has yielded cell populations with a greater metastatic potential than cells from the original cell population.[10-15]

Definitive evidence that malignant primary tumors contain subpopulations of cells with differing metastatic capabilities was first obtained in 1977 by Fidler and Kripke[16] using the B16 melanoma syngeneic to the C57BL/6 mouse. To investigate whether primary tumors contained cells of differing or uniform metastatic potential, they prepared a cell suspension from a subcutaneous primary tumor and divided it into two aliquots. One part was immediately assayed for its ability to form experimental pulmonary metastases after intravenous injection. From the second part of the original suspension, 17 clones were isolated and their progeny tested for their ability to produce experimental metastases. If the tumor contained cells of uniform metastatic potential, then the cloned sublines should each produce the same number of metastases as the uncloned parental population. This was not the case. The original uncloned parental tumor cell population produced similar numbers of metastases in different animals, but the cloned sublines differed markedly in their metastatic potential. Although the number of metastases produced by any given clone was constant, individual clones showed wide variation in their metastatic potential. Control subcloning experiments demonstrated that the cloning process was not responsible for the variability. These experiments thus demonstrated that the B16 tumor is heterogeneous and that highly metastatic tumor cell variants preexist in the parental tumor cell population.

The B16 melanoma line was established in 1954 and has been maintained by serial passage in either animals or in culture for many times the life span of its natural host. Metastatic diversity in this tumor might thus be an artefact of its antiquity. However, recent studies have revealed comparable metastatic heterogeneity in clonal subpopulations of another murine melanoma, the K-1735 melanoma, which is of much more recent origin.[17] This tumor arose in a C3H mouse subjected to ten 1-hour exposures to ultraviolet radiation followed by applications of 2.5% croton oil in acetone to the skin of the scapular region for 2 years. The primary tumor was removed and fragments were transplanted into immunodeficient animals to circumvent the possibility of immune selection. Several weeks later, a tissue culture line was established and cells from the fifth passage used to produce clones whose metastatic properties were assayed. The clones were found to differ dramatically from each other and also from the parent line in their production of lung metastases. Statistical analysis of the results indicated that only 2 of 22 K-1735 clones tested were indistinguishable from the heterogeneous polyclonal parent cell line. The K-1735 melanoma is thus no less heterogeneous than the B16 melanoma.

Clonal variation in metastatic properties is not peculiar to melanomas. Comparable, extensive heterogeneity in metastatic properties has been described in clones isolated from tumors of diverse histologic origin from the mouse,[18-22] the rat,[23] the chicken,[24] and the hamster.[25]

Analysis of metastatic heterogeneity in clonal subpopulations isolated from human tumors is only just beginning. Until recently, studies have been hindered by the lack of experimental systems for analyzing the *in vivo* behavior of human tumor cells. Transplantation into congenitally athymic nude mice has been used widely to assay the tumorigenic potential of human cells. However, a consistent finding has been that in the majority of reported examples the implanted tumors grew but failed to metastasize, including tumor cells isolated originally from metastases. Similar results have been obtained with animal tumors implanted into nude mice. However, it has been found recently that the failure of tumors to metastasize in nude mice is an age-dependent phenomenon. Tumors which are nonmetastatic in nude mice older than 10 weeks of age will metastasize at a high frequency if inoculated into 3-week-old animals.[26]

Recent studies in my laboratory have exploited this phenomenon to assay the metastatic properties of a series of clones isolated from a human melanoma. These experiments have revealed extensive heterogeneity in the metastatic properties of the clones.[6] These data thus indicate that clonal variation in metastatic ability is not a peculiarity of experimental animal tumors. Further studies are in progress to evaluate the clonal heterogeneity of other human melanomas and a series of human squamous cell lines isolated from squamous carcinomas of the head and neck.

The coexistence of clonal subpopulations with differing metastatic properties within the same tumor means that environmental selection pressures may have a different impact on individual subpopulations with resulting alteration in the balance between nonmetastatic and metastatic subpopulations and between subpopulations of low and high metastatic potential.

The growing body of experimental evidence showing that malignant tumors contain subpopulations of differing metastatic potential, including subpopulations that are nonmetastatic, has radically altered long-held views about the pathogenesis of metastases. Until the mid 1970s, dogma held that malignant neoplasms were populated by cells with identical metastatic abilities and metastasis was considered to represent a "random" process insofar as any cell from the primary cell was presumed to be capable of generating a metastatic lesion. The aforementioned studies demonstrating that tumors contain subpopulations with widely differing metastatic capabilities, including subpopulations that are tumorigenic, but nonmetastatic, indicates instead that metastasis is a nonrandom process caused by specific subpopulations of cells endowed with the properties needed to successfully complete each step in the metastatic process.

The concept that metastasis is a nonrandom process involving the selective survival of subpopulations of cells that possess the range of properties needed to complete each of the potentially destructive steps in the metastatic process does not mean that random (chance) events will not play any role. Subpopulations of tumor cells endowed with metastatic properties will be at constant risk throughout the metastatic process of perishing because of random events. For example, it is easy to envisage a situation in which a metastatic cell in transit in the circulation could easily be killed as a result of a random collision with a blood cell or the vessel wall; yet in a different situation in time and space, it might survive to complete the metastatic process and generate a metastatic tumor. Similarly, at any time, the competence of a tumor cell endowed with metastatic properties to complete a specific step in the metastatic process could be subject to reversible impairment imposed by the microenvironment in which it is residing.[7]

The exact number of phenotypically distinct subpopulations present in various tumors is not known. The number is undoubtedly high. Also, it is probably dynamic, fluctuating in the face of even small changes in growth conditions that may not even be detectable using our present crude assay systems.[27] It is considered likely that subpopulations that express metastatic capacity and subpopulations that are tumorigenic but noninvasive merely represent the two extremes of a broad spectrum of subpopulations present in heterogeneous tumors. The presence of tumor cell subpopulations that are invasive but are nonmetastatic has already been demonstrated.[15] The possibility must therefore be considered that additional subpopulations exist that can complete many, but not all, steps in the metastatic process (FIG. 1). For example, subpopulations may exist that can invade and enter the blood, but are not "fit" to survive their journey in the circulation. Other invasive subpopulations might survive transit in the circulation, but do not possess the properties needed for efficient arrest in the microcirculation. Consequently, a minimal number of subpopulations can probably be defined in terms of their competence to complete successive stages in the metastatic process (FIG. 1). Clearly, this is a minimal value. Coexisting with such subpopulations would be an unknown number of metastatic subpopulations of increasing aggressiveness that produce increasing levels of metastatic disease. At the other extreme, the tumorigenic but noninvasive phenotype may also represent a graded spectrum of phenotypic progression towards the eventual acquisition of invasive potential. Finally, subpopulations defined on the basis of their abilities to complete specific steps in the metastatic process can, in turn, be subdivided further on the basis of their heterogeneity for other phenotypes, including resistance to susceptibility to killing by host defense mechanisms and various therapeutic modalities (FIG. 2).

Malignant tumors in advanced progression may thus represent a remarkable mosaic of diverse cellular subpopulations that display almost limitless patterns of phenotypic variation.

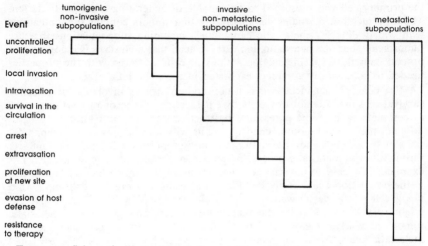

FIGURE 1. Schematic illustration of the possible minimal level of tumor cell subpopulation diversity that may exist within malignant neoplasms. Only metastatic subpopulations are "fit" to complete all of the indicated steps in the metastatic process. Other subpopulations are unable to complete one or more steps and are thus nonmetastatic.

The actual nature and the number of steps in the metastatic process that act as selection pressures to determine whether a subpopulation of cells is "fit" or "unfit" to proceed to the next step in the metastatic process may well differ from those listed in the ordinate. The steps listed represent those steps that can at least be studied experimentally in isolation with currently available techniques. (From Poste.[27] Reprinted by permission.)

THE EVOLUTION OF CELLULAR HETEROGENEITY IN MALIGNANT NEOPLASMS

Cellular diversity can arise in tumors by two, nonexclusive mechanisms. For tumors of multicellular origin, diversity is present from the outset (FIG. 3). However, even in these tumors, and certainly for tumors of unicellular origin, the available evidence suggests that additional diversity is generated by the emergence of cell variants during progressive tumor growth (FIG. 3). Striking evidence that tumors of unicellular origin can rapidly generate cell variants with differing phenotypes has been obtained by Fidler and Hart.[28] Individual colonies of BALB/c embryo fibroblasts produced by transformation of single cells by murine sarcoma virus were cultured as cell lines. Subclones were then isolated at intervals and their metastatic properties compared with the original parent lines. Remarkable diversity was detected in the metastatic properties of the subclones within as little as 42 days after transformation of the original parent cell.

Even though the kinetics with which cell variants are generated may vary in tumors of differing histologic origin and in tumors of common histologic origin in different patients, by the time of initial clinical presentation most tumors will exhibit extensive cellular heterogeneity for a wide range of phenotypes (see References 5, 6, and 27 for citations).

Nowell[29] has proposed that generation of cell variants is an inevitable and fundamental feature of progressive tumor growth. As discussed earlier, he proposes that tumor progression occurs via a series of multiple yet independent changes in many different cellular properties, resulting in rapid generation of clonal subpopulations with widely differing phenotypes. This diversity is amplified by the fact that tumor progression toward autonomy from host control may proceed simultaneously along many pathways and need not follow a set "program" of inevitable phenotypic progression. Under such circumstances a tumor would retain cellular uniformity only if all cells acquired (or lost) new characteristics simultaneously—a virtual impossibility!

At any time during progression, the number of subpopulations present in a tumor, and the extent of their phenotypic diversity, will thus reflect the selection pressures encountered during the lifetime of the tumor. Selection pressures can be natural (such as assault by host defense mechanisms or limiting nutritional conditions) or applied (therapy). Even though the kinetics for the generation of cell variants may vary in tumors of differing histologic origin, and in tumors of common histologic origin in different patients, the probability is high that by the time of initial clinical presentation most tumors will exhibit extensive cellular heterogeneity for a wide range of phenotypes.

Nowell's concept of tumor progression also proposes that as successive clonal subpopulations emerge they will display increasing genetic instability. This, coupled with the selection pressures imposed by host defense and/or therapy,

Anti-Tumor Agent

Chemotherapy																		
A	+	−	−	−	−	−	−	−	−	−	−	−	+	−	+	−	+	−
B	+	+	−	−	−	−	−	−	−	−	−	−	−	+	+	−	+	−
C	+	+	+	−	−	−	−	−	−	−	−	−	+	−	−	+	+	−
D	+	+	+	+	−	−	−	−	−	−	−	−	−	+	−	+	−	−
E	+	+	+	+	+	−	−	−	−	−	−	−	+	−	+	−	−	+
Radiotherapy	+	+	+	+	+	+	−	−	−	−	−	−	−	+	+	−	−	+
Hyperthermia	+	+	+	+	+	+	+	−	−	−	−	−	+	−	−	+	+	−
Antibodies	+	+	+	+	+	+	+	+	−	−	−	−	−	+	−	+	+	−
Lymphocytes	+	+	+	+	+	+	+	+	+	−	−	−	+	−	+	−	+	+
NK Cells	+	+	+	+	+	+	+	+	+	+	−	−	−	+	+	−	−	+
Macrophages	+	+	+	+	+	+	+	+	+	+	+	−	+	−	−	+	−	+
	S^n											R^n						

FIGURE 2. The effect of independent segregation of cellular phenotypes for susceptibility to killing by various natural (host defense mechanisms) and applied assaults (clinical therapy) on the range of subpopulation diversity present in a heterogeneous neoplasm ($+$ = susceptible; $-$ = resistant).

The pattern of cosegregation of phenotypes for susceptibility or resistance to multiple antitumor factors shown in the figure is entirely random and the number of different combinations of susceptible and resistant phenotypes that could be displayed by any particular subpopulation is, of course, far larger than that shown and for all practical purposes is infinite.

Within a heterogeneous population certain subpopulations will exist that are susceptible to a wide range of host defense mechanisms and therapeutic modalities (S^n = susceptibility to n cytotoxic factors). Conversely, other subpopulations may exist that are resistant to the same factors (R^n = resistance to n cytotoxic factors), and other subpopulations display various patterns of susceptibility and resistance. (From Poste.[27] Reprinted by permission.)

will favor relentless emergence of new subpopulations with enhanced metastatic capacities.

The relationship between genetic instability and metastatic ability has been studied recently using clones with low and high metastatic potential isolated from three murine tumors; the UV-2237 fibrosarcoma, the SF-19 fibrosarcoma and the K-1735 melanoma.[30] In all cases the rate of spontaneous cellular mutation to acquire resistance to ouabain or thioguanine was found to be significantly higher (5–7 times) in the highly metastatic clones.

Given the role of tumor progression as a mechanism for generating cellular diversity within tumors, and the apparent increasing genetic instability of the

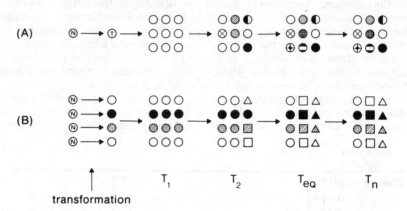

FIGURE 3. Schematic representation of possible events in the generation of cellular diversity and metastatic heterogeneity during tumor progression. After initial transformation of single (scheme **A**) or multiple (scheme **B**) normal cells (N), tumor cells are formed and undergo initial proliferation (T_1). In the case of tumors of multicellular origin (scheme **B**) cellular diversity is present from the outset. With time, progressive growth results in the generation of cell variants with different metastatic phenotypes. No time scale is implied for the different time intervals shown (T_1, T_2, T_3). The kinetics of the formation of metastatic variants will probably vary between tumors of different histologic origin and between tumors of similar histologic origin in different hosts in which tumors will be exposed to a different array of selection pressures imposed by host defense mechanisms and therapy. The formation of new variant subpopulations may not proceed indefinitely, and in populations containing multiple subpopulations the rate at which new metastatic variants emerge is lower than that in populations containing only a limited number of subpopulations. (From Fidler and Poste.[6] Reprinted by permission.)

new variants generated by this process, how is it that the metastatic properties of uncloned, polyclonal tumor cell lines can remain so constant? For example, the B16 melanoma cell lines, B16-F1 (low metastatic ability) and B16-F10 (high metastatic ability), have maintained their relative metastatic capacities during 8 years of serial passage *in vitro* and also after long periods of *in vivo* transfer.[31] What has prevented these differences from being obliterated by the generation of new variants with different metastatic properties? One reason may be that tumor cells within a polyclonal population do not behave as autonomous units, but are affected by the presence of other tumor cells. Support for this concept has been obtained in my laboratory on studies which show that different subpopulations of B16 melanoma cells isolated from the B16-F1 and B16-F10 cell lines can affect each other's behavior and influence the stability of the metastatic phenotype.[31]

Studies on individual clones isolated from the heterogeneous, polyclonal B16-F1 and B16-F10 lines revealed that their metastatic phenotypes were highly unstable during serial passage *in vitro* and *in vivo,* and variant subclones with diverse metastatic phenotypes emerged quickly.[31] In contrast, the metastatic properties of the uncloned parent cell lines were stable when exposed to the same culture conditions. The "destabilization" of the metastatic phenotype in the individual clones did not occur, however, when several clones were cocultivated together. The stability of the metastatic phenotype in individual clones during this experiment was verified by using clones bearing stable, drug-resistance markers and by showing that subclones exhibiting resistance to particular drugs had identical metastatic phenotypes to the original clones with the same drug-resistance phenotype.

These experiments suggest that in polyclonal tumors some form of "interaction" is occurring between the constituent clonal subpopulations. Thus, in a polyclonal population containing multiple subpopulations an apparent "equilibrium" exists which, in the absence of any further selection pressure, limits the emergence of new cell variants (or at least variants with altered metastatic properties) (FIG. 4).

Additional studies on the interaction between subpopulations have revealed that imposition of a selection pressure such as drug therapy can alter the "equilibrium" between the subpopulations and restrict subpopulation diversity by eliminating "unfit" subpopulations.[31] If the restriction in subpopulation diversity is substantial, then the "stabilizing" interactions involved in the "equilibrium" state are apparently lost and the surviving subpopulations exhibit marked phenotypic instability and quickly generate a new panel of variants with different metastatic properties (Ref. 31 and FIG. 4). With time, these variants, in turn, achieve a new equilibrium which persists until a new selection pressure again limits subpopulation diversity and the cycle is repeated (FIG. 4).

This phenomenon may also occur *in vivo*.[33] Isolation of multiple clones from individual lung metastases produced by the B16 melanoma has revealed that in "early" metastases, excised after 18 days, clones isolated from the same metastatic lesion typically show indistinguishable metastatic properties (that is, intralesional clonal homogeneity). This situation was found in approximately 80% of the early metastases tested, although the metastatic phenotypes of clones isolated from different metastases in the same animal do differ significantly (that is, interlesional clonal heterogeneity). In contrast, in "late" metastases excised after 40 days intralesional clonal homogeneity was found in only 30% of metastases and the remainder yielded two or more clonal subpopulations with differing metastatic properties (that is, intralesional heterogeneity). These data suggest that B16 melanoma metastases are populated initially by cells with a uniform metastatic phenotype. This is in agreement with data showing that the majority of experimental metastases result from the arrest and proliferation of a single tumor cell.[34] This *in vivo* situation is therefore analogous to the *in vitro* experiments described earlier in which individual B16 clones grown in isolation from other clones quickly generated variant subclones with altered metastatic properties. Studies are now in progress using B16 clones bearing drug-resistance markers to study the evolution of clonal heterogeneity within individual metastases *in vivo* in more detail.

Although these observations are the first to document an interaction between tumor cell subpopulations affecting metastatic behavior, work by Heppner and her colleagues has shown that cellular subpopulations isolated from the same mammary tumor exert growth-regulatory restraints on each other.[35] The interaction pattern is complex, however, with different patterns of uni- and bidirectional response occurring between different subpopulations. The same subpopulations also exhibit equally complex interactions affecting immunogenicity and sensitivity to cytotoxic drugs.[35] Similarly, nontumorigenic clones of B16 melanoma have been reported to suppress the tumorigenicity of other B16 clones when mixed together before implantation into mice.[36] The mechanism(s)

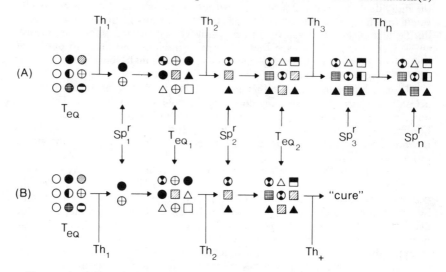

FIGURE 4. Schematic illustration of the possible effects of therapy on subpopulation diversity and stability of the metastatic phenotype in neoplastic lesions. By the time of initial clinical detection the lesion contains multiple tumor cell subpopulations. An "equilibrium" state (T_{eq}) exists in which "interaction" between the subpopulations limits the rate at which new metastatic variants are generated. On exposure to therapy (Th_1), susceptible subpopulations are killed and others survive (SP^r_1). This restriction of subpopulation diversity may render the surviving subpopulations phenotypically unstable and thus act as a stimulus for the generation of a new panel of tumor cell variants with widely differing metastatic properties. With increasing diversification, a new "equilibrium" state will again be imposed (T_{eq1}). On subsequent exposure to different treatment regimens (Th_2, Th_3), the cycle of subpopulation restriction and diversification will be repeated until either subpopulations resistant to all therapeutic efforts (SP^r_n) kill the patient (scheme **A**) or a therapeutic modality (Th_+) is identified that can kill all subpopulations within the lesion (scheme **B**). (From Fidler and Poste.[6] Reprinted by permission.)

underlying these fascinating events is not known. The numerous reports showing that the presence of the primary tumor can restrict the growth of metastases in certain tumors might also represent an analogous phenomenon (for a review, see Sugarbaker [37]).

    Irrespective of the mechanism involved, identification of these interactions between different subpopulations from the same tumor suggests that a full understanding of the role of tumor cell heterogeneity in determining the behavior of tumors and in predicting their response to therapy cannot be achieved by simple analysis of the individual component subpopulations, but will require more sophisticated analyses of subpopulation interactions.

Such interactions between different subpopulations also argue against anarchic progression of tumors. The apparent role of subpopulation diversity in regulating the rate at which new variant subpopulations of cells appear may be a mechanism whereby the tumor can maximize cellular diversity. Such a mechanism would serve two purposes: On the one hand, generation of new subpopulations under conditions where subpopulation diversity is restricted ensures that the tumor will not come to be dominated by a small number of subpopulations or even a single subpopulation. This has the advantage for the tumor that it reduces the likelihood that a destructive assault mounted against the tumor, either by host defense mechanisms or by the oncologist, will be successful in eliminating all of the subpopulations present. On the other hand, the apparent stimulation of subpopulation diversification caused by events that reduce subpopulation diversity provides a potentially potent mechanism for the relentless generation of new variants when the tumor is exposed to an assault that destroys a significant fraction of the subpopulations present.

We presently lack information about several fundamental questions concerning evolution of cellular diversity in malignant tumors. For example, when do metastatic variants first make their appearance in a tumor? Are they present very early in the life of a malignant tumor? Is metastatic potential present in certain tumors from the very outset of neoplastic conversion? Also, once metastatic subpopulations are present, do they have adaptive advantage over nonmetastatic subpopulations so that their contribution to the overall population will increase with progressive growth of the tumor? Answers to these questions are lacking and they represent obvious topics for future research.

The Phenotypic Heterogeneity of Malignant Tumor Cells and Therapy of Metastatic Disease

The findings that tumor cell subpopulations in polyclonal populations influence each other's behavior and that changes in subpopulation diversity can affect the rate at which new metastatic tumor cell variants emerge have potentitlly important implications for therapeutic practice. If we assume that similar regulatory interactions between tumor cell subpopulations occur *in vivo* and are common to most, if not all, tumors, then the timing of therapy and its effect on subpopulation diversity may be of crucial importance in determining whether a tumor can be destroyed.

For example, if a particular therapy were to kill the majority, but not all, of the subpopulations in a polyclonal tumor, the surviving subpopulations may be rendered phenotypically unstable because of loss of the regulatory interaction between constituent subpopulations which were previously in "equilibrium." By restricting subpopulation diversity, therapy may perturb this equilibrium and thus provide a stimulus for the rapid generation of new tumor cell variants from the surviving subpopulations (FIG. 4). Generation of variants would then continue until a sufficient level of subpopulation was achieved to again impose a new "equilibrium" via interaction between subpopulations and thus limit the rate at which new variants emerge (FIG. 5). Exposure of the tumor to subsequent treatment regimens would then repeat the cycle (FIG. 4, top panel) unless a therapeutic regimen was identified that was able to eliminate the surviving subpopulations before they had time to generate new variants (FIG. 4, lower panel).

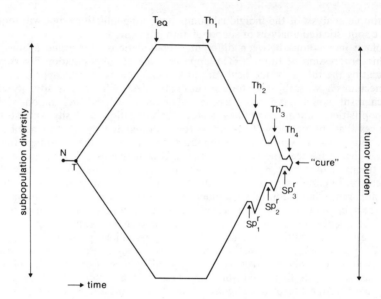

FIGURE 5. Schematic illustration of the possible effect of rapid sequential treatment of a neoplastic lesion with a series of different therapeutic regimens. After initial transformation of a normal cell (N) to establish an initial focus of tumor cells (T), new variants are generated to create a heterogeneous lesion populated by diverse subpopulations, which eventually establish an "equilibrium" state (T_{eq}) in which the generation of new variants is relatively low. When this population is exposed to therapy (Th_1), the subpopulation diversity and cell mass are reduced by the killing of susceptible subpopulations. The restriction of subpopulation diversity produced by therapy may provide a stimulus for surviving resistant subpopulations (Sp^r_1) to rapidly generate new metastatic variants. As depicted in this scheme, the second treatment regimen (Th_2) is given very shortly after the first treatment protocol, even though a residual tumor burden may not be evident clinically. By repeating the process and reducing the interval between successive treatment regimens (Th_1–Th_3), it is hoped that each successive treatment in the series will kill susceptible subpopulations in the tumor fractions (SP^r_{1-3}) that survive the preceding treatment(s) before they are able to generate a large number of new variants which may include variant phenotypes that will prove resistant to all available therapies. By truncating successive treatment regimens into a limited time period, it may be possible either to eradicate tumor cells entirely or to reduce the residual tumor burden to a sufficiently low level where host defense mechanisms, perhaps augmented by biological response-modifier therapy, can kill any remaining cells. (From Fidler and Poste.[6] Reprinted by permission.)

If the scheme in FIGURE 4 is correct, new experimental strategies will need to be explored with the objective of overcoming the problem of phenotypic instability in those tumor cell subpopulations that survive a previous treatment protocol. To achieve this it would be necessary to reduce the time between successive treatment with different therapeutic regimens (FIG. 5). The aim of using a series of different treatment protocols in rapid succession would be to attempt not only to kill those subpopulations that have survived the previous treatment before they are able to generate large numbers of new variants, but also to kill new variant subpopulations as soon as they emerge (FIG. 5). This contrasts with the practice in which subsequent treatment regimens using different agents are often not employed if the first treatment protocol appears successful in eliminating clinically detectable tumor burden. In this situation, additional treatment regimens are implemented only when evidence of a recurrent tumor is detected (FIG. 6). By the time such recurrent lesions become detectable clinically, phenotypic diversification of the surviving subpopulations may well

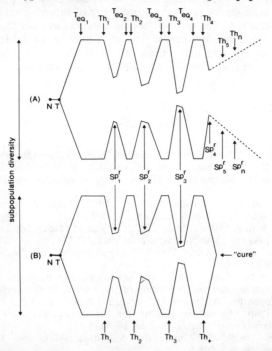

FIGURE 6. Schematic illustration of the possible effects of extended staging of successive treatment regimens on subpopulation diversity in neoplastic lesions. After initial transformation of a normal cell (N) to establish an initial focus of tumor cells (T), extensive phenotypic diversity is generated within the lesion, creating a heterogeneous lesion populated by diverse subpopulations that interact to establish an "equilibrium" state (T_{eq}) in which emergence of new variant subpopulations is limited. Treatment of such a lesion (Th_1) destroys some, but not all, subpopulations. Restriction in subpopulation diversity perturbs the preexisting equilibrium and stimulates the surviving subpopulation (SP^r_1) to generate new variants. This diversification process culminates in the establishment of a new "equilibrium" state between the new variants (T_{eq2}). By this time, recurrent tumor growth is detectable clinically and a second, different treatment regimen (Th_2) is initiated and another cycle of subpopulation restriction and diversification ensues. This process will continue until either the patient dies from a tumor burden (SP) that is refractory to multiple successive treatments (Th_5–Th_n) (scheme A) or a therapy is identified that is able to eradicate the entire remaining tumor burden (scheme B; Th_+). In contrast to the treatment strategy shown in FIGURE 5, the extended intervals between successive treatments shown in this figure may allow residual tumor cells to undergo extensive phenotypic diversification between treatments and thus increase the likelihood that new variants refractory to therapy will emerge.

have taken place and the lesion is populated by a diverse set of new subpopulations which may have widely differing therapeutic sensitivities (FIG. 5).

Research is only just beginning to examine the validity of these concepts and to establish whether the issues discussed here are of limited or general significance in the behavior of metastatic tumors. Further work is now needed to address two important questions: The first is whether therapy, by restricting subpopulation diversity within a heterogeneous neoplastic lesion (primary tumor or metastases), increases the phenotypic instability of surviving subpopulations, as proposed in FIGURE 4. The second question concerns whether the phenotypic diversification of the residual tumor burden surviving an initial treatment protocol (single or multiple modalities) can be blocked by treatment with a series of additional treatment modalities applied in rapid succession, as proposed in FIGURE 5.

REFERENCES

1. STEELE, G. G. 1977. Growth Kinetics of Tumors. Clarendon Press. Oxford.
2. SKIPPER, H. E. 1978–1980. Cancer Chemotherapy. Vols. 1–4. Southern Research Institute Monographs. University Microfilms International. Dallas, TX.
3. FREI, E., III & G. P. CANELLOS, G. P. 1980. Dose: A critical factor in cancer chemotherapy. Am. J. Med. **69:** 585–597.
4. FIDLER, I. J. & R. J. WHITE, Eds. 1982. Design of Models for Testing Cancer Therapeutic Agents. Van Nostrand. New York, NY.
5. POSTE, G. & I. J. FIDLER. 1980. The pathogenesis of cancer metastasis. Nature **283:** 139–146.
6. FIDLER, I. J. & G. POSTE. 1982. The heterogeneity of metastatic properties in malignant tumor cells and regulation of the metastatic phenotype. *In* Tumor Cell Heterogeneity. A. Owens, Ed. Academic Press, New York, NY. In press.
7. WEISS, L. 1980. Metastasis: Differences between cancer cells in primary and secondary tumors. Pathobiol. Ann. **10:** 51–81.
8. KOCH, F. E. 1939. Zur Frage der Metastasenbildung bei Impftumoren. Krebsforsch. **48:** 495–505.
9. KLEIN, E. 1955. Gradual transformation of solid into ascites tumors. Evidence favoring the mutation-selection theory. Exp. Cell Res. **8:** 188–199.
10. FIDLER, I. J. 1973. Selection of successive tumor lines for metastasis. Nature New Biol. **242:** 148–149.
11. BRUNSON, K. W., G. BEATTIE & G. L. NICOLSON. 1978. Selection and altered tumour cell properties of brain-colonising metastatic melanoma. Nature **272:** 543–545.
12. KERBEL, R. S., R. R. TWIDDY & D. M. ROBERTSON. 1978. Induction of a tumor with greatly increased metastatic growth potential by injection of cells from a low-metastatic H-2 heterozygous tumor cell line into an H-2 incompatible parental strain. Int. J. Cancer **22:** 583–594.
13. HART, I. R. 1979. The selection and characterization of an invasive variant of the B16 melanoma. Am. J. Pathol. **97:** 587–600.
14. SCHIRRMACHER, V., G. SHANTZ, K. CLAUER, D. KOMITOWSKI, H.-P. ZIMMERMANN & M.-L. LOHMANN-MATTHES. 1979. Tumor metastases and cell-mediated immunity in a model system in DBA/2 mice. I. Tumor invasiveness in vitro and metastasis formation in vivo. Int. J. Cancer **23:** 233–244.
15. POSTE, G., J. DOLL, I. R. HART & I. J. FIDLER. 1980. In vitro selection of murine B16 melanoma variants with enhanced tissue invasive properties. Cancer Res. **40:** 1636–1644.

16. FIDLER, I. J. & M. L. KRIPKE. 1977. Metastasis results from pre-existing variant cells within a malignant tumor. Science **197:** 893–895.
17. FIDLER, I. J., E. GRUYS, M. A. CIFONE, Z. BARNES & C. BUCANA. 1981. Demonstration of multiple phenotypic diversity in a murine melanoma of recent origin. J. Natl. Cancer Inst. **67:** 947–956.
18. DEXTER, D. L., H. M. KOWALSKI, B. A. BLAZAR, A. FLIGIEL, R. VOGEL & G. H. HEPPNER. 1978. Heterogeneity of tumor cells from a single mouse mammary tumor. Cancer Res. **38:** 3174–3181.
19. KRIPKE, M. L., E. GRUYS & I. J. FIDLER. 1978. Metastatic heterogeneity of cells from an ultraviolet light-induced murine fibrosarcoma of recent origin. Cancer Res. **38:** 2962–2967.
20. SUZUKI, N., M. WILLIAMS, M. HUNTER & H. R. WITHERS. 1980. Malignant properties and DNA content of daughter clones from a mouse fibrosarcoma: differentiation between malignant properties. Br. J. Cancer **42:** 765–771.
21. CHAMBERS, A. F., R. P. HILL & V. LING. 1981. Tumor heterogeneity and stability of the metastatic phenotype of mouse KHT sarcoma cells. Cancer Res. **41:** 1368–1372.
22. TALMADGE, J. E., J. R. STARKEY & D. R. STANFORD. 1981. In vitro characteristics of metastatic variant subclones of restricted genetic origin. J. Supramol. Struct. Cell Biochem. **15:** 139–151.
23. READING, C. L., K. W. BRUNSON, M. TORRIANNI & G. L. NICOLSON. 1980. Malignancies of metastatic murine lymphosarcoma cell lines and clones correlate with decreased cell surface display of RNA-tumor virus envelope glycoprotein gp70. Proc. Natl. Acad. Sci. USA **77:** 5943–5947.
24. SHEARMAN, P. J. & B. M. LONGENECKER. 1981. Clonal variation and functional correlation of organ-specific metastasis and an organ-specific metastasis-associated antigen. Int. J. Cancer **27:** 387–395.
25. ENDERS, J. F. & G. T. DIAMANDOPOULOS. 1969. A study of variation and progression in oncogenicity in an SV 40-transformed hamster heart cell line and its clones. Proc. Roy. Soc. Ser. B **171:** 431–443.
26. HANNA, N. 1980. Expression of metastatic potential of tumor cells in young nude mice is correlated with low levels of natural killer cell-mediated cytotoxicity. Int. J. Cancer **26:** 675–680.
27. POSTE, G. 1982. Experimental systems for analysis of the malignant phenotype. *In* Cancer Metastasis Reviews. I. J. Fidler, Ed. Nijhoff. Amsterdam. In press.
28. FIDLER, I. J. & I. R. HART. 1981. The origin of metastatic heterogeneity in tumors. Eur. J. Cancer **17:** 487–494.
29. NOWELL, P. C. 1976. The clonal evolution of tumor cell populations. Acquired genetic lability permits stepwise selection of variant sublines and underlies tumor progression. Science **194:** 23–28.
30. CIFONE, M. & I. J. FIDLER. 1981. Increasing metastatic potential is associated with increasing genetic instability of clones isolated from murine neoplasms. Proc. Natl. Acad. Sci. USA **78:** 6949–6952.
31. POSTE, G., J. DOLL & I. J. FIDLER. 1981. Interactions between clonal subpopulations affect the stability of the metastatic phenotype in polyclonal populations of B16 melanoma cells. Proc. Natl. Acad. Sci. USA **78:** 6226–6230.
32. NICOLSON, G. L. 1981. Personal communication.
33. POSTE, G., J. TZENG, J. DOLL, R. GREIG & I. ZEIDMAN. 1981. Unpublished observations.
34. POSTE, G., J. DOLL, A. E. BROWN, J. TZENG & I. ZEIDMAN. 1982. A comparison of the metastatic properties of B16 melanoma clones isolated from cultured cell lines, subcutaneous tumors and individual lung tumors. Cancer Res. In press.

35. MILLER, B. E., F. R. MILLER, J. LEITH & G. H. HEPPNER. 1980. Growth interaction in vivo between tumor subpopulations derived from a single mouse mammary tumor. Cancer Res. **40:** 3977–3981.
36. NEWCOMB, E. W., S. C. SILVERSTEIN & S. SILAGI. 1978. Malignant mouse melanoma cells do not form tumors when mixed with cells of a non-malignant subclone: relationships between plasminogen activator expression by the tumor cells and the host's immune response. J. Cell Physiol. **95:** 169–177.
37. SUGARBAKER, E. V. 1979. Cancer metastasis: a product of tumor-host interactions. Current Problems in Cancer **III:** 3–59.

STEM CELLS VERSUS STEM LINES

C. S. Potten and L. G. Lajtha

Paterson Laboratories
Christie Hospital & Holt Radium Institute
Withington, Manchester M2O 9BX, England

The hematopoietic system is perhaps the most complex of the interlinked hierarchical cell populations in the adult organism. Because of its accessibility to sampling, and to recent developments in experimental techniques, it is the best understood system. This is fortunate, because what we are learning from the study of the hematopoietic system is clearly going to be applicable to other cell systems, as we will discuss in this paper.

PLURIPOTENTIALITY

The concept of the three-tier system in erythropoiesis and granulopoiesis is well known (FIG. 1) and implies a stem cell population which is pluripotential in the sense that it can give rise to further differentiated descendants.[1] These descendants form two transit populations: the first differentiation step producing a progenitor population such as the "committed" erythroid progenitors, experimentally defined as *in vitro* erythroid burst-forming units (BFU-E) or erythropoietin-responsive cells (ERC). These give rise by a second differentiation step to the morphologically recognizable erythroblasts. In the case of granulopoiesis, the first differentiation step produced the committed granulocytic-macrophage progenitor (experimentally defined as *in vitro* granulocytic-macrophage colony-forming cells [GMCFC]), which gives rise to the recognizable granulocytes and monocytes–macrophages.

The hematopoietic system is, of course, more "pluripotential" than simply generating erythrocytes and granulocytes. Apart from giving rise to thrombopoiesis via megakaryocytes, there is evidence that the hematopoietic stem cell gives rise to lymphoid cells,[2] osteoclasts (but apparently not osteoblasts),[3] and at least some other "stromal" cells.[4] The differentiation pathways, kinetics, and regulation of these progeny are, however, as yet unclear. Similarly, it remains unclear precisely how the decision-making regarding pluripotentiality is achieved, that is, whether an individual stem cell has several options open and is committed to a particular line in response to external factors or alternatively whether it passes through a few binary (bipotential) cell cycles.[5]

In other systems such as that of the intestinal epithelium there is some, largely circumstantial, evidence to support the idea that the putative stem cells are at least tripotential, generating columnar, mucus-secreting, and Paneth cells. There is a suggestion that epidermal stem cells may also possess a certain pluripotentiality in that they may be capable of regenerating cells containing either epidermal or hair keratin, cells undergoing ortho- or para- types of keratinization, sebum-secreting cells, and possibly even mucus-secreting cells (for example, vitamin-A-induced metaplasia).

49

0077–8923/82/0397–0049 $01.75/0 © 1982, NYAS

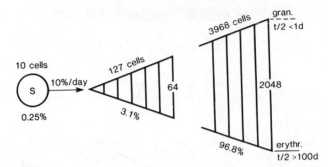

FIGURE 1. Scheme of two interlinked transit populations arising from a self-maintaining (stem) cell population. Two distinct differentiation steps induce the first and second transit populations with 6 and 5 cycles of amplification (64 and 32 times), respectively. The *upper numbers* represent the total number expected in each compartment, which are expressed as a percentage of the total population *below*. If 10% of the stem cell population is induced to differentiate per day, the proportion of stem cells in the total cells will be approximately 10: 4000.

COLONY FORMATION; CLONOGENICITY

While the pluripotentiality of the hematopoietic stem cell is well established on sound cytogenetic evidence,[6] it is important to remember that the only method with which hematopoietic stem cells could be quantitatively studied (at least until very recently) was the spleen colony-forming method,[7] which is essentially restricted to one species: the mouse. That the pluripotent spleen colony-forming cells in mouse (CFU-S or CFC-S) are stem cells is not doubted. However, it is clear that in other species the stem cells cannot form splenic colonies, neither can they in the WW^v mutant mouse).[8] In other words, the mouse CFU-S is a stem cell, but not all stem cells are CFU-S!

One should qualify this even further for the hematopoietic system: it is not certain that *every* splenic nodule in an irradiated and bone-marrow-grafted mouse is the result of a pluripotent stem cell. It is conceivable that some very early, already "committed" progenitors may produce a small visible colony in a mouse spleen. Hence, if we wish to equate stem cells with CFU-S, it should be remembered that not every splenic colony originates from a pluripotent stem cell! The only proof for the stem cell's being the CFU-S is the demonstration that the colony is transplantable, forming erythroid as well as granulocytic secondary colonies and, which is an even more stringent proof, that it can restore hematopoiesis in a lethally irradiated animal.

In epithelial systems these detailed experimental approaches have not as yet been adopted. However, simple clonal regeneration techniques similar to the CFU-S assay have been developed for some epithelial systems, such as those of the intestine, the epidermis, and even the spermatogenic epithelium. Perhaps the best understood is the epithelial system of the intestines, where similar but more extensive limitations and problems exist. In the steady-state crypt, it appears that not all stem cells are clonogenic (a few are very radio-sensitive and hence stand little chance of ever making regeneration foci) and not all clonogenic cells are stem cells in the steady-state crypt (there are many more clonogenic cells than steady-state stem cells, about 60 to about 16)[9] (FIG. 2).

SELF-MAINTENANCE

This then leads to the second cardinal property of the hematopoietic stem cell: self-maintaining capacity (the first was its pluripotentiality).

The terms "self-maintenance," "self-renewal," and "self-reproduction" are being used interchangeably in the literature, to the detriment of clarity. Self-renewal or self-reproduction may well apply to a cell that divides and produces two daughter cells that are operationally identical with the mother cell. This, in fact, happens, for example, with every division of early normoblasts or granulocytes, but these cells are clearly transit cells in the sense that an apparently inexorable maturation process gradually changes them, through 5 or 6 cell cycles, into a fully mature end-cell incapable of proliferation. At any one division the change is imperceptible (= apparent self-reproduction), yet the cell line is clearly not self-maintaining. Certainly most transit cell divisions are symmetric, producing two identical daughters. However, in the highly polarized epithelial tissues, the daughter cells occupy a higher position between the mature functional and proliferative "poles" and could be regarded as distinct from their mother by virtue of position, past division history, or future division potential.

The hematopoietic stem cells, however, are *self-maintaining* in the sense

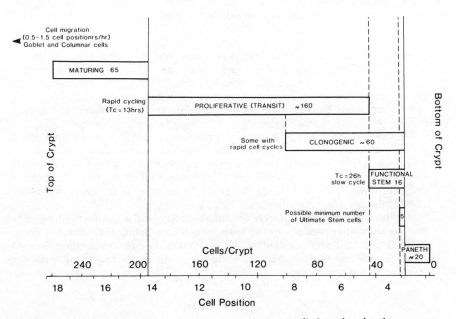

FIGURE 2. Cell populations in the crypt of the small intestine in the mouse. The population size, degree of overlap, and the various cell lineages (pluripotency) are shown.

that they divide some 200 times on the average in a mouse life span (probably some 2000 times in a human life span) [10] and they can be transplanted from an old animal into a young one in which virtually the same number of cell cycles will be completed. In the mouse this process may be repeated through 3 or 4 life spans. In the small intestine the stem cells may undergo as many as 1000 cell divisions in a mouse's lifetime (perhaps several thousands of divisions for humans), while in skin, in the mouse, the stem cells might divide some 150 times in the life of the animal. Generally serial transplant experiments have not been conducted using epithelial stem cells.

It would be futile to argue whether such cells, with their large division potential, are "immortal" in the sense that they could divide for ever and ever. Tissue culture cell lines are customarily termed "immortal," yet few if any of them have been carried through 2000 cell cycles—some 5½ years at daily doublings—*maintaining their identity*, that is, without demonstrable genetic changes. Hematopoietic and epithelial stem cells, however, appear to do just that: they maintain their operationally definable properties throughout hundreds (in some species maybe even thousands) of cell cycles.

For purposes of clarity—especially in view of the varying degrees of amplification in transit populations—we would suggest the criterion for self-maintenance be hundreds of cell cycles, probably five hundred at least.

STEM CELL NUMBER AND DEGREE OF AMPLIFICATION

One stem cell per day differentiating (input into the amplification compartment) could maintain some 4000 cells in amplifying transit maturation, and about 1000 granulocytes, or 200,000 erythrocytes in the peripheral blood (FIG 1).

With a 10% per day turnover (that is, 10% of stem cells differentiating per day) the total stem cell population would represent about 0.25% of the marrow cellularity. This may sound a rather low percentage, but to bring it up to 2.5% one would have to assume less than 1% turnover per day and the experimental data in the mouse suggest that the figure is close to 10% (cells in S as measured by thymidine suicide experiments).[11] Whichever is the case, the stem cells are a small minority in the bone marrow cell population.

In the surface epithelial systems the number of amplifying cell divisions is considerably less at 3 or 4 (that is, an 8–16-fold amplification). Hence, the stem cells, which, at least in the intestine, are probably all cycling, albeit slightly more slowly than the transit cells, constitute about 10% of the total proliferative cell pool, that is, about 10% of the proliferative zone of the crypt and about 10% of the basal layer in epidermis (FIG. 3).

In the stratified epithelium on the dorsal surface of the tongue the frequency may be somewhat similar. In the testis, about 10 amplification divisions occur (a total potential amplification of about 1000-fold). However, there is considerable cell loss so that the stem cells constitute up to about 1–2% of the spermatogonial population.

AGE STRUCTURE

This problem of "age structure of stem cells" has been raised in the past. The question involves a subpopulation of aging stem cells, originating from some "early" or "primary" stem cells. An "aging" subpopulation, however, with a limited amplification, represents another transit population.

To produce a spleen colony with 1–2 million differentiated cells and 10–100 further CFU-S might require a minimum of say 20 cell cycles, assuming a 40% removal to differentiation per cycle. If we assume that a similar 20 cell cycles occur in normal bone marrow hematopoiesis, most of which would occur within a transit stem cell compartment, then the number of ultimate "real" or "primary" stem cells might be unacceptably low—perhaps only a few per mouse or a few tens per man (with the more likely 30-cell-cycle amplification capacity). Even if this were increased by one or two orders of magnitude, it still might be an unacceptable "risk" to rely upon a few hundred stem cells in the mouse for all the hematopoietic cell replacement throughout the life of the animal, that is, without the cells' showing any evidence of aging and yet also being capable of coping with hematopoietic repopulation during transplantation experiments.

The number of cell cycles that have been assumed is taken from the mouse.

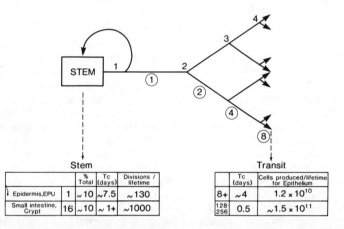

FIGURE 3. Proliferative organization of the proliferative units in epidermis (EPU)[26] and intestine (crypt).

That this number is somewhat elastic is well known. It should be remembered that 3–4 extra divisions during transit means an increase in output 8–16 times. Consequently, a one-tenth normal stem cell population can be compensated for by 3.3 average extra divisions during transit (as in the case of chronic irradiation conditions, for example).[12] The same number of extra amplifying divisions over normal may provide a 10 times normal output (as in hemolytic anemia), without any increased differentiation demand on the stem cells.

The niche hypothesis,[13] as well as the more general spatial configuration within the bone marrow of CFU-S and early differentiated cells,[14] suggests that different microenvironmental milieus might exist for cells of different hierarchical positions. These differing milieus might impose differing functional capabilities on the stem cells and hence impose an operational heterogeneity on the cell population. This seems likely to be the case in the surface epithelia, where topographic considerations are more evident and more easily studied. In the small intestine a steady progressive movement (displacement) of cells up the crypt can be seen. Here, the primary stem cells (to which all other cell replacement can be traced) occur at a specific cell position within the tissue (a circumferential ring of about 16–18 cells located just above the Paneth cells) (FIG. 2). Whether all these cells are in fact equipotential primary stem cells is not clear. Clonal regeneration studies suggest that about four times as many crypt cells can act as tissue regenerators as can act as "primary" stem cells. These clonogenic cells presumably occupy the four cell positions immediately above the Paneth cells (four circumferential rings of cells, three of which must be regarded as cells in transit that retain the property of clonal regeneration). Again this may merely be a reflection of the cell position (micromilieu) imposing a form of operational heterogeneity.

In epidermis the distribution of stem cells is such that each unit of proliferation apparently contains a single stem cell, which largely precludes any question of age structure. However, even here there is the question whether or not the hair follicles contain some primitive stem cells (highly efficient tissue regenerators).

PROLIFERATION CONTROL

Information is rapidly accumulating about factors controlling cell proliferation in the hematopoietic system. Factors involved in the control of the committed progenitors and recognizable maturing cells will not be discussed in this paper (recent reviews include those of Burgess and Metcalf,[15] Moore,[16] Lord,[17] and Testa [18]). Two points can be made, however: first, several of these factors have been investigated entirely with *in vitro* systems and hence their relevance to *in vivo* control is open to question. Second, there are a number of cell-line-specific proliferation modulators that act by slowing down (but not stopping) the cell cycle progression. These have been demonstrated to act *in vivo* and hence their physiologic role is more firmly established.

Proliferation control in the stem cell population appears to be different. First, the mechanism appears to be local, at least in the sense that a part of the femur, if shielded, will take little part in the regeneration of the rest of the irradiated bone marrow.[19] Second, two substances with different molecular weights have been demonstrated to be present in hematopoietic tissue: a stem-cell-specific proliferation inhibitor (fraction IV, more than 50,000 mol wt) and a stem cell proliferation stimulator (fraction III, 30–50,000 mol wt).[17] The specificities of these materials have been rigorously checked: the inhibitor (fraction IV) acts only on the pluripotent stem cells and not even on their immediate descendants, such as CFU-C (TABLE 1). Similarly, the stimulator (fraction III) does not appear to stimulate BFU-E. These factors are not produced by the stem cells, but by cells of different densities (FIG. 4) in the "stromal" fraction of the hematopoietic cell population.[20] Both the inhibitor and the stimulator are freely released from and are actively synthesized by their producer cells. Washed cells resuspended in serum-free medium will continue to release these factors for many hours.[17]

The mode of action of these stem cell proliferation regulators is also different from that of the erythroblast or granulocyte proliferation modulators. The modulators do not completely stop the proliferation of the cells, but the stem cell inhibiting "fraction IV" shuts down stem cell cycling completely. Indeed the action is more than a complete shutdown, it is a switch-off in the sense

TABLE 1

	CFU-S /10⁶ BM Cells	Per- centage in S *	CFU-C/ Plate	Per- centage in S *
Control	20.6 ± 1.7	31.0 ± 1.0	74.5 ± 4.5	45.8 ± 10
Fraction IV from normal bone marrow	18.7 ± 1.4	4.5 ± 1	73.5 ± 5.5	43.6 ± 7.2
Fraction IV from regenerating bone marrow or any other fraction from normal or regenerating bone marrow	20 ± 2	33 ± 5		

* ³H-thymidine kill.

that after a brief incubation with the inhibitor the cells may be washed thoroughly and then resuspended in medium—they remain in a noncycling state. The same switch, in this case to "on," happens after brief incubation with the fraction III stem cell stimulator: cells washed and resuspended will then continue cycling.[17]

A further intriguing aspect was in the interrelationships between the producer cells for fraction III and the inhibitor fraction IV and vice versa. The available evidence indicates that incubation of the stimulator-producing (fraction III) cells with an excess of the inhibitory fraction IV prevents the continued production of the stimulatory fraction III, and vice versa.

"NICHE" OR MICROMILIEU

While the picture of stem cell proliferation control is by no means complete, some features emerge from which at least a provisional sketch can be made. FIGURE 5 illustrates what has been mentioned earlier about stem cell

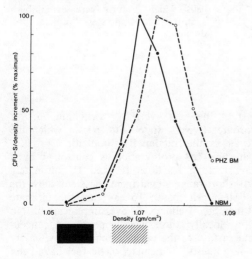

FIGURE 4. Density distribution of CFU-S in normal (NBM) (●) and regenerating (○) bone marrow (phenylhydrazine-treated, PHZ BM). The *solid block* indicates the density region in which the inhibitor-(fraction IV)-producing cells are concentrated. This represents only 3% of the total CFU-S population in normal marrow; the *hatched block* that of the stimulator-(fraction III)-producing cells, which represent only 22% of the CFU-S in stimulated marrow.[20]

proliferation control—the stem cells "signalling" their presence to the inhibitor-(fraction IV)-producing cells; these, in turn, inhibit stem cell cycling and also stimulator (fraction III) production. Removal (for differentiation or otherwise) of a stem cell will result in a decrease in the local strength of the signal to the fraction IV-producing cells. This results in a decrease of the local inhibitor production; consequently, the repressed stimulator (fraction III)-producing cells become active, and the stimulation produced by them can trigger another stem cell into the proliferative cycle.

It has been mentioned also that there is a time lag between administration of the inhibitor and cessation of cycling of stem cells. This is interpreted by postulating that the inhibition does not stop the stem cells which are in cycle

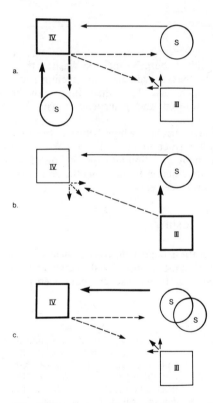

FIGURE 5. Scheme illustrating the interactions between CFU-S(s)/inhibitor-producing cells (IV) and stimulator-producing cells (III) in the regulation of stem cell proliferation. The relative intensities of the various signals are illustrated by the weights of the lines drawn. *Broken lines* are inhibitory signals; *full lines* are stimulatory signals except for those going from S to IV, which represent the signal that a stem cell is present. (a) The presence of a full complement of stem cells results in inhibitor production, which suppresses cell division in S and also stimulator production; (b) a deficiency in stem cells results in less inhibitor, which in turn permits stimulator production; (c) the result of (b) is an increase in stem cells, which in turn increases inhibitor synthesis and suppresses stimulator production.

(G_1-S-M), but prevents the onset of the next cycle by "switching on," or diverting the cells into, the nonproliferative G_0 state (FIG. 6), in which the cells remain until triggered into cycle by the fraction III stimulator.

It is envisaged, therefore, that stem cell proliferation is controlled by a balance of two short-range acting factors; fractions III and IV ultimately regulated themselves by a similarly short-range signal from the stem cells, the signal strength depending on the stem cell mass. To say that the ultimate regulation is the "local" stem cell mass is, of course, an oversimplification. No attempt is being made to define how "locally" these signals operate. A concentration gradient from the endosteal surface to the center of the marrow cavity has been noted [14] (FIG. 7), and micro "nests" of hematopoietic foci have been

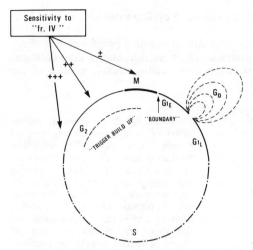

FIGURE 6. Possible mechanism of action of the inhibitory fraction IV factor. It is assumed that it eliminates the effect of a "trigger mechanism," which enables the cell to enter into proliferation after it has completed a mitotic cycle. As a consequence, after mitosis, the cell will be held in (switched into) a nonproliferating state (the stimulatory factor [fraction III] would reverse the effect of the inhibitor).

seen in bone marrow sections, and to some extent in the long-term marrow culture as well. Although it may be said that the ultimate signal comes from the local stem cell mass, the appropriate balance between inhibitor and stimulator concentrations must depend on the local number and functional state of the fraction-III- and fraction-IV-producing cells. A hypothetical microhabitat is illustrated in FIGURE 8 which shows varying distances between stem cells and factor-producing cells. On this basis, stem cell 4 is further from fraction-IV-producing cells and nearer to fraction-III-producing cells. The reverse is true for stem cell 3, hence the probability that stem cell 4 is going to cycle is greater than that of stem cell 3. Clearly, if in various regions of the hematopoietic system the relative proportions (or factor-producing capacities) of the inhibitor-versus stimulator-producing cells differ, the probability of cycling (turnover)

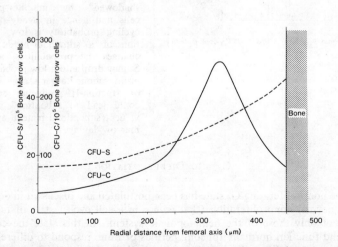

FIGURE 7. Distribution of the pluripotential CFU-S and the committed granulocyte precursor cells, CFU-C, across a radius of the cylindrical section of a mouse femur. (From Lord.[27] Reprinted by permission.)

of stem cells may differ too. Such difference in cycling rates has, in fact, been described by Lord.[14]

Regrettably, there are no hard *in vivo* data concerning proliferation modulation or control within epithelial systems. However, speculative considerations favor the idea of extremely local (over a few cell positions) control in the crypt.[21]

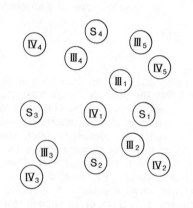

Order of distance to the 3 nearest

$$\left[\begin{array}{l} S \rightarrow IV : 1 < 2 < 3 < 4 \\ S \rightarrow III : 4 < 1 < 2 < 3 \end{array}\right.$$

∴ P (prolif.) : 4 > 2 (> 1 > 3)

[If III₁ elimin. P (prolif.) : 4 (> 3 > 2 > 1) = "subopt. plateau"]

FIGURE 8. A hypothetical micromilieu showing spatial relationships between stem cells (S), inhibitor-producing cells (IV), and stimulator-producing cells (III). The proximities are exaggerated. The average distance between each stem cell and the three nearest fraction IV- and fraction-III-producing cells can be estimated and the stem cell ranked in order of closeness to fraction-IV- or fraction-III-producing cells. The probability of proliferation (P.prolif) will depend on the balance between the proximity of fraction IV and fraction III producers. S_4 stem cell is the furthest from its inhibitor-producing neighbors (IV_4 and IV_5) and closest to its stimulator-producing neighbors (III_4 and III_5)—hence its probability of entering into proliferation is the highest. The stem cell with the next highest probability for cycling is S_2 (on the average nearer to stimulator-producing cells than inhibitor producers); S_1 and S_3 are more "overshadowed" by inhibitor-producing cells and hence in steady-state their cycling probability is low. Elimination of a stimulator-producing cell changes the probabilities, and even S_2 may drop into a low probability for proliferation. Larger scale elimination of fraction-III-producing cells thus could lead to suboptimal stem cell values (suboptimal plateau after bone marrow damage).

G_0 AND DIFFERENTIATION

The nonproliferating G_0 state has been postulated and discussed in detail [22, 23] as the normal nonproliferating (that is, not in a cell cycle) state of most stem cells, not only those of the hematopoietic system. In this state the cells may exist and function normally for long periods of time, respond to differentiation-inducing stimuli (if applicable to the stem cell line in question), and from this true resting stage (in respect of proliferation) they can be triggered into the cycling stage. In the case of the CFU-S of mice, the normal steady-state cycling rate is low, and mean turnover times of 3–4 days have been estimated.[10] Since the cycle times of cycling stem cells is considerably shorter than that, probably not much more than 7–8 hours in the mouse, the implication is that the majority of the stem cells at any given time are in a G_0 state.

A similar line of reasoning could be applied to the epidermis where the duration of the cycle $(S + G_2 + M)$ is about 20 hours, while the average inter-mitotic time might be of the order of 100 hours. On stimulation the system responds with a temporal reaction very similar to that of liver or salivary glands or indeed the adjacent, closely related, resting (G_0) hair follicles.[24] In the intestine the situation is less clear. No unequivocal evidence for resting (G_0) cells exists.

Nothing is known as yet about the stimuli or mechanisms whereby pluri-potent hematopoietic cells are induced to differentiate into one or other of the "committed" progenitor lineages. The term "committed" is imprecise—it would be more correct to say "more restricted in commitment" since even the pluri-potent hematopoietic stem cells are committed to produce a progeny, albeit one more "colorful" than that of their more restricted descendants. However, since differentiation (as opposed to maturation) is a qualitative change in the cells [1] a stem cell that is induced to differentiate ceases to remain a stem cell. In this sense differentiation "removes" stem cells from the population by turning them into some other cell, which thus ceases to signal its presence as a stem cell; it is thus the differentiation process that is the primary steady-state regulator of the stem cell population turnover (but not of the stem cell mass).

The biological significance of relatively long noncycling states in stem cells can only be surmised. The suggestion has been put forward [23] that this is a period required for "genetic housekeeping" in these cells that have a lifelong self-maintaining capacity, that is, cells in which errors in the genome, if not corrected, would be perpetuated and amplified. This would not apply to the relatively short-lived dividing transit populations with transit times measured in days, or 1 or 2 weeks. The stem cells—*because* of their long proliferation potential—are potential hazards for the organism if the integrity of their genome is not protected (maintained).

Accepting, for argument's sake, that the G_0 state represents necessary periods of nonproliferation (nonDNA synthesis), we have to consider how the optimal length of this state is maintained. To say that in the hematopoietic stem cells of the mouse the mean G_0 period (turnover time minus cell cycle time) is about 3 days is clearly a superficial approximation; the overall random-ness of removal of cells for differentiation—and the consequent cycling of stem cells—would result in a spectrum of G_0 periods ranging from perhaps hours only to months. Furthermore, it may be that what is significant for the cell is its "G_0 history," that is, the total time spent in G_0 state during a given period. If this is so, it may be considered that cells with a "short overall G_0 history" (for example, during the previous days) are more "at risk" than those with a long G_0 history. To eliminate cells "at risk" would be of some advantage and an "economical" way to do it would be to remove them for differentiation. As maturing transit cells they will only undergo a limited number of cell cycles and will be eliminated from the body as fully mature end cells.

Consequently, we would propose that stem cells with short G_0 histories (that is, higher cycling rate than average) have a higher sensitivity to differ-entiation-inducing stimuli, that their probability for removal to differentiation ("p diff.") thus increases, and that they are preferentially removed from the stem cell population. This also implies that their probability for self-maintenance ('p prolif.') is decreased. The application of this concept (FIG. 9) to various tissues including epithelia has been reviewed elsewhere.[25] The changes in "p diff." and "p prolif." can also be speculatively related to the tissue micro-milieu.

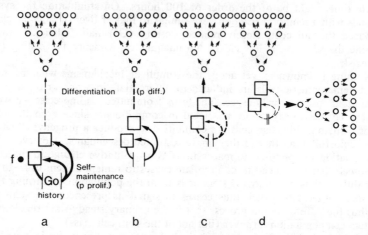

FIGURE 9. Schematic representation of cell replacement in adult tissues.[25] Stem cells of variable G_0 history may be located at specific positions (a–d) within the tissue relative to a hypothetical focal point (f) or niche. With increasing displacement from the focal point, the G_0 history may decrease, while the probability of removal to differentiation (p diff.) increases. The probability of self-maintenance (p prolif.) is the inverse of p diff.; the thicker the line the greater the probability.

REFERENCES

1. LAJTHA, L. G. & R. SCHOFIELD. 1974. On the problems of differentiation in hemopoiesis. Differentiation 3: 313–320.
2. WU, A. M., J. E. TILL, L. SIMINOVITCH & E. A. McCULLOCH. 1968. Cytological evidence for a relationship between normal hematopoietic colony forming cells and cells of the lymphoid system. J. Exp. Med. 127: 455–464.
3. ASH, P., J. F. LOUTIT & K. M. S. TOWNSEND. 1980. Osteoclasts derived from haemopoietic stem cells. Nature 282: 699–670.
4. KEATING, A. & J. SINGER. 1981. Personal communication.
5. HOLTZER, H. 1979. Comments. Differentiation 14: 33–34.
6. FORD, C. E., J. L. HAMERTON, D. W. H. BARNES & J. F. LOUTIT. 1956. Cytological identification of radiation-chimaeras. Nature 177: 452–454.
7. TILL, J. E. & E. A. McCULLOCH. 1961. A direct measurement of the radiation sensitivity of normal mouse bone marrow cells. Radiat. Res. 4: 213–222.
8. McCULLOCH, E. A., L. SIMINOVITCH & J. E. TILL. 1964. Spleen-colony formation in anemic mice of genotype WW. Science 144: 844–846.
9. POTTEN, C. S. & J. H. HENDRY. 1983. Stem cells in murine small intestine. In Stem Cells: Their Identification and Characterisation. C. S. Potten, Ed. Churchill Livingstone. Edinburgh. In press.
10. SCHOFIELD, R. & L. G. LAJTHA. 1976. Cellular kinetics of erythropoiesis. In

Congenital Disorders of Erythropoiesis. Ciba Foundation Symposium **37:** 3–24.
11. BECKER, A. J., E. A. McCULLOCH, L. SIMINOVITCH & J. E. TILL. 1965. The effect of differing demands for blood cell production on DNA synthesis by hemopoietic colony-forming cells of mice. Blood **26:** 296–308.
12. LAJTHA, L. G., L. V. POZZI, R. SCHOFIELD & M. FOX. 1969. Kinetic properties of haemopoietic stem cells. Cell Tissue Kinet. **2:** 39–49.
13. SCHOFIELD, R. 1978. The relationship between the spleen colony-forming cell and the haemopoietic cell: A hypothesis. Blood Cells **4:** 7–25.
14. LORD, B. I., N. G. TESTA & J. H. HENDRY. 1975. The relative spatial distributions of CFU-S and CFU-C in the normal mouse femur. Blood **46:** 65–72.
15. BURGESS, A. W. & D. METCALF. 1980. The nature and action of granulocyte-macrophage colony stimulated factors. Blood **56:** 947–958.
16. MOORE, M. A. S. 1979. Humoral regulation of granulopoiesis. Clin. Haematol. **8** (2): 287–309.
17. LORD, B. I. 1979. Proliferation regulators in haemopoiesis. Clin. Haematol. **8:** 435–451.
18. TESTA, N. G. 1979. Erythroid progenitor cells—their relevance for the study of haematological disease. Clin. Haematol. **8:** 311–334.
19. GIDALI, J. & L. G. LAJTHA. 1972. Regulation of haemopoietic stem cell turnover in partially irradiated mice. Cell Tissue Kinet. **5:** 147–157.
20. WRIGHT, E. G., B. I. LORD, T. M. DEXTER & L. G. LAJTHA. 1979. Mechanisms of haemopoietic stem cell proliferation control. Blood Cells **5:** 247–258.
21. POTTEN, C. S. 1982. Spatial inter-relationships in surface epithelia: Their significance in proliferation control. *In* The Functional Integration of Cells in Animal Tissues. M. E. Finbow and J. D. Pitts, Eds.: 285–300. Cambridge University Press. Cambridge.
22. LAJTHA, L. G. 1963. On the concept of the cell cycle. J. Cell. Comp. Physiol. **62** (Suppl. 1): 143.
23. LAJTHA, L. G. 1979. Stem cell concept. Differentiation **14:** 23–24.
24. POTTEN, C. S. 1971. Tritiated thymidine incorporation into hair follicle matrix and epidermal basal cells after stimulation. J. Invest. Derm. **56:** 311–317.
25. POTTEN, C. S., R. SCHOFIELD & L. G. LAJTHA. 1979. A comparison of cell replacement in bone marrow, testis and three regions of surface epithelium. Biochim. Biophys. Acta **560:** 281–299.
26. POTTEN, C. S. 1974. The epidermal proliferative unit: The possible role of the central basal cell. Cell Tissue Kinetics **7:** 77–88.
27. LORD, B. I. 1978. Cellular and architectural factors influencing the proliferation of hemopoietic stem cells. *In* Cold Spring Harbor Conference on Cell Proliferation **5:** 775–788. B. Clarkson, P. A. Marks and J. E. Till, Eds.

GLUTATHIONE AND AFLATOXIN-B₁-INDUCED LIVER TUMORS: REQUIREMENT FOR AN INTACT GLUTATHIONE MOLECULE FOR REGRESSION OF MALIGNANCY IN NEOPLASTIC TISSUE *

A. M. Novi,† R. Flörke, and M. Stukenkemper

Department of Pathology
Düsseldorf University
Düsseldorf, Federal Republic of Germany

INTRODUCTION

Previous results from this laboratory demonstrated that reduced glutathione (GSH) administered to rats bearing aflatoxin-B₁-induced liver tumors caused regression of tumor growth.[1] These findings in animals have raised the question as to whether the GSH treatment might be applied to humans.

With regard to the practical use of GSH as an antitumor drug, evidence should first be provided that the intact molecule is required by the neoplastic tissue for regression of malignancy. A reason for this is the findings of Hahn et al.,[2] who demonstrated that undegraded GSH does not enter normal liver tissue. In this paper, the question was approached by identifying the chemical form of the radioactive product recovered in neoplastic liver after administration of labeled GSH. In our previous experiments [1] the antitumor effect of GSH was investigated after administering a high dose (0.4 g/kg) by gastric intubation, an exogenous load that may influence the absorption of GSH from the gastrointestinal tract and/or its uptake by the neoplastic liver. It was therefore of interest to compare the amounts of radioactivity in livers of rats given a low or a high dose of labeled GSH.

The results reported here show that under both experimental conditions most of the radioactivity recovered in the liver was that of GSH, a result favoring the assumption that GSH itself is the active agent in producing regression of malignancy.

MATERIALS AND METHODS

Animals

Details on treatment of the animals and dosage of carcinogen were given in previous papers.[1, 3] Briefly, tumors were induced in the liver of female Wistar rats by an 8-week carcinogenic regimen of aflatoxin B₁ (AFB₁) (25 μg AFB₁ in 40 doses). Two experiments were carried out for comparison of the

* This work was supported by Research Grant IV B5–FA 8804 from the Ministerium für Wissenschaft und Forschung des Landes Nordrhein-Westfalen.

† Address for correspondence: Dr. A. M. Novi, Pathologisches Institut der Universität Düsseldorf, Moorenstrasse 5, 4000 Düsseldorf, Federal Republic of Germany.

0077–8923/82/0397–0062 $01.75/0 © 1982, NYAS

presence of radioactivity in tissues of rats given a single intragastric administration of [^{35}S]GSH. In the first experiment (the low-dose experiment) control and tumor-bearing animals were each given 0.26 μg GSH containing 18 μCi ^{35}S label (specific activity 21.3 Ci/mmol; New England Nuclear Corp., Boston, MA). In the second experiment (the high-dose experiment) the dose was 100 mg GSH containing 50 μCi of ^{35}S label (final specific activity: 0.15 mCi/mmol; New England Nuclear Corp., Boston, MA). All rats were killed 30 min after GSH administration, when peak levels of radioactivity were observed in both control and neoplastic liver (results to be reported in details elsewhere). Sacrifice took place between 10 A.M. and 2 P.M. All rats were fasted for 48 hours before intragastric administration of labeled GSH.

Tissue Preparation

The rats were killed by decapitation. After exanguination of the animals, tissues from control and tumor-bearing rats were quickly removed, weighed, rapidly frozen in a hexane dry-ice bath, and homogenized in 3 vols of 0.1 M phosphate buffer, pH 7.0, containing 0.1 M dithiothreitol. For determination of total organ radioactivity, aliquots of the total homogenate were solubilized and counted in Protosol/Econofluor (New England Nuclear Corp., Boston, MA). The radioactivity in the acid-soluble and acid-insoluble fraction of total homogenate was determined by precipitating aliquots of samples with 10% trichloroacetic acid and digesting the residual pellet with 1 N NaOH at 60° C for 30 min. Both fractions were counted in Aquasol. Packed blood cells were washed by resuspension in 0.9% NaCl solution and then lysed by addition of distilled water. Aliquots from each sample (whole blood or fractions) were solubilized and counted in Protosol/Biofluor (New England Nuclear Corp., Boston, MA).

Thin-Layer Chromatography of Acid-Soluble Sulfhydryl Compounds

To identify the cellular radioactive acid-soluble sulfhydryl compounds, liver homogenates were treated with a final concentration of 10% trichloroacetic acid to yield protein-free supernatants, aliquots of which were extracted with ether, concentrated by evaporation, and applied to a Dowex 50(H$^+$) column (3 × 1 cm). The bound fraction was eluted with 1.7 M NH$_4$OH and dried under N$_2$, and the residue was dissolved in 1 M dithiothreitol to which carrier GSH (0.016 M) and cysteine (0.04 M) were added. One μl aliquot of this solution was applied to cellulose thin-layer plates (E. Merck, Darmstadt, FRG), which were developed in one dimension [4] by 1-butanol/pyridine/acetic acid/water (30/20/6/18), or in two dimensions by 1-butanol/ethyl acetate/ acetic acid/water (20/10/10/7) (first dimension), followed by water-saturated 1-butanol. All running systems contained β-mercaptoethanol (20 μl/ml). Areas corresponding to sulfur-containing compounds, located by reference to unlabeled standards stained with ninhydrin and nitroprusside, were scraped into a glass counting vial containing 0.5 ml water. After heating for 60 min at 60° C, 10 ml Aquasol was added and the sample counted in a Beckmann LS 7500 scintillation counter. The purity of labeled GSH was established by rechromatography followed by exposure of the plates to X-ray film.

*Effect of Dose on the Amount of Radioactivity in Tissues of
Normal and Tumor-Bearing Rats 30 Minutes After a Single
Intragastric Administration of [^{35}S]-Glutathione*

To our knowledge, data thus far are lacking on absorption of glutathione after oral administration of this compound. It was therefore of interest to investigate whether the low or the high dose of GSH used in this study might be absorbed differently in normal and in tumor-bearing animals. Absorption was indirectly measured by estimating the amount of radioactivity that had disappeared from the gastrointestinal canal at 30 min. Data in FIGURE 1 show that at this time interval after a single intragastric administration of the low or the high dose of labeled GSH, the amount of radioactivity in the gastro-intestinal canal and its distribution in the stomach and intestine was quite similar in control and tumor-bearing animals.

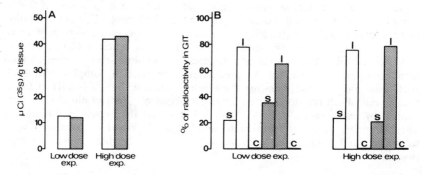

FIGURE 1. Comparison of the total radioactivity content (**A**) and distribution (**B**) in the gastrointestinal tract (GIT) of normal rats (□) and rats bearing aflatoxin-B₁-induced liver tumors (▨) after intragastric administration of a low or a high dose of labeled glutathione. Rats were given labeled GSH (as described in the MATERIALS AND METHODS section) and were killed 30 min later. S = stomach; I = small intestine; C = colon.

TABLE 1 compares the distribution of radioactivity in tissues of control rats and rats bearing AFB₁-induced liver tumors after a single administration of the low or the high dose of GSH. Under both experimental conditions the liver contained a greater amount of ^{35}S than any other organ. However, the relative amount of radioactivity taken up by the neoplastic liver was highly influenced by the dose of GSH: at the low dose, the specific activity of the neoplastic tissue was only 14% that of control animals, but control values were again reached with the high dose. While ruling out the possibility that the relative decrease in ^{35}S uptake by the neoplastic tissue with the low dose reflects the difficulty of the compound to penetrate tumor tissue, these results suggest that the uptake mechanism of the labeled compound by the neoplastic liver cells may be different after an intragastric load of GSH. Autoradiographic investigations carried out in parallel (results to be published elsewhere) have shown that the radioactivity is present in parenchymal and nonparenchymal

TABLE 1

EFFECT OF DOSE ON THE DISTRIBUTION OF RADIOACTIVITY IN TISSUES OF NORMAL RATS AND OF RATS BEARING AFLATOXIN-B₁-INDUCED LIVER TUMORS

	Experiment 1 (Low Dose)				Experiment 2 (High Dose)			
	Percentage of Absorbed Dose		Specific Activity (dpm/100 mg tissue)		Percentage of Absorbed Dose		Specific Activity (dpm/100 mg tissue)	
Tissue	Control	AFB₁	Control	AFB₁	Control	AFB₁	Control	AFB₁
Liver	68.0	22.0	123,360	16,880	4.0	11.0	11,102	11,610
Kidney	5.2	5.0	37,960	35,850	0.12	2.7	2,310	23,335
Spleen	0.85	0.6	14,030	12,350	0.05	0.08	2,080	2,520
Blood	11.9	9.4	103,350 *	86,910 *	1.84	2.4	38,870 *	46,675 *

NOTE: For details of the experimental conditions see text and FIGURE 1. Each value is the mean of two determinations, each consisting of four animals.
* dpm/ml blood.

liver cells. Since only 5.8% of the total liver population is composed of non-parenchymal cells,[5] the differences mentioned above should reflect different concentrations of radioactivity inside the parenchymal cells. Of interest was the observation that for the kidney the amount of radioactivity in AFB_1-treated rats was ten times that in control animals with the high dose of GSH. At present we have no explanation for these findings. However, the observation that the amount of ^{35}S in the blood and its fractions (TABLES 1 and 2) in the systemic circulation was about the same in control as in tumor-bearing rats rules out the possibility that the aforementioned variations resulted from a different distribution of radioactivity in the systemic blood.

For the spleen, no significant differences were observed between control and AFB_1-treated animals under either experimental condition.

TABLE 2

EFFECT OF DOSE ON THE DISTRIBUTION OF RADIOACTIVITY IN BLOOD FRACTION OF NORMAL RATS AND RATS BEARING AFLATOXIN-B_1-INDUCED TUMORS

	Percentage of ^{35}S in Blood (dpm/ml blood)			
	Low-dose Experiment		High-dose Experiment	
Fraction	Control	AFB_1	Control	AFB_1
Plasma	50	48	55	50
	(50%)	(50%)	(70%)	(65%)
Packed cells	13	14	12	11

NOTE: For details of the experimental conditions see text and FIGURE 1. Blood samples were taken just prior to sacrifice and analyzed for radioactivity as described in the MATERIALS AND METHODS section. Figure in parenthesis gives percentage of ^{35}S label in TCA-insoluble fraction of plasma. Each value represents the mean of two experiments, each consisting of four animals.

Effect of Dose on the Recovery of Glutathione by Normal or Neoplastic Liver 30 Minutes after a Single Intragastric Administration of This Compound

Independent of the absolute amount of ^{35}S label taken up by the liver, the distribution pattern of radioactivity into the acid-soluble and acid-insoluble fraction of control and neoplastic liver was approximately the same, with 70–85% of the label in the acid-soluble fraction. As shown in TABLE 3, 82–87% of this label was found in glutathione and 3–4% in cysteine in both normal and neoplastic liver, a result demonstrating that GSH administered intragastrically is mostly recovered as the intact molecule in both control and neoplastic liver. Data in TABLE 4 show that the level of GSH in both normal and neoplastic tissue is highly increased after an intragastric load of the compound. For the neoplastic liver, the relative amount of GSH was 10% of control values with the low dose while it reached control values with the high dose. Of interest is the observation that these variations paralleled the ones reported above for the liver uptake of radioactivity, a result suggesting that the level of GSH in the neoplastic cells is regulated at the cell membrane.

TABLE 3

AMOUNT OF RADIOACTIVITY DETECTED IN GLUTATHIONE AND CYSTEINE BY THIN-
LAYER CHROMATOGRAPHY OF THE ACID-SOLUBLE POOL OF NORMAL AND NEOPLASTIC
LIVER CELLS

Experiment	Radioactivity in the Acid-soluble Pool (dpm/g tissue)	Percentage of Soluble Pool Radioactivity in:	
		Glutathione	Cysteine
Low Dose			
Control liver	807,260	87	3
Neoplastic liver	94,750	85	4
High dose			
Control liver	91,400	85	4
Neoplastic liver	90,000	82	4

NOTE: For details of the experimental conditions, see text and FIGURE 1. Livers
were processed for detection of radioactive label in glutathione and cysteine as
outlined in the MATERIALS AND METHODS section. Average dpm spotted was 500,
except for control livers with the low dose (2000 dpm).

DISCUSSION

While providing no information on the mechanism of either GSH absorption from the gastrointestinal canal or uptake by the liver, the results of this
study demonstrate that GSH administered intragastrically is mostly recovered
as the intact molecule by the normal and neoplastic liver. With regard to the
practical use of GSH as an antitumor agent, it is of interest that the amount
of GSH recovered by the neoplastic liver is influenced by the administered dose,
a result suggesting that the antitumor effect of this compound may be dose-
dependent. A comparison of our findings in control rats with those of Hahn

TABLE 4

EFFECT OF DOSE ON THE RECOVERY OF GLUTATHIONE (GSH) IN CONTROL AND
NEOPLASTIC LIVER

Experiment	GSH Concentration (ng/g tissue)	Percentage of Variation of Control Values
Low Dose		
Control liver	2,5	100
Neoplastic liver	0,25	10
High Dose		
Control liver	28,500	100
Neoplastic liver	29,000	100

NOTE: For details of the experimental conditions, see text and FIGURE 1. Livers
were processed for detection of GSH in the cellular acid-soluble pool as described
in MATERIALS AND METHODS section. Each value is the mean of two experiments,
each consisting of four animals.

et al.[2] indicates that the route of GSH administration is determinant for the recovery of this compound by the liver. When 0.26 μg of GSH was given intragastrically to control rats (this study), up to 6% of the administered dose was recovered by the liver as the intact molecule. At variance[2] with our findings, no glutathione or only traces could be detected in the liver after intravenous administration of an amount of GSH more than 10×10^3 times that given intragastrically in this study (low-dose experiment). It is thus likely that the route of GSH administration (oral) may be determinant for the antitumor effect of this compound.

This study has shown that GSH administered intragastrically is mostly recovered as the intact molecule in the neoplastic liver, a finding consistent with the assumption that the undegraded tripeptide is required for regression of malignancy in the neoplastic liver. However, the mechanism whereby this compound causes regression of aflatoxin-B_1-induced liver tumors is presently unknown.

Glutathione is probably the most abundant natural low molecular weight thiol. Many roles have been ascribed to this ubiquitous tripeptide, and recent studies have begun to delineate its metabolism and physiologic function.[6-9] Hepatic GSH reacts with a variety of oxidized metabolites of organic compounds, giving rise to GSH conjugates that may be further metabolized and excreted as mercapturic acid.[10, 11] Most of the cellular GSH is present in the cytosol.[12] Occurrence of GSH bound to protein by mixed disulfide linkages is also reported.[13] Being a strong nucleophile,[14] GSH protects essential nucleophilic sites on vital macromolecules from electrophilic attack by "reactive" metabolites of toxicants that otherwise would initiate cell damage.[15] For AFB_1, this is supported by the finding of Mgbodile *et al.*,[16] who showed that the reduction of GSH levels in the livers of rats makes these animals more sensitive to the effect of the toxicant. Of interest is that a decrease in GSH content is also reported in rapidly growing hepatomas.[17, 18]

Carcinogens like AFB_1, which generate epoxides, have been reported to conjugate readily with GSH.[19-21] The formation of an AFB_1–GSH conjugate was found to occur concomitantly with the inhibition of AFB_1–DNA binding.[22] Glutathione-transferase B, or ligandin, has been isolated as a covalent adduct with carcinogens,[23] and an increased binding was found coincident with a decrease in the susceptibility of hepatocytes to carcinogenic insult.[24] GSH conjugation with ultimate carcinogens is therefore thought to be a very important detoxication reaction modulating AFB_1 carcinogenicity in various species.

If the classic assumption is made that the carcinogenic effect of AFB_1 is due to its covalent binding to DNA,[25] then GSH should protect against AFB_1 carcinogenesis only when administered at the very early phase of the neoplastic process, that is, before fixation of genotypic changes occurred.

Previous reports from this laboratory[1] have offered direct evidence that GSH protects against AFB_1-induced carcinogenesis when administered at the late stages of tumor progression. More recently, Brada and Bulba have reported that GSH administered to rats with palpable liver tumors induced by ethionine resulted in survival of the animals.[26] These findings are quite difficult to understand on the basis of the dominant concept of chemical carcinogenesis that tumor is brought about by an irreversible and incontrollable mutation.

Our recent experiences with the aflatoxin model of carcinogenesis has led us to view the carcinogenic process with a different perspective. Combined morphologic and biochemical observations during the development of liver tumors induced by AFB$_1$ have raised the level of complexity of the problem of determining which effect of AFB$_1$ is a nonspecific toxic one and which is necessarily related to carcinogenesis. By correlated light and electron microscopic studies [3] we have shown that the lag time preceding the appearance of cancer by histologic standards (up to 32 weeks after AFB$_1$ withdrawal) is characterized by a constant spectrum of ultramicroscopic changes which are usually considered either manifestation of a toxic injury or an adaptive response to a toxic agent. Both types of changes were essentially the same during and after AFB$_1$ administration, and they also characterized the hepatocytes within the hyperplastic foci, hyperplastic nodules, and neoplastic areas.[27] Biochemically, the carcinogenic activity of AFB$_1$ (between 7 and 66 weeks after cessation of AFB$_1$ forced feeding) resulted in a biphasic increase of liver weight due to a combination of hypertrophy and hyperplasia,[28] a pattern of liver growth usually observed during drug detoxication.[29] A reasonable interpretation of these morphologic and biochemical experiments was that the carcinogen might persist within the liver once its exogenous supply is stopped. Subsequent experiments with labeled AFB$_1$ proved this to be true.[30] These results are compatible with the hypothesis that aflatoxin-B$_1$-dependent neoplasia is a special case of reaction to toxicity, the characteristic of which is that the toxicant instead of immediately injuring the target cells will be stored into them. As a logical consequence of this hypothesis one could propose that the therapeutic effect of glutathione consists in "trapping" the reactive aflatoxin B$_1$ metabolites, a process leading to decreased toxicity. Experiments in this direction are currently under way in this laboratory.

ACKNOWLEDGMENT

We thank Prof. W. Hort for suggestions, criticism, and encouragement.

REFERENCES

1. Novi, A. M. 1981. Regression of aflatoxin B$_1$-induced hepatocellular carcinomas by reduced glutathione. Science **212:** 541–542.
2. Hahn, R., A. Wendel & L. Flohé. 1978. The fate of extracellular glutathione in the rat. Biochim. Biophys. Acta **539:** 324–337.
3. Novi, A. M. 1977. Liver carcinogenesis in rats after aflatoxin B$_1$ administration. *In* Current Topics in Pathology. E. Grundmann & W. H. Kirsten, Eds. Vol. 65: 105–163. Springer Verlag. Berlin-Heidelberg, Germany.
4. States, B. & S. Segal. 1969. Thin layer chromatographic separation of cystine and the N-ethylmaleimide adducts of cysteine and glutathione. Anal. Biochem. **27:** 323–329.
5. Van de Werve, G. 1980. Isolation and characteristics of hepatocytes. Toxicology **18:** 179–185.
6. Kosower, N. S. & E. M. Kosower. 1976. The glutathione–glutathione disulfide system. *In* Free Radicals in Biology. W. E. Pryor, Ed. Vol. **2:** 55–84. Academic Press. New York, NY.
7. Meister, A. 1975. Biochemistry of glutathione. *In* Metabolic Pathways, 3rd ed. D. M. Greenberg, Ed. Vol. **7:** 101–188. Academic Press. New York, NY.
8. Orrenius, S. & D. P. Jones. 1978. Functions of glutathione in drug metabolism. *In* Functions of Glutathione in Liver and Kidney. H. Sies and A.

Wendel, Eds.: 163–175. Springer Verlag. Berlin-Heidelberg-New York.

9. SIES, H., A. WAHLLÄNDER, C. WAYDHAS, S. SOBOLL & D. HÄBERLE. 1980. Functions of intracellular glutathione in hepatic hydroperoxide and drug metabolism and the role of extracellular glutathione. *In* Advances in Enzyme Regulation. G. Weber, Ed. Vol. **18:** 303–320. Pergamon Press. Oxford-New York.

10. CHASSEAUD, L. F. 1979. The role of glutathione and glutathione S-transferases in the metabolism of chemical carcinogens and other electrophilic agents. *In* Advances in Cancer Research. G. Klein & S. Weinhouse, Eds. Vol. **29:** 175–274. Academic Press. New York, NY.

11. WOOD, J. L. 1970. Biochemistry of mercapturic acid formation. *In* Metabolic Conjugation and Metabolic Hydrolysis. W. H. Fishman, Ed. Vol. **2:** 261–299. Academic Press. New York, NY.

12. WAHLLÄNDER, A., S. SOBOLL & H. SIES. 1979. Hepatic mitochondrial and cytosolic glutathione content and the subcellular distribution of GSH-S-transferases. FEBS Lett. **97:** 138–140.

13. HARRAP, K. R., R. C. JACKSON, P. G. RICHES, C. A. SMITH & B. T. HILL. 1973. The occurrence of protein-bound mixed disulfides in rat tissues. Biochim. Biophys. Acta **310:** 104–110.

14. WIELAND, T. 1954. Chemistry and properties of glutathione. *In* Glutathione. S. Colowick, A. Lazarow, E. Racker, D. R. Schwartz, E. Stadtman and A. Waelsch, Eds.: 45–57. Academic Press. New York, NY.

15. REID, W. D. 1973. Relationship between tissue necrosis and covalent binding of toxic metabolites of halogenated aromatic hydrocarbons. *In* Proceedings of the 5th International Congress on Pharmacology. Vol. **2:** 187–202. Karger. Basel.

16. MGBODILE, M. U. K., M. HOLSCHER & R. A. NEAL. A possible protective role for reduced glutathione in aflatoxin B_1 toxicity: Effect of pretreatment of rats with phenobarbital and 3-methylcholanthrene on aflatoxin toxicity. Toxicol. Appl. Pharmacol. **34:** 128–142.

17. FIALA, S., A. MOHINDRU, W. G. KETTERING, A. E. FIALA & H. P. MORRIS. 1976. Glutathione and gamma glutamyl transpeptidase in rat liver during chemical carcinogenesis. J. Natl. Cancer Inst. **57:** 591–598.

18. WIRTH, P. J. & S. S. THORGEIRSSON. 1978. Glutathione synthesis and degradation in fetal and adult rat liver and Novikoff hepatoma. Cancer Res. **38:** 2861–2865.

19. DEGEN, G. H. & H. G. NEUMANN. 1978. The major metabolite of aflatoxin B_1 in the rat is a glutathione conjugate. Chem.-Biol. Interact. **22:** 239–255.

20. JERINA, D. M. & J. W. DALY. 1974. Arene oxides: A new aspect of drug metabolism. Science **185:** 573–583.

21. RAJ, H. G., K. SANTHANAM, R. P. GUPTA & T. A. VENKITASUBRAMANIAN. 1975. Oxidative metabolism of aflatoxin B_1: Observations on the formation of epoxide-glutathione conjugate. Chem.-Biol. Interact. **11:** 301–305.

22. LOTLIKAR, P. D., S. M. INSETTA, P. R. LYONS & E. C. JHEE. 1980. Inhibition of microsome-mediated binding of aflatoxin B_1 to DNA by glutathione S-transferase. Cancer Lett. **9:** 143–149.

23. LITWACK, G., B. KETTERER & I. M. ARIAS. 1971. Ligandin: A hepatic protein which binds steroids and bilirubin carcinogens and a number of exogenous organic anions. Nature **234:** 466–467.

24. SMITH, G. J., V. SAPICO OHL & G. LITWACK. 1977. Ligandin, the glutathione S-transferase, and chemically induced hepatocarcinogenesis: A review. Cancer Res. **37:** 8–14.

25. WOGAN, G. N. 1973. Aflatoxin carcinogenesis. *In* Methods in Cancer Research. H. Busch, Ed. Vol. **7:** 309–344. Academic Press. New York, NY.

26. BRADA, Z. & S. BULBA. 1982. The regression of dl-ethionine induced hepatocellular carcinoma in rats by glutathione treatment. Presented at the Fifth

Annual Seminar of Cancer Researchers in Florida, Tampa, Florida, February 6, 1982.

27. Novi, A. M. 1981. Phenotypic identity of preneoplastic and neoplastic hepatocytes during aflatoxin B_1 (AFB_1)-induced liver carcinogenesis. J. Cancer Res. & Clin. Oncol. **99:** A39.

28. Novi, A. M. 1979. Sequential biochemical and morphological study of the rat liver during the early phase of aflatoxin B_1-induced carcinogenesis. Verh. Dtsch. Ges. Path. **63:** 476–477.

29. Shenoy, S. T. & C. Peraino. 1977. Changes in liver composition in phenobarbital-induced hepatomegaly. Exp. Mol. Pathol. **27:** 134–141.

30. Novi, A. M. 1980. Covalent interaction of ^{14}C-aflatoxin B_1 with macromolecules of rat liver during aflatoxin B_1 carcinogenesis. Toxicol. Lett. **1** (special issue): 0.109.

AN EXPERIMENTAL BIOLOGICAL BASIS FOR INCREASING THE THERAPEUTIC INDEX OF CLINICAL CANCER THERAPY

Bridget T. Hill

Imperial Cancer Research Fund Laboratories
London WC2A 3PX, England

L.A. Price

Head and Neck Unit
Royal Marsden Hospital
London, England

INTRODUCTION

After several decades during which antitumor drugs were considered predominantly, if not exclusively, for use in palliation of advanced disease, the role of chemotherapy is now being reassessed. Integration of chemotherapy with surgery and/or radiotherapy as first-line treatment is becoming more widely accepted for several tumors, particularly certain tumors in children, testicular teratomas and small-cell lung cancers.[1, 2] It is hoped that this approach, predominantly initiated in centers in North America, will be more widely adopted and extended to treatment of other common "solid" tumors. However, most of these clinical advances have arisen from the empirical design of therapies. Results of experimental laboratory studies published in the 1950s and early 1960s did provide a basis for adjuvant chemotherapy,[3, 4] although their clinical application was not tested until many years later. Experimental data were also available which emphasized the importance of full dose and optimal scheduling of drugs.[3-6] The reluctance of clinicians often to use chemotherapy is based on a widely held but mistaken belief that intensive chemotherapy automatically produces severe or even life-threatening toxic side effects.

The more logical design of safe and effective chemotherapy programs remains the joint aim of both clinicians and experimental laboratory scientists. Extrapolation of experimental data to the clinical management of malignant disease is often highly speculative and can even be misleading. In particular, the value of cell cycle kinetics in designing clinical chemotherapy protocols frequently has been questioned and criticized.[7-10] However, before we dismiss any valuable clinical application of cell cycle kinetic concepts, it is essential to distinguish between measurements of traditional cell cycle parameters on heterogeneous tumor cell populations and those concerned with "stem" cell kinetics, as originally described by the Toronto School.[11-13]

Experimental studies by Bruce and his colleagues [11] in 1966 provided the first demonstration that antitumor agents could be used selectively to destroy malignant as opposed to normal stem cells. We have extended the original experimental animal studies using human tumor cell lines and human tumor biopsy material *in vitro*. In particular, we have investigated in detail the influence of the duration of drug exposure on cytotoxicity. These experimental

72

0077–8923/82/0397–0072 $01.75/0 © 1982, NYAS

data have provided the basis for our kinetically based method of administering cancer chemotherapy over approximately 24 hours, thereby permitting the use of full-dose intensive drug combinations with greatly reduced side effects and no loss of therapeutic efficacy. The background experimental studies and their clinical applications are described in this presentation.

RESULTS AND DISCUSSION

Original Experimental Animal Studies

Successful chemotherapy depends on antitumor drugs exerting their differential effects on malignant and normal cells. In particular the maximal number of malignant *stem* cells must be destroyed with minimal damage to normal *stem* cells. It is the stem cells that are considered responsible for maintaining the integrity and continued survival of any population and they are capable of an indefinite number of cell divisions.[14, 15] In 1966 Bruce and his colleagues [11] were one of the first groups to highlight a kinetic difference between normal and malignant stem cells. They then showed, using lymphoma-bearing mice,

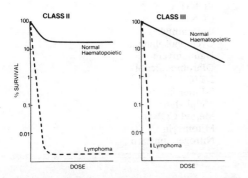

FIGURE 1. Kinetic classification of antitumor drugs based on the survival of normal hematopoietic and lymphoma colony-forming cells from mice treated with the drugs over 24 hours. (After Bruce et al.[11])

that by administering drugs over 24 hours this difference could be exploited, resulting in increased selective toxicity against the malignant cells. The drugs used fell into two main classes on the basis of shape of the survival curves obtained, as shown in FIGURE 1: Class II consisted of those drugs that after some initial kill did not further increase bone marrow stem-cell kill irrespective of dose while Class III included drugs which increased the bone marrow stem-cell kill with higher dose. In both classes there was marked selectivity against malignant stem cells. This specificity appeared to be based on the fact that in untreated mice most of the hematopoietic stem cells were resting, while most of the lymphoma stem cells appeared to be proliferating.[16] However, the time-dependence of these observations is important. Prolonged exposure beyond 48 hours or on a daily schedule resulted in increased damage to normal stem cells and a loss of selectivity.[17, 18] Similarly, if mice were treated after previous injury to the marrow, when hematopoietic stem cells were being recruited to a proliferating state so as to repair the damage, the selecitvity of these agents for malignant cells was lost, that is, the kinetically exploitable difference between normal and malignant stem cells applied only over a limited time of approximately 24 hours.

These studies formed the basis for the Kinetic Classification of Antitumor Drugs and have since been extended by various investigators to include other agents, as listed in TABLE 1.

Clinical Implications of these Experimental Studies

We proposed that a knowledge of this Kinetic Classification of Antitumor Agents might enable the effects of drugs on the bone marrow to be predicted. In this way toxicity could be reduced and safer cancer chemotherapy achieved. Therefore from these experimental data we made certain predictions, detailed in TABLE 2 and then tested them clinically.

TABLE 1

KINETIC CLASSIFICATION OF ANTITUMOR DRUGS *

Class II	Class III
Azaserine	Actinomycin D
Cytosine arabinoside	Adriamycin
Hydroxyurea	BCNU
6-Mercaptopurine	CCNU
Methotrexate	Chlorambucil
Procarbazine	Cyclophosphamide
Vinblastine	Daunomycin
Vincristine	Dibromodulcitol
	DTIC
	5-Fluorouracil
	Melphalan
	Methyl CCNU
	Mitomycin C
	Nitrogen mustard

* Reviewed by Hill.[19]

Clinical Verification of Experimental Predictions

Scheduling drugs over approximately 24 hours in man rather than treatment over a prolonged period of several days has been shown to reduce the toxicity but not the effectiveness of chemotherapy, provided certain standard medical precautions listed in TABLE 3 are routinely observed. TABLE 4 provides examples of how the administration of several antitumor drugs has been rescheduled. For example, a total dose of 40 g of hydroxyurea can be administered as 10 g every 6 hours for 24 hours and repeated every 14 days, as opposed to the conventional daily administration of approximately 1.5 g over 15 days. Similarly, actinomycin D at approximately comparable total dosage can be administered safely as an intravenous "stat" dose, as we recommend, rather than by daily administration for 5 days. In all cases problems of bone marrow toxicity have been reduced, and when nausea and vomiting occurred, their duration was significantly shortened. It has also been shown that the marrow toxicity of combination chemotherapy can be significantly reduced if the drugs are given over 24 hours only rather than over several days. For example, in

TABLE 2

EXPERIMENTAL PREDICTIONS OF CLINICAL RELEVANCE *

1. Optimal tumor cell kill can be achieved *without* severe bone marrow toxicity.
2. Marrow toxicity will be less if drugs are given over 24–36 hours in man.
3. Marrow toxicity of Class II agents is related more to duration of exposure than to dose.
4. Class III agents in combination will be additively toxic to the marrow, and doses should be reduced proportionately.
5. The practice of giving small daily doses of drugs from either class should be avoided.

* After Hill [19] and Price.[20]

breast cancer,[24] testicular teratomas,[25] and nonsquamous cell lung cancer,[26] in the treatment of advanced disease, the response rates achieved have been comparable with those reported using alternative and more toxic drug scheduling.

Prediction 3 in TABLE 2 was first tested clinically with methotrexate. In 1969 we showed [27] that 20,000 mg of methotrexate (a Class II agent) could be given safely over 24 hours and that this was associated with no additional toxicity, provided the precautions listed in TABLE 3 were rigorously observed. However, when the dose was reduced to 7,000 mg, but the infusion time was increased to 48 hours, there was a significant decrease in both platelet and neutrophil counts. This illustrates that the toxicity was proportional to the time

TABLE 3

PRECAUTIONS TO BE OBSERVED IN ALL CASES WHEN CHEMOTHERAPY
IS BEING ADMINISTERED

1. *Never* give another treatment cycle unless the peripheral white cell and platelet counts have returned to their original level. If in doubt, postpone treatment for 1 week.
2. Patients with impaired renal function receiving methotrexate *must* have an extended folinic acid "rescue" (that is, three times longer than normal). Patients with a creatinine clearance of less than 60 ml/min should not be given methotrexate at all.
3. Doses of all Class III drugs, such as cyclophosphamide, adriamycin, 5-fluorouracil and cis-platinum, should be halved in patients who have had extensive thoracic, pelvic, or abdominal irradiation.
4. Adriamycin should not be given to patients with a history of cardiac failure. The total dose of adriamycin should never exceed 550 mg/m². The dose of adriamycin should be halved in patients who have impaired hepatic function.
5. *All* patients, especially those receiving drugs that are excreted in the urine, such as methotrexate, hydroxyurea and cis-platinum, *must be adequately hydrated* and passing urine while they are receiving the drugs (that is, passing at least 2 liters of urine in 24 hours).
6. Bleomycin should not be given to any patient with impaired respiratory function.
7. Combinations containing nitrosoureas, melphalan, or mitomycin C should be given only every 6 to 8 weeks because these drugs have a delayed effect on the bone marrow.

of the infusion and not to the dose of methotrexate used. The data in FIGURE 2 show the effects on the peripheral blood count of a child with leukemia given similar doses of methotrexate on two different schedules: (a) twice weekly, as in a 1972 Medical Research Council Trial; and (b) over 24 hours as an infusion. The effect on the blast count was the same on each occasion. However, the twice-weekly schedule was associated with a profound decrease in platelet and neutrophil counts, in contrast to the lack of toxicity accompanying the 24-hour schedule. Thus, prediction 3 appears valid for methotrexate. We have also shown (1) that the high doses of hydroxyurea listed in TABLE 4 can be given safely provided the time of treatment does not exceed 30 hours, and

TABLE 4

CLINICAL RESCHEDULING OF DRUGS OVER 24 HOURS

Drug	Class	Conventional Dose and Schedule *	Modification Using the 24-Hour Method
Hydroxyurea	II	20–30 mg/kg orally daily for 15 days or to toxicity	40 g (total dose) over 24 hr (10 g q 6 hr $\times$ 4) every 2 weeks
Procarbazine	II	70–140 mg/m² daily for 14 days; 100–200 mg daily for 7 days, then 300 mg daily to toxicity	800 mg (total dose) over 24 hr (200 mg q 6 hr $\times$ 4) every 3 weeks
Cytosine arabinoside	II	2 mg/kg daily for 10 days; 0.5–1 mg/kg infused for 10 days	400 mg (total dose) infused over 24 hr every 3 weeks
VP–16–213	II	60 mg/m² intravenously daily for 5 days; 120 mg/m² orally daily for 5 days	1200 mg (total dose) infused over 16 hr every 2–3 weeks
Actinomycin D	III	0.5 mg daily for 5 days; 0.015 mg/kg daily for 5 days	2 mg (total dose) intravenously statim every 3 weeks
Dibromodulcitol	III	4–6 mg/kg daily over 15 days; 2.5–3 mg/kg daily for 30–42 + days	2 g (total dose) orally every 3 weeks

* These data were obtained from Goodman and Gilman,[21] except for VP–16–213 and dibromodulcitol, where Arnold and Whitehouse [22] and Michler et al.,[23] respectively, are quoted.

(2) that the high doses of cytosine arabinoside and procarbazine given over 24 hours are much less toxic than similar doses divided and administered over several days.[28]

When Class II drugs are administered over fewer than 48 hours they can be added to other drug combinations in full dosage without enhancing bone marrow toxicity. For example, in advanced bronchogenic carcinoma 200 mg methotrexate was added to adriamycin (80 mg/m²) and 5-fluorouracil (1200 mg), without reducing their dose levels. Toxicity was not increased and in this case a markedly superior response rate resulted.[26] The conventional "MOPP"

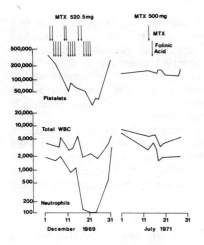

FIGURE 2. Peripheral blood chart of a patient receiving similar doses of methotrexate (see text). Note the marked toxicity with the twice-weekly regimen and no toxicity with the 24-hour regimen. (After Price.[20])

treatment for Hodgkin's disease has also been modified to include procarbazine over 2 days only, and patients have tolerated total dosages of procarbazine of 1700 mg without side effects other than nausea.[29]

The inclusion of more than one Class III agent in a combination, however, requires a proportionate reduction in dosage for safety, as pointed out in prediction 4 (TABLE 2). Our original protocol for treating breast cancer, designed in 1971, included cyclophosphamide (600 mg/m²), 5-fluorouracil (500 mg/m²), vincristine (1 mg/m²), and methotrexate (100 mg/m² infused over 16 hours) followed at 20 hours by a standard folinic acid rescue. This resulted in a 67% response rate in advanced disease with minimal toxicity [24] compared with that reported when the same drugs were given over 5 days. With the advent of adriamycin, we have now incorporated this Class III agent into our protocol, but observing the same kinetic principles we have reduced the doses of cyclophosphamide and 5-fluorouracil, as shown in FIGURE 3. This protocol has produced a response rate of 70% in advanced disease with minimal toxicity other than alopecia.[30] It is now being used as an adjuvant treatment for Stage II breast cancer in a randomized, prospective, controlled trial by the West Midlands Oncology Breast Cancer Group (WMOBCG) in the United Kingdom. Survival data are not yet available. However, toxicity data have been presented

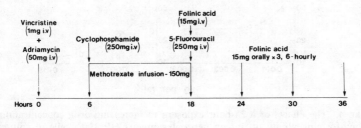

(Price-Hill, 1977)

FIGURE 3. The West Midland Oncology Breast Cancer Group trial protocol for node-positive breast cancer patients. (Designed by Price and Hill, 1977.)

for patients entered by 33 surgeons in 24 collaborating hospitals.[31] In 667 cycles of treatment no serious bone marrow toxicity and no overt cardiac damage have been observed. Alopecia occurred in all patients. Nausea complicated 66% of treatment cycles and vomiting occurred in 48%. Both symptoms were usually of short duration (2 of 21 days) and quality of life between treatment cycles has been very satisfactory. This small number of adverse side effects compares very favorably with those of other previously reported and ongoing adjuvant studies in breast cancer.

In summary, therefore, these experimental animal studies have provided a basis for safer cancer chemotherapy involving minimal toxicity to normal bone marrow without compromising antitumor effectiveness. We have now extended the original experimental studies and are working with human tumors predominantly *in vitro*. We continue to test our laboratory observations for clinical value and some examples are discussed below.

Recent Experimental and Clinical Studies with Human Tumor Material

Evaluation of Newer Antitumor Agents

Experimental Data. Working with established human tumor cell lines, we have evaluated drug sensitivities using 24-hour exposure times and we have assessed effects on survival using colony-forming assays. The data in FIGURES 4 and 5 using neuroblastoma (CHP 100) cells [32] show that using these straightforward *in vitro* assays we are able to reproduce the two types of survival curves originally described by Bruce *et al.*[11] Similar observations have also been made

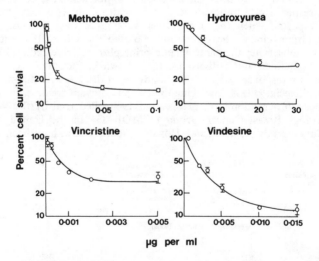

FIGURE 4. The effects of a 24-hour exposure to increasing drug concentrations on the colony-forming ability of human neuroblastoma (CHP 100) cells in culture. A plateau in these survival curves is always observed with these drugs. Each point represents the mean of four estimations and the experiments were repeated at least twice. Only standard errors in excess of 5% have been included on the figures. (From Hill and Whelan.[32] Reprinted by permission.)

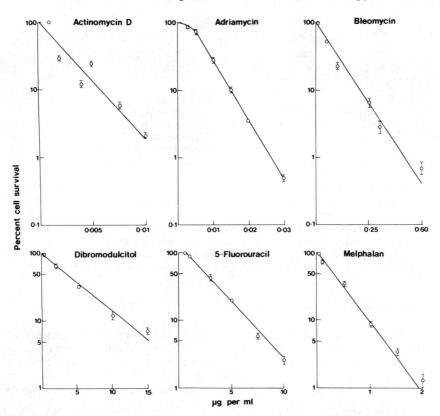

FIGURE 5. Same experiment as that described in FIGURE 4, but with all these drugs, tumor cell kill increased exponentially wtih increasing drug concentrations.

in our laboratory using lines of human colon carcinoma (COLO 205 and LoVo cells). We have therefore used this simple model system to examine and classify newer antitumor agents. Examples from our recent studies are listed in TABLE 5 and data for four of these drugs are shown in FIGURE 6.

Clinical Application. This ability to classify the newer antitumor agents provides information for their clinical scheduling. If drugs are administered over 24 hours, any myelotoxicity of Class III drugs would increase with increasing dose, but this would not be the case for Class II agents. This information is valuable for testing new drugs as single agents and is important if they are to be incorporated safely into drug combinations. For example, (1) a dose of 1200 mg of VP–16–213 can be infused safely over 16 hours without marrow toxicity or any changes in patients' routine biochemical profiles; and (2) the demonstrated additional value of cisplatin in testicular teratomas led to our rescheduling the valuable protocol originally proposed by Einhorn.[33] We also included further drugs and our modified schedule is as follows: at time zero, cyclophosphamide 500 mg intravenously immediately, vinblastine 10 mg intravenously immediately and actinomycin D 2 mg intravenously immediately; from zero to 6 hours, a methotrexate infusion of 200 mg in 2 liters of normal saline

TABLE 5

KINETIC CLASSIFICATION OF NEWER ANTITUMOR AGENTS

Class II	Class III
DDMP	mAMSA
ICRF 159	Cis-Platinum
Pyrazofurin	4'-epiadriamycin
Vindesine	4'-deoxyadriamycin
VP–16–213	Ellipticinium
	Spirogermanium

solution, followed by a 6-hour infusion from 6 to 12 hours of bleomycin 60 mg; then from 12 to 16 hours, 100 mg cisplatin in 1 liter of dextrose-saline solution; and finally a folinic acid rescue commencing at 16 hours (15 mg orally or intramuscularly, 8 doses 6-hourly). This modified protocol can be administered safely, with antiemetic cover, and requires hospitalization for only three days for each treatment cycle. In this pilot study in a small number of patients it is also effective, but of course long term follow-up data are not yet available.

Establishment of Time-Dependent Cytotoxicity of Antitumor Agents

Experimental Data. The animal studies of Bruce *et al.*[11, 17, 18] emphasized the critical time-dependence of selectivity with the antitumor drugs against malignant cells, since selectivity was reduced or lost after prolonged exposure beyond 48 hours. We have investigated the importance of the time factor in scheduling drug exposures using our *in vitro* model system. FIGURE 7 shows

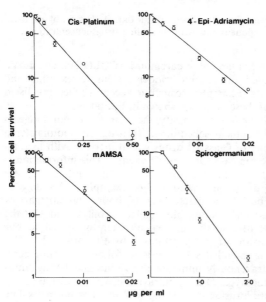

FIGURE 6. The effects of a 24-hour exposure to increasing concentrations of certain newer antitumor agents on the colony-forming ability of human neuroblastoma (CHP 100) cells in culture. Data were obtained and analyzed as detailed for FIGURE 4.

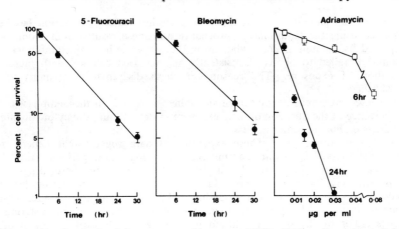

FIGURE 7. Survival of human neuroblastoma (CHP 100) cells estimated by colony-forming assays after treatment *in vitro* with a fixed concentration of either 5-fluorouracil (5000 ng/ml) or bleomycin (250 ng/ml) for a variable exposure time (1–30 hours) or a range of adriamycin concentrations for either 6 or 24 hours. Data were obtained and analyzed as detailed in FIGURE 4.

that for Class III drugs there is increasing kill both with increased duration of exposure and increased drug concentration. However, for Class II drugs (FIG. 8) negligible kill occurs after a 1-hour exposure, even to very high drug concentrations, but by increasing the exposure time, further cell kill can be achieved. A plateau in the survival curves is always obtained, however, for methotrexate, irrespective of any increase in drug concentration, but the level of this plateau is dictated by the length of drug exposure. Similar data are also available for the colon carcinoma COLO 205 cells and with human ovarian tumor cells obtained

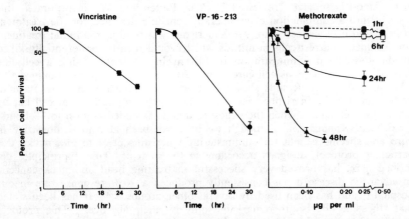

FIGURE 8. Survival of human neuroblastoma (CHP 100) cells estimated by colony-forming assays after treatment *in vitro* with a fixed concentration of either vincristine (5 ng/ml) or VP–16–213 (500 ng/ml) for a variable exposure time (1–30 hours) or a range of methotrexate concentrations for 1, 6, 24 or 48 hours. Data were obtained and analyzed as detailed in FIGURE 4.

directly from patients.[34, 35] In these latter studies, colony formation has been assessed using the Courtenay [36] procedure and these results differ from those reported by Salmon et al.,[37] who, using the assay method of Hamburger and Salmon,[38] failed to observe consistently an increased cell kill with increased duration of exposure. The reason for these discrepancies remains to be established.

These more recent experimental studies therefore further emphasize the importance of the duration of drug exposure in determining the cytotoxic effects of drugs on human tumor cells.

Clinical Application. These experimental data suggest that benefit may accrue if Class II agents are administered over longer time periods rather than as "stat" doses. This provides a rationale for infusing these drugs over approximately 24 hours, a procedure being tested now, for example, with VP–16–213 (see earlier) and vindesine.[39] Indeed, if one follows the original data of Bruce et al.[11] precisely, there may well be benefit in administering all drugs either by infusion or split dosage over 24 hours rather than in using "stat" doses. Further knowledge of pharmacokinetics would help to achieve a constant dose during a 24-hour drug exposure in man. It will then be necessary to set up randomized studies to establish which treatment strategy proves most effective clinically.

Value of Sequencing Drugs in Combinations

Experimental Data. We have investigated the possibility that the effectiveness of combination chemotherapy may be improved by specifically spacing and sequencing drugs. For example, in the early 1970s, it was often proposed that attempts should be made to exploit the principle of synchronization and recruitment to enhance tumor cell kill. The validity of this procedure had been demonstrated in a few *in vitro* systems and was implicated in several experimental models *in vivo* (reviewed by Van Putten [40]). We incorporated this concept into a combination chemotherapy schedule designed for the treatment of head and neck cancer (FIG. 9). Vincristine was used as the initial treatment which aimed to arrest cells in mitosis which would then be preferentially killed by the subsequent administration of bleomycin. Recently, using a cell line derived from a squamous cell carcinoma of the tongue, we have examined this scheduling *in vitro*. Results shown in TABLE 6 demonstrate no advantage to pretreatment with vincristine. However, they again emphasize that cell kill by the drugs is enhanced when the exposure time is extended from 6 to 18 hours.

Clinical Application. Although we have not been able to demonstrate *in vitro* any specific benefit for administering vincristine prior to bleomycin, this particular protocol, designed according to the stem cell kinetic principles described here, has proved very successful in treating head and neck cancers. In advanced disease it has consistently produced a 70% response rate in our hospital [41] and has been used by several other groups.[42–44] It has been stated that "the side effects are remarkable only by their absence." This protocol therefore has proved highly acceptable to both clinicians and patients.

We have shown that prior radiation significantly reduces response to scheduled A chemotherapy.[41, 45] However, we have now used schedule A chemotherapy as initial treatment on days 1 and 14 prior to definitive local therapy. Of 195 patients evaluated on day 28 for chemotherapy response, 131 (67%)

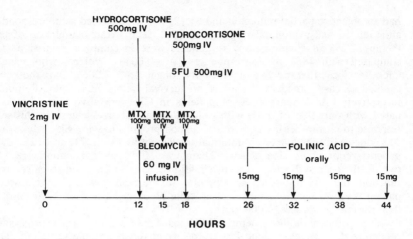

HOURS

FIGURE 9. Schedule A chemotherapy for the treatment of head and neck cancer. (After Price and Hill.[41])

TABLE 6

INFLUENCE OF DURATION OF EXPOSURE AND SEQUENCING OF A COMBINATION OF VINCRISTINE, METHOTREXATE AND BLEOMYCIN ON THE *in Vitro* SENSITIVITY OF A HUMAN CELL LINE DERIVED FROM A SQUAMOUS CELL CARCINOMA OF THE HEAD AND NECK (HN-1)

Drugs Used	Exposure Duration *in Vitro* at 37°	Percent Survival *
Single Agents		
Vincristine (1.5 ng/ml)	6 hr	83.0 ± 8.5
	18 hr	56.0 ± 3.4
Methotrexate (0.4 μg/ml)	6 hr	100 ± 5.3
	18 hr	24.0 ± 2.3
Bleomycin (0.75 μg/ml)	6 hr	65.0 ± 3.9
	18 hr	17.1 ± 2.2
Combinations		
"Simultaneous"		
Vincristine, methotrexate,	All drugs for 6 hr	61.0 ± 3.2
and bleomycin	All drugs for 18 hr	6.5 ± 0.6
"Sequential"		
Vincristine, methotrexate,	VCR at zero, then	
and bleomycin	add MTX + BLM at	
	6 hr; assess	35.0 ± 4.1
	survival at 18 hr	

* Survival was assessed by colony-forming assays, using soft agar.[35] Each point represents the mean of four estimations ± standard error of the mean. The experiment has been repeated three times.

had an objective partial remission and 64 (23%) were classed as nonresponders, although 16 had a minimal response of 20–30%.[46] After completion of local therapy, 72% of chemotherapy responders were in complete remission (CR) compared with 48% of nonresponders (p > 0.001). Patients who achieved CR after local therapy live significantly longer (p > 0.001) than those with residual disease: median durations of survival being 52.4 and 7.8 months, respectively. At 5 years 46% of patients in CR were alive (FIG. 10) compared with only 9% of those with residual disease at assessment. In this series response to chemotherapy is therefore a good prognostic sign. Side effects from 412 courses of schedule A are minimal (as shown in TABLE 7), and 125 (63%) patients reported *no* side effects. There was 100% patient compliance. The two deaths occurred after protocol violations: One patient had impaired renal function and was not given an extended folinic acid "rescue," and a second patient received chemotherapy with a white blood cell count of 3000 mm³ *but* their normal count was 10,000 mm³.

This protocol is now being considered for evaluation in a prospective, randomized, controlled clinical study designed to answer the question: Does the addition of effective cancer chemotherapy significantly improve overall survival compared with local therapy alone?

FUTURE PROSPECTS

The kinetically based approach to cancer chemotherapy, which we have advocated over the past 11 years, and which has now been confirmed by many different investigators over several thousand treatment cycles, shows that chemotherapy can be given intensively but safely. It can also be integrated safely with radiotherapy and surgery, provided the timing is right. This removes the main objection to integrating local and systemic therapy in a combined attack. This approach to cancer chemotherapy therefore has major implications for cancer treatment in the next 10 years.

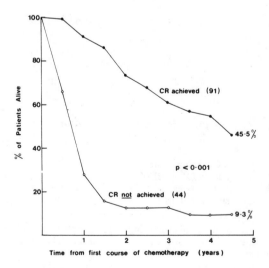

FIGURE 10. Actuarial survival of 135 patients with advanced head and neck cancer receiving schedule A chemotherapy (see FIGURE 9) prior to "curative" local therapy. The survival of those 91 patients achieving a complete remission at assessment is compared with those 44 patients with residual disease at assessment.

TABLE 7

SIDE EFFECTS FROM 412 COURSES OF SCHEDULE A CHEMOTHERAPY

Side Effect	Number
Bone marrow depression	
white blood cell count < 3000 mm^3	5 (1%)
white blood cell count < 2500 mm^3	1
Serositis (no intubation required)	17 (4%)
Peripheral neuropathy	11 (3%)
Pulmonary complications	2
Cardiovascular complications	1
Skin rash/pigmentation	14 (4%)
Anorexia, nausea, vomiting	31 (8%)
Alopecia (partial)	12 (3%)
Malaise or lethargy	14 (4%)
Death from treatment (protocol violations)	2
Other (headache, 2; constipation, 4; indigestion,	20
1; eye-watering, 1; exacerbation of peripheral vascular	
disease, 1; exacerbation of gout, 1; abdominal	
distention, 1; earache, 1; pyrexia, 2; diarrhea, 1; muscular	
ache in inguinal region, 1; ankle edema, 1; dizziness, 3)	

Implications for the Treatment of Advanced Disease

1. Full-dose chemotherapy protocols can be administered on a regular basis.

2. Patients spend much less time in hospital (usually only 1 night every month).

3. Provided that the usual precautions are observed, toxicity to normal tissues, especially the bone marrow, is markedly reduced.

4. The need for intensive supportive therapy such as platelet transfusions, isolation techniques, and antisepticemia regimens is drastically lessened.

5. There is no loss of therapeutic effect.

6. Intensive chemotherapy can now be offered to patients without ruining the quality of their lives.

Implications for Adjuvant Chemotherapy

This kinetically based approach has the following advantages for adjuvant chemotherapy:

1. Full-dose intensive combination chemotherapy can be given early and safely.

2. Intervals between courses of chemotherapy can be the minimum consistent with clinical tolerance, especially for the first 4 or 5 cycles, since there is no severe myelosuppression.

3. These chemotherapy protocols can be integrated successfully and safely with surgery and/or radiotherapy.

4. These are the necessary requirements for increasing survival.

The principles outlined here and our verification that they work clinically enable us to meet these requirements, and, provided there is more cooperation between surgeons, radiotherapists and chemotherapists, there is a significant chance that in the next decade increased cure rates can be achieved in certain common tumors for which effective drugs are available, such as tumors of the breast, lung (small cell), and head and neck, and perhaps for bladder, prostate, and ovarian tumors as well.

ACKNOWLEDGMENTS

The support and encouragement given to us throughout these studies by Dr. P. E. Thompson Hancock, Professor F. Bergel, Dr. R. Baserga, Dr. J. H. Goldie, Dr. L. M. Franks, Mr. J. D. Griffiths, and Dr. D. Geraint James has and continues to be very much appreciated. We are grateful to members of the Cellular Chemotherapy Laboratory at the Imperial Cancer Research Fund— H. T. Rupniak, Angela S. Bellamy, and R. D. H. Whelan—for allowing us to quote some of their unpublished experimental data, and we thank our colleagues Mr. H. J. Shaw and Dr. V. M. Dalley in the Head and Neck Unit, The Royal Marsden Hospital, London, for entering their patients into these head and neck cancer studies. We would like to thank Dr. J. R. W. Masters for his comments during the preparation of the manuscript. We are pleased to acknowledge the secretarial assistance of Mrs. E. Simmons, the artwork of Mrs. A. Symons, and the facilities of the I.C.R.F. Photographic Department.

REFERENCES

1. ZUBROD, C. G. 1979. Semin. Oncol. **6:** 490–505.
2. SALMON, S. E. & S. E. JONES, Eds. 1981. Adjuvant Therapy of Cancer. III. 1–603. Grune and Stratton. New York, NY.
3. SKIPPER, H. E., F. M. SCHABEL, JR. & W. S. WILCOX. 1965. Cancer Chemother. Rep. **45:** 5–28.
4. SHAPIRO, D. M. & R. A. FUGMANN. 1957. Cancer Res. **17:** 1098–1101.
5. GRISWOLD, D. P. 1975. Cancer Chemother. Rep. (Part 2) **5:** 187–204.
6. GOLDIN, A., J. M. VENDITTI & S. R. HUMPHRIES. 1956. J. Natl. Cancer Inst. **17:** 203–212.
7. HALL, T. C. 1971. Natl. Cancer Inst. Monogr. **34:** 15–19.
8. VAN PUTTEN, L. M. 1974. Cell Tissue Kinet. **7:** 493–505.
9. HART, J. S., R. B. LIVINGSTON, W. K. MURPHY, B. BARLOGIE, E. A. GEHAN & G. P. BODEY. 1976. Semin. Oncol. **3:** 259–270.
10. TATTERSALL, M. H. M. & J. S. TOBIAS. 1977. Lancet **1:** 141–142.
11. BRUCE, W. R., B. E. MEEKER & F. A. VALERIOTE. 1966. J. Natl. Cancer Inst. **37:** 233–245.
12. McCULLOUGH, E. A., L. SIMINOVITCH & J. E. TILL. 1964. Science **144:** 844–846.
13. McCULLOUCH, E. A. & J. E. TILL. 1971. Am. J. Pathol. **65:** 601–619.
14. LAJTHA, L. G., G. R. OLIVER & C. W. GURNEY. 1962. Br. J. Haematol. **8:** 442–460.
15. TILL, J. E., E. A. McCULLOUGH, R. A. PHILLIPS & L. SIMONOVITCH. *In* The Proliferation and Spread of Neoplastic Cells: 21st Annual Symposium on Fundamental Cancer Research at M.D. Anderson Hospital & Tumor Institute at Houston, Texas.: 235–244. Williams & Wilkins Baltimore, MD.
16. BRUCE, W. R. & F. A. VALERIOTE. 1968. *In* The Proliferation and Spread of Neoplastic Cells, 21st Annual Symposium on Fundamental Cancer Research at M.D. Anderson Hospital & Tumor Institute at Houston, Texas.: 409–420. Williams & Wilkins Co. Baltimore, MD.

17. BRUCE, W. R. & B. E. MEEKER. 1967. J. Natl. Cancer Inst. **38:** 401–405.
18. BRUCE, W. R., B. E. MEEKER, W. E. POWERS & F. A. VALERIOTE. 1969. J. Natl. Cancer Ints. **42:** 1015–1025.
19. HILL, B. T. 1978. Biochim. Biophys. Acta **516:** 389–417.
20. PRICE, L. A. 1973. *In* Proceedings of the 3rd Eli Lilly Symposium on the Vinca Alkaloids in the Chemotherapy of Malignant Disease. W. I. H. Shedden, Ed.: 35–40. Sherraff. Cheshire, UK.
21. GOODMAN, L. S. & A. GILMAN, Eds. 1980. *In* The Pharmacological Basis of Therapeutics, 5th ed.: 1–1843. Macmillan. New York, NY.
22. ARNOLD, A. M. & J. M. A. WHITEHOUSE. 1981. Lancet **2:** 912–915.
23. MISCHLER, N. E., R. H. EARHART, B. CARR & D. C. TORMEY. 1979. Cancer Treat. Rev. **6:** 191–204.
24. GOLDIE, J. H. & L. A. PRICE. 1977. Br. Med. J. **2:** 1064.
25. ATKINSON, N. K. & T. J. McELWAIN. 1973. *In* The Proceedings of the 3rd Eli Lilly Symposium on the Vinca Alkaloids in the Chemotherapy of Malignant Disease, W. I. H. Shedden, Ed.: 77–99. Sherraff. Cheshire, U.K.
26. ANDERSON, G., G. THOMAS & J. STUART-JONES. 1977. Br. J. Dis. Chest. **71:** 179–182.
27. GOLDIE, J. H., L. A. PRICE & K. R. HARRAP. 1972. Eur. J. Cancer **8:** 409–414.
28. PRICE, L. A. & B. T. HILL. 1981. *In* Safer Cancer Chemotherapy. L. A. Price, B. T. Hill, and M. W. Ghilchik, Eds.: 9–18. Bailliere Tindall. London, UK.
29. KITCHEN, G. 1981. *In* Safer Cancer Chemotherapy. L. A. Price, B. T. Hill, and M. W. Ghilchik, Eds.: 103–104. Bailliere Tindall. London, UK.
30. PRICE, L. A., B. T. HILL, P. MARKS, I. MONEYPENNY, A. HOWELL & J. M. MORRISON. 1982. In preparation.
31. MORRISON, J. M. 1981. *In* Safer Cancer Chemotherapy. L. A. Price, B. T. Hill, and M. W. Ghilchik, Eds.: 24–30. Bailliere Tindall. London, UK.
32. HILL, B. T. & R. D. H. WHELAN. 1981. Pediat. Res. **15:** 1117–1122.
33. EINHORN, L. H. 1979. Cancer Treat. Rep. **63:** 1659–1662.
34. HILL, B. T., H. T. RUPNIAK, R. D. H. WHELAN & S. A. METCALFE. 1982. *In* Proceedings of the 3rd Conference on Human Tumor Cloning, Tucson, Arizona. Abstract No. 44.
35. RUPNIAK, H. T. & B. T. HILL. 1982. Proc. of the 23rd Annual Meeting of the British Association for Cancer Research, Edinburgh, Scotland. Abstract No. P23.
36. COURTENAY, V. D. & J. MILLS. 1978. Br. J. Cancer. **37:** 261–268.
37. SALMON, S. E., F. L. MEYSKENS, JR., D. S. ALBERTS, B. SOEHNLEN & L. YOUNG. 1981. Cancer Treat. Rep. **65:** 1–12.
38. HAMBURGER, A. & S. E. SALMON. 1977. Science **197:** 461–463.
39. YAP, H.-Y., G. R. BLUMENSCHEIN, G. P. BODEY, G. N. HORTOBAGYI, A. U. BUZDAR & A. DISTEFANO. 1981. Cancer Treat. Rep. **65:** 775–779.
40. VAN PUTTEN, L. M., H. J. KEIZER & J. H. MULDER. 1976. Eur. J. Cancer **12:** 79–85.
41. PRICE, L. A. & B. T. HILL. 1980. J. Laryngol. Otol. **94:** 89–90.
42. BEZWODA, W. R., N. G. DeMOOR & D. D. DERMAN. 1979. Med. Pediat. Oncol. **6:** 353–357.
43. MALAKER, K., F. ROBSON & H. SCHIPPER. 1980. J. Otolaryngol. **9:** 24–30.
44. SERGEANT, R. & G. DEUTSCH. 1981. J. Laryngol. Otol. **95:** 69–74.
45. PRICE, L. A., B. T. HILL, A. H. CALVERT, V. M. DALLEY, A. LEVENE, E. R. BUSBY, M. SCHACHTER & H. J. SHAW. 1978. Oncology **35:** 26–28.
46. PRICE, L. A. & B. T. HILL. 1982. Proc. Am. Soc. Clin. Oncol. **1:** 202.

KINETIC PERTURBATIONS DURING CANCER THERAPY *

L. Simpson-Herren †

Southern Research Institute
Birmingham, Alabama 35255

Successful treatment of widely metastasized cancer usually depends on a multimodality approach to eliminate both primary and metastatic foci. Numerous attempts have been made to utilize growth kinetics as a guide to design of protocols and a predictor of drug response, but results have often been less than successful. Frei and Hart [1] reported that the pretreatment thymidine-labeling index (TLI) of leukemia blast cells in AML correlated positively with the likelihood of complete remission and negatively with the duration of remission. However, other investigators disagreed with this observation. Hall [2] and Tannock [3] claimed that pretreatment kinetic information was of no practical value in choosing drugs or predicting response. Norton [4] stated that "with or without our direct intention, kinetic principles continually exert an important influence in everyday therapeutic decisions."

The controversies over the value of kinetic information may result from oversimplification of the kinetics of growth of a widespread, multifocal tumor and the perturbations that take place during therapy. Kinetic measurements made on untreated primary tumors may have little relevance for designing efficacious protocols for (1) metastatic foci in the presence of the primary tumor or (2) the residual primary or secondary foci following the initial perturbation that results from "debulking" the tumor by surgery, irradiation, or drug treatment.

Perturbing effects of therapy may range from suppression of cell proliferation in residual tumor tissue from hours to days to stimulation of proliferation that may persist from hours to the lifetime of the host. In view of the diversity of effects and the time frame in which they occur, perhaps the kinetics of tumor recovery may prove to be the most useful parameter for scheduling multiple modality therapy or combination chemotherapy. [5-7]

There is no longer a question that activity of the majority of drugs available to the oncologist today is related to the proliferative state of the target cell population. [8-10] "What is surprising is that there is so little evidence for *cycle-independent* or *phase-independent* drug effect." [11] It thus becomes advisable to evaluate the existing evidence for fluctuations in cell proliferation in the target population that occur during the course of therapy and to determine the efficacy of drug therapy that utilizes information on the periods of high and low proliferation.

* Previously unpublished data were obtained under Grant RO1–CA25313–03 and DCT Contract NO1–CM–97309 from the National Cancer Institute.

† Address for correspondence: Southern Research Institute, 2000 Ninth Avenue South, P.O. Box 3307–A, Birmingham, Alabama 35255.

0077–8923/82/0397–0088 $01.75/0 © 1982, NYAS

POPULATION KINETICS OF TUMORS IN DIFFERENT ANATOMIC SITES

Although most of the currently available kinetic data on experimental and clinical cancer were obtained on primary tumors, the diversity of growth kinetics that may occur when a tumor becomes widespread is becoming evident.

Secondary tumors grow more rapidly with a higher thymidine-labeling index (TLI) and a shorter cell cycle time than do the primary tumors in the same hosts in some experimental tumor models.[12-14]

For example, this was observed in the spontaneous pulmonary metastases in our studies of the subcutaneously implanted primary Lewis lung carcinoma (FIG. 1). The TLIs in both sites decrease with tumor age and time post implant, but the TLI of the pulmonary metastases was higher than the TLI of the corresponding primary tumor in every mouse where both sites could be evaluated (FIG. 2).[12] A higher labeling index in secondary tumor foci was reported in spontaneous C3H mammary tumors, in spontaneous mammary tumors of

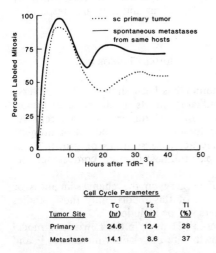

FIGURE 1. Computer-fitted PLM curves for primary subcutaneous Lewis lung tumors and spontaneous lung metastases in the same hosts. Values for Tc and Ts were estimated from the computer analysis.

Cell Cycle Parameters

Tumor Site	Tc (hr)	Ts (hr)	TI (%)
Primary	24.6	12.4	28
Metastases	14.1	8.6	37

Sprague-Dawley rats, and in human mammary tumors.[13-15] A similar observation was made in the transplantable C3H/16C mammary adenocarcinoma in the presence of spontaneous lung metastases (FIG. 3) and in pulmonary, ovarian, and kidney metastases of the ovarian M5076 tumor cell (FIG. 4).

These data are consistent with observations on other tumor systems that the growth kinetics of a tumor are influenced by anatomic site. Preliminary data suggest that the tissue of origin may provide near optimal conditions for growth of cells.[16]

Further evidence for a difference in growth kinetics in different sites may be found in studies of the TLI of leukemia L1210 cells inoculated by different routes (FIG. 5). The relative TLIs in this study correspond to the response to drugs of L1210 cells implanted by these routes.[17, 18]

Kawaguchi et al.[19] compared the TLI of rat ascites hepatoma AH7974 cells that lodged in the choroid plexus and in the brain after injection into the carotid artery and found TLIs in the choroid plexus as much as two-fold higher.

The preceding results clearly indicate that the kinetic state of the target

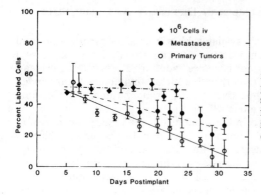

FIGURE 2. Thymidine-labeling index versus time post implant of primary Lewis lung tumors and spontaneous lung metastases. Data for artificial lung metastases after intravenous implant are shown for comparison.

tumor population prior to perturbation may provide widely differing sensitivity or resistance to drugs that are proliferation-dependent and may also respond in diverse ways to perturbation.

Effects of Surgery on Residual Tumor

Surgical excision of a large primary tumor has been shown to have diverse and, in some instances, apparently contradictory effects on the residual tumor. Perturbation may be due to (1) reduction of total tumor mass that removes the suppressive effects of a large growing tumor; (2) the rebound of immune competence after tumor removal that may act as a stimulus of growth[20]; or (3) the surgical procedure per se may impair the host immune competence and permit rapid growth of residual tumor.[21]

Extensive data exist on the effects of surgery on the changes in mass or number of metastases, but for the purposes of this report, only those studies that quantitate changes in kinetic parameters will be included.

Surgical excision of large primary tumors (21-day) in the Lewis lung model results in stimulation of the TLI and growth rate of residual metastases[22] and

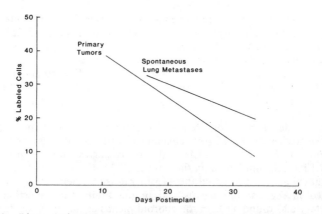

FIGURE 3. Lines derived from linear regression analysis of thymidine-labeling index data versus time post implant in the mammary adenocarcinoma C3H/16C tumor and spontaneous lung metastases.

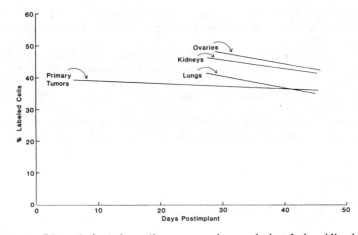

FIGURE 4. Lines derived from linear regression analysis of thymidine-labeling indexes versus time for M5076 ovarian tumors and spontaneous metastases to the ovaries, lungs, and kidneys.

no change in the length of the cell cycle (FIG. 6). However, if the primary tumor is removed at an earlier stage (day 14), before the decrease with post-implant time occurs in the metastases, then minimal elevation of TLI is evident, but the usual decrease with time does not occur.[22] This suggests that each tumor system may have a maximal growth rate and TLI that may be approached under ideal conditions in an unsynchronized cell population and that this rate represents the limit for stimulation. If the TLI of the residual tumor is close to the maximal value for the system under study (as in early Lewis lung

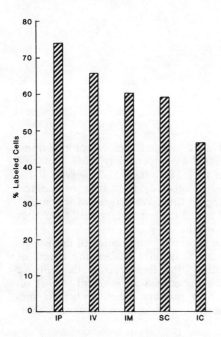

FIGURE 5. Pulse thymidine-labeling indexes of L1210 cells implanted by different routes.

tumors), then surgery does not result in a stimulation of TLI, but prevents the suppression that occurs in the intact host. The net result is continuation of rapid growth.

Increases in TLI of residual tumor tissue within 24–48 hours after surgical excision of a tumor mass have been reported after removal of one tumor from a mouse bearing multiple spontaneous C3H mammary tumors,[13] and after removal of one tumor from mice bearing doubly-implanted C3H mammary tumors [14] (TABLE 1).

The work of Eccles and Alexander [23] with a transplanted rat sarcoma suggests the presence of an immunologically mediated mechanism whereby latent

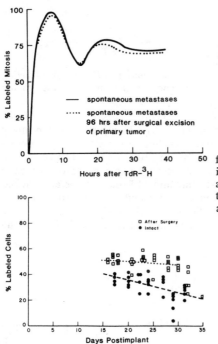

FIGURE 6. Computer-fitted PLM data for spontaneous Lewis lung metastases in untreated mice and data 96 hours after surgical removal of the primary tumor, and thymidine-labeling indexes as a function of tumor age.

tumor metastases were held in restraint after surgical removal of the transplanted primary tumor. In those rats treated by surgery only, 90% remained tumor-free for the 18-month observation period (TABLE 2). However, if the immune system was challenged by either whole-body irradiation or thoracic duct drainage, then 42 to 70% (depending on time post surgery of treatment) died of distant metastases. In this tumor model the immune system, even after surgery, restrained growth of residual tumor cells.

Some experimental data do support the concept of suppression of metastastic growth by removal of the primary tumor. Schatten [24] studied the effects of trauma on metastases following amputation of a limb bearing the primary tumor and concluded that removal of the tumor had an inhibitory effect on metastases. Repeated laparotomies and liver massage increased hepatic metastases from a mouse tumor, suggesting the activation of dormant tumor cells.[25]

TABLE 1

EFFECTS OF SURGICAL EXCISION OF A PRIMARY TUMOR ON LABELING
OF THE RESIDUAL TUMOR

| Tumor System | Thymidine-labeling Indexes | | Investigators |
	Intact (0 hr)	Surgery (24-hr post surgery)	
Spontaneous C_3H tumors (double)			Schiffer, Braunschweiger, and Stragand (1978)
Resect 1	4.5	9.1	
Bisect 1	3.7	11.5	
Doubly implanted C_3H tumors			Gunduz, Fisher, and Saffer (1979)
Surgery day			
14	30	36	
21	25	35	
28	20	25	
	$^{125}IUdR$ Uptake (cpm)		
Lewis lung tumor (10 days after surgery)			Gorelick, Segal, and Feldman (1980)
1×10^6 cells	3,306	2,605	
1×10^5 cells	3,022	14,026	

EFFECTS OF RADIATION ON THE SURVIVING CELL POPULATION

Measurement of perturbation of kinetic parameters as a result of ionizing radiation is complicated by continued cell cycle traverse of lethally damaged cells for several generations. Hermens and Barendsen [26] reviewed the effects of radiation on a variety of experimental and clinical tumors and found the observed kinetic responses to be highly variable. Kallman [27] utilized an *in vitro* assay to evaluate the changes in TLI that occurred in the clonogenic cell population of a EMT6 sarcoma after irradiation *in vivo* (TABLE 3). The

TABLE 2

APPEARANCE OF LATENT METASTASES *

Control	Day	Death due to Metastases
Surgery only	14	10%
Surgery and thoracic duct drainage	14	
	1–7	53%
	7–14	44%
	30–37	38%
Surgery and whole-body irradiation	14	
	1	58%
	7	37%
	30	30%

* Data of Eccles and Alexander.[23]

TABLE 3

EFFECTS OF IRRADIATION ON THE THYMIDINE-LABELING INDEXES OF EMT6 TUMORS USING AN *in Vitro* ASSAY *

	24-Hour Thymidine-Labeling Indexes			
	Days After Irradiation			
Irradiation Dose	0	2	4	5
300 rads	80	62	77	66
600 rads	80	62	65	75

* From Kallman.[27]

observed TLI following 24-hr exposure to ^{3}H-TdR decreased for a period, then approached the pretreatment value, and the time frame depended on the dose. After 300 rads the nadir occurred on day 2, with maximal recovery by days 3 or 4. After 600 rads, the nadir also occurred on day 2, but maximal recovery was delayed until day 6 or later.

Braunschweiger *et al.*[28] described the perturbing effects of ionizing radiation on the cell kinetics of T1699 transplantable mouse tumors utilizing ^{3}H-TdR labeling and the primer-dependent DNA polymerase (PDP) assay. A summary of the results is shown in TABLE 4. These investigators used the kinetic data to plan fractional dose protocols (1000 r) and found the most efficacious schedules were those in which the fractions were given just prior to full proliferative recovery and the least effective to be those in which fractions coincided with the time of maximal proliferative activity.

PERTURBATION OF GROWTH KINETICS BY CHEMOTHERAPY

Within the past 15 to 20 years, conclusive evidence has been obtained on the importance of schedule on the therapeutic index of drugs administered in experimental models and in man.[29] Since the schedule-dependency of methotrexate in leukemia L1210 was demonstrated by Goldin,[30] the need for cytotoxic drug levels of phase-specific drugs during the sensitive phase of the cell cycle has been clear. However, therapeutic schedules for multiple courses of the same drug, for multiple drugs, or for multiple modalities have been largely empirical. There is a large body of qualitative data that support the concept

TABLE 4

CYTOKINETIC CHANGES IN T1699 MOUSE MAMMARY TUMORS FOLLOWING IRRADIATION *

Time	TLI	PDPI	Ts
First phase (within 24 hr)	↓	↑	↑
Second phase (dose-dependent interval)	↓	↓	↑
Third phase	↑	↑	↓ (normal)
Fourth phase	normal	normal	normal

* From Braunschweiger *et al.*[28]

that drugs perturb the cell population kinetics and that this perturbation influences the sensitivity of the surviving cells to subsequent therapy. However, the available studies that measure directly the kinetic perturbation or the kinetics of recovery, and particularly the studies that attempt to relate kinetic effects to efficacy of schedules are limited. Perturbation due to drugs may be in the form of (1) reversible or irreversible cell cycle arrest of sensitive cells, depending on dose and duration of exposure, and (2) continued cell cycle traverse of lethally damaged cells, in addition to cell death. Cell cycle related effects are studied primarily *in vitro* and the results are difficult, if not impossible, to translate directly to design of therapeutic protocols *in vivo*.

However, the kinetics of tumor recovery *in vivo*, particularly the TLI or growth fraction, appear to be useful parameters for design of protocols. In

TABLE 5

CELL-KINETICS-DIRECTED CHEMOTHERAPY *

Tumor System	Host	Drug	Sequencing Interval	Second Drug	Therapeutic Endpoint
T1699 mammary tumor	DBA mouse	AD	3 days	CP	Tumor regression and cure
		CP	7 days	CP	
13762 mammary tumor	Rat (Fischer)	AD	5 days	CP	Tumor regression and cure
		CP	9 days	CP	
C₃H spontaneous mammary tumors	C₃H mouse	CP	4 days	AD	Tumor regression and life-span
C₃H spontaneous mammary tumors	C₃H mouse	Dexamethasone	42–48 hr	Vincristine or 5-FU	Tumor regression
		Methylprednisone	18–24 hr	Vincristine or 5-FU	

* From Braunschweiger and Schiffer.[33, 34]

experimental systems, the relevance of kinetics to optimal scheduling has been demonstrated. The antileukemic activity of arabinosylcytosine and methotrexate against a slow-growing acute myeloid leukemia of the rat correlates well with changes in the thymidine-labeling index.[31] Tumor cell kinetics reflect the inhibitory effects of *Corynebacterium parvum* in combination with cyclophosphamide used in treatment of spontaneous C3H mammary tumors.[32]

Braunschweiger and Schiffer [33, 34] utilized changes in the TLI and primer-dependent DNA polymerase index (PDPI) to schedule cyclophosphamide and adriamycin therapy in T1699 mouse mammary tumors and in 13762 rat mammary tumors (TABLE 5). Changes in the cell kinetic parameters after perturbation could be used to design efficacious as well as nonefficacious schedules. In studies of perturbation of kinetic parameters in the high-growth-fraction 13762 rat mammary tumors and the low-growth-fraction spontaneous C3H tumor models, cell proliferation was slightly elevated in both tumors by 24 hours. An interval of subnormal cell proliferation that was longer in the high-growth-fraction tumor than in the low-growth-fraction tumor followed cytotoxic chemotherapy.[35] The PDP index of the high-growth-fraction tumor recovered to the pretreatment value, but the PDP index exceeded the pretreatment value in the low-growth-fraction tumor.

Preliminary results of a study designed to measure the effects of surgical excision as well as treatment with (MeCCNU) on the TLI and tissue mass in the M5076 ovarian tumor are shown in FIGURE 7. Treatment by surgical excision or MeCCNU was given on day 21 and mice from each group were taken for evaluation at frequent intervals thereafter. Inadequate numbers of tumor cells were found in the ovaries to evaluate TLI until day 35, but outgrowth of the metastases in this organ was similar both in TLI and time in both the surgically treated and the control groups. Proliferative activity was still suppressed by the MeCCNU on day 49. The TLI of primary tumors recurring after surgery or MeCCNU was not significantly different from the control value. These results suggest that surgical excision of the primary M5076 tumor had little influence on time of appearance or the TLI of ovarian metastases. The suppression of proliferative activity in the residual tumor or the ovarian metastases is evident as long as 10 days after treatment. Efforts to define the recovery kinetics of the M5076 tumor and evaluate therapy based on these data are still in progress.

Hormones are frequently used as one component of multiple drug therapy in a hormone-sensitive tumor and the effects on cell proliferation may range

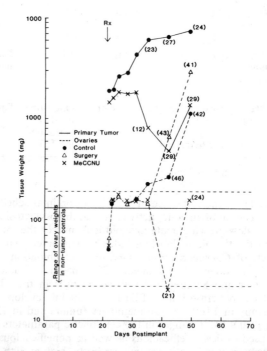

FIGURE 7. Growth data for M5076 ovarian tumors and ovaries after no treatment, surgical excision of the primary tumor on day 21, or a single dose of MeCCNU (40 mg/kg) given on day 21. Values for thymidine-labeling indexes at selected points are shown in parentheses. Dotted lines indicate range of weights for normal ovaries.

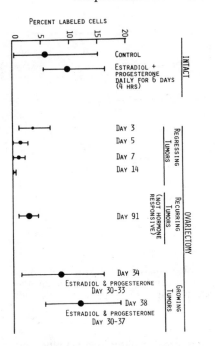

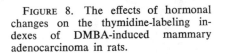

FIGURE 8. The effects of hormonal changes on the thymidine-labeling indexes of DMBA-induced mammary adenocarcinoma in rats.

from suppression to stimulation, depending on the hormone-sensitivity of the tumor cell populations. In the dimethylbenzanthracene-induced mammary adenocarcinoma of the rat, hormonal manipulation may suppress or stimulate the proliferative activity of a subpopulation of the tumor (FIG. 8) to produce an outgrowth of a hormone-sensitive or -insensitive population; however, there is little evidence for elimination of the sensitive or insensitive population from the tumor.

CONCLUSIONS

The lines that result from a linear regression analysis of TLI data as a function of time post implant for several experimental tumor models are shown in FIGURE 9. These data demonstrate the diversity of growth kinetics that may be found in a single tumor system as well as in multiple tumor systems. We propose a hypothesis for interpretation of the effects of perturbation by surgery, irradiation, and drugs on tumors with a range of growth fractions. Implicit in the hypothesis is the assumption that for each tumor system there is a maximal TLI that exists under optimal growth conditions and will not be exceeded in the absence of synchronization of cell cycle progression.

From this schema, we postulate the following working hypotheses (FIG. 10):

1. In a high-growth-fraction tumor, surgery does not increase proliferative activity significantly; irradiation and chemotherapy produce a high cell kill, a prolonged period of low proliferative activity, and a recovery to the pretreatment value.

2. In a low-growth-fraction tumor, surgery stimulates proliferative activity to a value higher than the pretreatment value; chemotherapy and irradiation

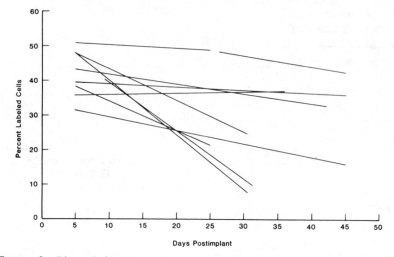

FIGURE 9. Lines derived from linear regression analysis of thymidine-labeling index data versus time post implant for a variety of transplantable experimental tumors and spontaneous metastases to illustrate the range of changes in index with time that may be expected.

produce a low cell kill, a short period of subnormal proliferative activity, and a recovery to a proliferative rate in excess of the pretreatment value.

The time frame for the proliferative effects should be tumor-dependent. These working hypotheses may provide a framework for interpretation of existing data and further investigation of protocol design.

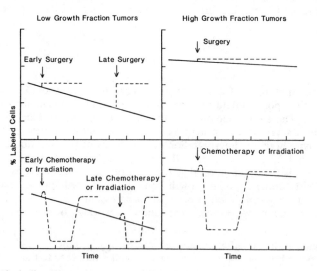

FIGURE 10. A diagrammatic representation of a working hypothesis that incorporates the currently available data on kinetic effects and recovery kinetics after surgery, irradiation, and chemotherapy.

REFERENCES

1. FREI, E., III & J. S. HART. 1973. Cytokinetic studies and treatment response in adult leukemia. Recent Results Cancer Res. **43:** 81–87.
2. HALL, T. C. 1971. Limited role of cell kinetics in clinical cancer chemotherapy. *In* Production of Response in Cancer Therapy Vol. **34:** 15–17. NCI Monograph. Washington, DC.
3. TANNOCK, I. 1978. Cell kinetics and chemotherapy. A critical review. Cancer Treat. Rep. **62**: 1117–1133.
4. NORTON, L. 1978. Thoughts on a role for cell kinetics in cancer chemotherapy. *In* Controversies in Cancer. Design of Trials and Treatments. H. J. Tagon and M. J. Staquet, Eds.: 105–115. Masson. New York, NY.
5. SIMPSON-HERREN, L. 1977. Kinetics and multiple modality therapy. Presented at the First Annual Meeting of the Cell Kinetics Society, March 11–13, Birmingham, Alabama.
6. AMADORI, S., M. C. PETTI, A. DEFRANCESCO, A. CHIERICHINI, C. MASTROVINCENZO, M. G. TESTA & F. MANDELLI. 1976. Lack of prognostic significance of the pretreatment labeling and mitotic indices of marrow blasts in acute nonlymphocytic leukemia (ANLL). Cancer **41:** 1154–1160.
7. DETHLEFSEN, L. A. 1979. Cellular recovery kinetic studies relevant to combined-modality research and therapy. Int. J. Radiat. Oncol. Biol. Phys. **5:** 1197–1203.
8. STEEL, G. G. & T. C. STEPHENS. 1979. The relation of cell kinetics to cancer chemotherapy. Adv. Pharmacol. Ther. Proc. 7th Int. Congr. Pharmacol. **10:** 137–145.
9. BHUYAN, B. K. 1977. Cell cycle-related cellular lethality. *In* Growth Kinetics and Biochemical Regulation of Normal and Malignant Cells. B. Drewinko and R. M. Humphrey, Eds.: 373–375. Williams and Wilkins. Baltimore, MD.
10. MADOC-JONES, H. & F. MAURO. 1974. Site of action of cytotoxic agents in the cell life cycle. *In* Antineoplastic and Immunosuppressive Agents. I. Handbook of Experimental Pharmacology. XXXVIII. A. Sartorelli and D. G. Johns, Eds.: 205–219. Springer-Verlag. New York, NY.
11. STEEL, G. G. 1977. The Growth Kinetics of Tumours. Oxford University Press.
12. SIMPSON-HERREN, L., A. H. SANFORD & J. P. HOLMQUIST. 1974. Cell population kinetics of transplanted and metastatic Lewis lung carcinoma. Cell Tissue Kinet. **7:** 349–361.
13. SCHIFFER, L., P. G. BRAUNSCHWEIGER & J. J. STRAGAND. 1978. Tumor cell population kinetics following non-curative treatment. *In* Fundamentals in Cancer Chemotherapy. Antibiot. Chemother. F. M. Schabel, Ed. Vol. **23:** 148–156. Karger. Basel.
14. GUNDUZ, N., B. FISHER & E. A. SAFFER. 1974. Effect of surgical removal on the growth and kinetics of residual tumor. Cancer Res. **39:** 3861–3885.
15. SCHIFFER, L. M., P. G. BRAUNSCHWEIGER, J. J. STRAGAND & L. POULAKOS. 1979. The cell kinetics of human mammary cancers. Cancer **43**(5): 1707–1719.
16. SIMPSON-HERREN. 1982. Relationship of thymidine labelling indices of metastatic tumours to site and tissue of origin. Cell Tissue Kinet. **15:** 114.
17. SKIPPER, H. E., F. M. SCHABEL, JR., W. S. WILCOX, W. R. LASTER, JR., M. W. TRADER & S. A. THOMPSON. 1965. Experimental evaluation of potential anticancer agents. XVIII. Effects of therapy on viability and rate of proliferation of leukemia cells in various anatomic sites. Cancer Chemother. Rep. **42:** 41–64.
18. WODINSKY, I., P. E. MERKER & J. M. VENDITTI. 1977. Responsiveness to chemotherapy of mice with L1210 lymphoma implanted in different anatomic sites. J. Natl. Cancer Inst. **59:** 405–408.
19. KAWAGUCHI, T., M. ENDO, S. YOKOYA & K. NAMURA. 1981. Influence of

lodgement site on the proliferation-kinetics of tumor cells. Experientia **37**: 414–415.

20. PARANJPE, M. S. & C. W. BOONE. 1974. Kinetics of the anti-tumor delayed hypersensitivity response and more with progressively growing tumors: Stimulation followed by specific suppression. Int. J. Cancer **13**: 179–184.

21. GORELICK, E., S. SEGAL & M. FELDMAN. 1980. Control of lung metastatis progression in mice: Role of growth kinetics of 3LL Lewis lung carcinoma and host immune reactivity. J. Natl. Cancer Inst. **65**: 1257–1264.

22. SIMPSON-HERREN, L., A. H. SANFORD & J. P. HOLMQUIST. 1976. Effects of surgery on the cell kinetics of residual tumor. Cancer Treat. Rep. **60**: 1749–1760.

23. ECCLES, S. A. & P. ALEXANDER. 1975. Immunologically-mediated restraint of latent tumour metastases. Nature **257**: 52–53.

24. SHATTEN, W. E. 1958. An experimental study of the postoperative tumor metastases. I. Growth of pulmonary metastases following total removal of primary leg tumor. Cancer **11**: 455–459.

25. FISHER, B. & E. R. FISHER. 1959. Experimental evidence in support of the dormant cell. Science **130**: 918–919.

26. HERMENS, A. F. & G. W. BARENDSEN. 1977. Effects of ionizing radiation on the growth kinetics of tumors. *In* Growth Kinetics and Biochemical Regulation of Normal and Malignant Cells. B. Drewinko and R. M. Humphrey, Eds.: 531–545. Williams and Wilkins. Baltimore, MD.

27. KALLMAN, R. F. 1977. Discussion presented after paper presented by A. J. Hermens. *In* Growth Kinetics and Biochemical Regulation of Normal and Malignant Cells. B. Drewinko and R. M. Humphrey, Eds.: 545–546. Williams and Wilkins. Baltimore, MD.

28. BRAUNSCHWEIGER, P. G., L. L. SCHENKEN & L. M. SCHIFFER. 1979. The cytokinetic basis for the design of efficacious radiotherapy protocols. Int. J. Rad. Oncol. Biol. Phys. **5**: 37–47.

29. BLUM, R. J. & E. FREI, III. 1979. Combination chemotherapy. *In* Methods in Cancer Research. V. T. DeVita, Jr. and H. Busch, Eds. Vol. **XVII**: 215–257.

30. GOLDIN, A., N. MANTEL, S. W. GREENHOUSE, J. M. VENDITTI & S. W. HUMPHREY. 1954. Effect of delayed administration of citrovorum factor on the antileukemic effectiveness of aminopterin in mice. Cancer Res. **14**: 43–48.

31. AGLIETTA, M. & P. SONNEVELD. 1978. The relevance of cell kinetics for optimal scheduling of 1-β-D-arabinofuranosyl cytosine and methotrexate in a slow growing acute myeloid leukemia (BNML). Cancer Chemother. Pharmacol. **1**: 219–223.

32. FISHER, B. & N. GUNDUZ. 1979. Further observations on the inhibition of tumor growth by *Corynebacterium parvum* with cyclophosphamide. X. Effect of treatment on tumor cell kinetics in mice. J. Natl. Cancer Inst. **62**: 1545–1551.

33. BRAUNSCHWEIGER, P. G. & L. M. SCHIFFER. 1980. Effect of adriamycin on the cell kinetics of 13762 rat mammary tumors and implications for therapy. Cancer Treat. Rep. **64**: 293–300.

34. BRAUNSCHWEIGER, P. G. & L. M. SCHIFFER. 1980. Cell kinetic-directed sequential chemotherapy with cyclophosphamide and adriamycin in T1699 mammary tumors. Cancer Res. **40**: 737–743.

35. BRAUNSCHWEIGER, P. G. & L. M. SCHIFFER. 1978. Therapeutic implications of cell kinetic changes after cyclophosphamide treatment in "spontaneous" and "transplantable" mammary tumors. Cancer Treat. Rep. **62**: 727–736.

CONTROL OF THE INITIATION OF
DNA SYNTHESIS IN MAMMALIAN CELLS *

David M. Prescott

*Department of Molecular, Cellular and Developmental Biology
University of Colorado
Boulder, Colorado 80309*

Cell reproduction is regulated by modulation of the transit of the cell from mitosis to the initiation of DNA synthesis. Thus, the slower a cell reproduces, the longer it remains in the G_1 period; at the same time the sum of the lengths of S, G_2, and M remains roughly constant, changing little even with large changes in growth rate.

These observations point clearly to the presence of an on/off switch that ultimately controls entry of the cell into DNA synthesis. We know in a general way how the switch is operated; lack of essential nutrients or growth factors turn the switch to the off position, and the cell remains arrested in G_1 until the switch is turned on after provision of the missing nutrient or growth factor. Alternatively, the arrest of the cell in G_1 by inhibitors, including naturally occurring inhibitors,[1, 2] must represent the operation of an on/off switch. Possibly all G_1-arresting conditions or factors, specific and nonspecific, ultimately impinge on the same on/off switch, although this hypothesis is difficult to test. Some observations have suggested the presence of more than one switch in G_1, for example, different ones for various growth factors and nutrient deprivation. The idea of multiple switches is supported primarily by experiments that attempt to define the location of switches within G_1 or by experiments that attempt to define an order for two or more switches operated by different limiting conditions. Several difficulties, including particularly the possibility of remote connection between the immediate target of a blocking condition and the eventual operation of a switch, make interpretation of such experiments somewhat uncertain. The number and location of on/off switches in G_1 are crucial parts of the eventual study of the molecular nature of the switch mechanism and its operation and how it regulates the cell cycle.

Any hypothesis dealing with regulation of cell reproduction must also account for the reproductive behavior of cells in cleavage stage embryos. Early embryo cells of a wide variety of species ranging from insects and sea urchins to mammals have cell cycles that entirely lack a G_1 period. Such rapidly reproducing cells appear to multiply without restraint; any control switch(es) must be continuously in the "on" position. The cycles of cleavage stage cells may perhaps be regarded as archtype cycles uncomplicated by effects of regulating rates of cell reproduction. In subsequent embryonic development G_1 periods appear and cell reproduction slows down, particularly in connection with differentiation, reflecting active regulation of the cell cycle.

Almost all lines of cultured cells used to study cell reproduction and its regulation have G_1 periods in their cell cycles. Much attention has been given

* This work is supported by Grant CD–139 to D. M. Prescott from the American Cancer Society.

0077–8923/82/0397–0101 $01.75/0 © 1982, NYAS

to the analysis of G_1 in such cells, particularly with regard to events that might occur specifically and uniquely in G_1 and which might lead to some insight about the mechanism of cell cycle arrest. There are two cultured cell lines of Chinese hamster cells (DON and V79–8) that lack G_1 periods in the cycles, and reproduce with generation times of 9.5 hours or less. Studies of one of these (V79–8) have yielded information that bears on questions about G_1 and the presence of a control switch. A review of this work occupies the remainder of this paper.

THE V79–8 CELL

The origin of this cell is somewhat unclear. It is a subclone of a cell line isolated from Chinese hamster lung.[3] It was first reported by Robbins and Scharff[4] to have a G_1-less cell cycle. The circumstances of its origin by subcloning are unknown to us. Other subclones of the original V79–8 line have G_1 periods.

When grown on a plastic surface in Dulbecco's modified Eagle's medium containing 10 to 15% fetal calf serum and buffered at pH 7.4 with 25 mM Tricine, the cells have an average generation time of 9.5 to 10.0 hours.[5, 6] In Ham's F-12 medium supplemented with 10% fetal calf serum, V79–8 cells have an average generation time of about 8 hours. At both generation times no G_1 period is detectable by the labeled mitosis method and the difference in generation times is accounted for entirely by a corresponding change in the length of the S period. A 5-minute pulse with ^{3}H-labeled thymidine (50 Ci/mM; 10 μCi/ml) results in labeling of 90 to 95% of the cells in an asynchronously dividing population.

When mitotic cells (mixture of prometaphase, metaphase, and anaphase cells) are collected by the mechanical dislodging from a monolayer, more than 40% are in DNA synthesis within 10 minutes, more than 80% have entered S by 20 minutes, and ~95% are in S at 30 minutes. Most cells in late telophase have already entered DNA synthesis. Careful autoradiographic analysis has shown that V79–8 cells also lack a G_2 period.[5]

CYTOPLASMIC INITIATOR OF DNA SYNTHESIS IN V79–8 CELLS

S-phase cells contain a cytoplasmic factor(s) that induces DNA synthesis in a G_1-phase nucleus, as first shown by Rao and Johnson.[7] Fusion of a mitotic cell with an interphase cell induces premature mitotic condensation of the interphase chromosomes,[8] indicating the presence of a chromosome-condensing factor(s) in the cytoplasm of a mitotic cell. The appearance of the initiation factor for DNA synthesis and the chromosome-condensation factor are cell-cycle-specific events. In several cell types (all with G_1 periods) the DNA synthesis initiation factor is absent in G_2 and mitotic cells and either accumulates in G_1[9] or is synthesized specifically at the end of the G_1 period. In any case, it is demonstrable by cell fusion in the cytoplasm of *only* S-period cells. How the initiation factor works is not known. It initiates DNA synthesis, but apparently does not influence the temporal program of replication of replicon families within the S period.[10] It is without effect on the DNA of G_2 and mitotic cells, indicating that the molecular organization of the chromatin in these cycle stages is somehow fundamentally different from the chromatin organization of G_1 cells.

Fusion of a mitotic G_1^- V79–8 cell with a HeLa cell in G_1 causes simultaneous premature chromosome condensation and induction of DNA synthesis.[9] Thus, unlike G_1^+ cells such as HeLa or CHO, the V79–8 cell contains the cytoplasmic inducer of DNA synthesis *during mitosis*. Hence, the inducer is present in the cytoplasm throughout the cell cycle of the V79–8 cell. The "constitutive" presence of the inducer may account for the entry of cells into DNA synthesis without delay at the end of mitosis.

DOMINANCE OF THE G_1^- PHENOTYPE

V79–8 cells were fused with cells that have G_1 periods (G_1^+ cells), and the cell cycles of resulting hybrid cells were analyzed. When V79–8 cells were fused with CHO cells ($G_1 = 3.0$ hours),[11] all resulting hybrids had G_1^- cell cycles. The data in TABLE 1 illustrate the results of fusion of V79–8 cells with embryonic, diploid fibroblasts.[17] All seven hybrid cells analyzed were G_1^-. (In addition, all seven hybrids have generation times and S periods shorter than those of either parent.) From this we concluded [11] that the G_1^- cell supplies some factor or gene activity that is limiting in a G_1^+ cell so as to cause a G_1 period, that is, that the G_1^- state is dominant over the G_1^+ state. Conceivably, the factor so provided could be the constitutive synthesis of the DNA synthesis initiator discussed earlier.

MUTATION OF G_1^- CELLS TO G_1^+ CELLS

We next asked whether V79–8 cells could be converted into G_1^+ cells by mutation.[6] V79–8 cells were treated with N-methyl-N'-nitro-N-nitrosoguanidine (MNNG). The survivors were cultured and subjected to a ³H-thymidine procedure that would select for cells that now spent more time in non-S parts of the cell cycle. The selection scheme consisted of a series of 2-hour incubations with ³H-thymidine separated by 10-hour intervals without ³H-thymidine. Since V79–8 cells spend less than 2 hours of each cycle in non-S (in mitosis), all should be killed by incorporation of ³H-thymidine. Multiple 2-hour treatments were used to assure this result. Mutated cells that had acquired either a G_2 period, a prolonged mitotic period, or a G_1 period would have a higher probability of surviving the ³H-thymidine incubations.

Among 15 clones raised from survivors that were analyzed all had generation times longer than those observed in the original V79–8 parent cell.[6, 18] In each case the addition of a G_1 period accounted for the increase in generation time, with no induction of a G_2 period or change in the length of S + M (TABLE 2). We have no direct evidence that the appearance of a G_1 period is the result of gene mutation. However, the G_1^+ phenotype in these clones has remained stable during up to 7 months of culture. In addition, the G_1 phenotype is temperature-sensitive in at least one cell clone, with a G_1 period present at 37° and 39° C but absent at 33° C. We assume therefore that the conversions from G_1^- to G_1^+ are probably the result of mutation.

TABLE 1

LENGTHS OF THE CELL CYCLE PHASES (IN HOURS) FOR THE G_1^- V79–8 CELL, FOR EMBRYONIC FIBROBLASTS IN CULTURE, AND FOR SEVEN HYBRID LINES CREATED BY FUSING A V79–8 CELL WITH A FIBROBLAST *

	G_1	S	$G_2 + M$	GT
V79–8	0	8.75	.75	9.5
Chinese Hamster Embryo Fibroblasts	5	8.0	2.25	15.2
Hybrids				
1	0	6.6	1.5	8.0
2	0	5.7	1.5	7.3
3	0	6.8	1.25	8.0
4	0.25	5.3	2.25	7.8
5	0	6.8	2.0	8.8
6	0	6.4	1.25	7.7
7	0.25	6.5	1.75	8.6

* Data of R. M. Liskay.

COMPLEMENTATION AMONG G_1^+ MUTANT CELLS

To determine whether the G_1^+ clones derived by treatment with MNNG are the result of mutation in different genes, five of the different mutant cells were fused with one another in all possible combinations (TABLE 3).[6] The process of fusion itself did not change the G_1 status of a cell; for example, fusion of one mutant G_1^+ cell with another G_1^+-1 cell produced only G_1^+ hybrids. However, with one exception all combinations of fusion of mutants G_1^+-1 through G_1^+-5 resulted in complementation, that is, production of G_1^- hybrids. Only fusion of G_1^+-4 with G_1^+-5 gave G_1^+ hybrids. Thus, four complementation groups were defined for the five mutant lines. Therefore, the basis or reason for the existence of a G_1 period is different in the four complementation groups.

TABLE 2

CELL CYCLE VALUES FOR SEVEN G_1^+ MUTANT CELL LINES DERIVED FROM THE G_1^- V79–8 CELL LINE *

Mutant Cell Line	G_1	S	M	Generation Time
G_1^+-1	4.25	9.5	0.75	14.5
G_1^+-2	2.5	9.0	0.5	12.0
G_1^+-3	2.0	9.5	0.5	12.0
G_1^+-4	3.5	9.0	0.5	13.0
G_1^+-5	4.0	9.5	0.5	13.5
G_1^+-9	5.0	9.0	0.5	14.5
G_1^+-13	7.5	9.0	0.5	17.0

* From Liskay and Prescott.[6]

TABLE 3

FUSION OF MUTANT CELLS WITH ONE ANOTHER TO TEST FOR COMPLEMENTATION *

	G_1^+-1	G_1^+-2	G_1^+-3	G_1^+-4	G_1^+-5
G_1^+-1	nc	c	c	c	c
G_1^+-2	c		c	c	c
G_1^+-3	c	c		c	c
G_1^+-4	c	c	c		nc

NOTE: c = complementation, which means that the hybrid cells formed by fusion were G_1^-; nc = no complementation, that is, hybrid cells with G_1 periods.
* From Liskay and Prescott.[6]

THE G_1^+ MUTANTS MAY HAVE MUTATIONS AFFECTING CELL GROWTH

The observation that mutation of any one of apparently many genes causes delay in initiation of S indicates that the cellular process being affected required many genes. One such process requiring the proper functions of hundreds of different genes is cell growth. Thus, any mutation that slows growth might cause the appearance of a G_1 period. This possibility is based on experiments (for example, those of Killander and Zetterberg [12]) that a cell somehow senses its own size or growth state and uses the information to control the operation of an on/off switch that in turn controls entry into DNA synthesis. It is a common observation that agents or conditions that *slow* growth lengthen G_1, and agents or conditions that *prevent* growth cause cells to remain blocked in G_1.

The growth-impairment hypothesis was tested by measuring rates of protein synthesis in V79–8 cells and in G_1^+ mutants.[13] In three of four mutants tested the rates of protein synthesis were reduced compared with those of the parent G_1^- cell (TABLE 4). The degree by which protein synthesis was inhibited was roughly in proportion to the length of the G_1 period induced in a particular mutant cell. In one G_1^+ mutant the rate of protein synthesis was not reduced. This cell could have suffered from a mutation that reduced some component of cell growth without reducing the rate of protein synthesis.

If the G_1^- cell is converted to a G_1^+ cell by mutations that reduce the rate

TABLE 4

RELATIVE RATES OF PROTEIN SYNTHESIS IN THE PARENTAL G_1^- LINE V79–8 AND G_1^+ MUTANT LINES *

Cell	G_1	GT	Relative Rate of Protein Synthesis
V79–8	0	9	100%
G_1^+-1	2.9	13.2	68%
G_1^+-5	3.1	13.0	108%
G_1^+-6	4.9	15.0	59%
G_1^+-7	4.0	14.0	63%

* From Liskay et al.[13]

of cell growth, then it should be possible to induce a G_1 period in the G_1^- cell by slowing protein synthesis by other means. G_1^- cells were grown continuously in the presence of a low level of the inhibitor cycloheximide; the concentration of cycloheximide chosen was sufficient to slow the rate of protein synthesis by about 40%.[13] Under this condition the generation time of the G^{1-} cell increased by 4.2 hours; the increase was accounted for by the appearance of a 4.2-hour G_1 period.

These two sets of experiments strongly support but do not prove that the mutations cause G_1 periods by slowing cell growth.

FUSION OF SOME STANDARD G_1^+ CELL LINES WITH EACH OTHER PRODUCES G_1^- HYBRID CELLS

All of the foregoing observations deal with the G_1^- cell and G_1^+ mutants derived from it. The conclusions that were developed could also be tested with cell lines that normally possess G_1 periods in their cell cycles. Almost all of the cell lines derived from various animals proliferate in culture with G_1 periods. Four standard Chinese hamster cell lines known as DeDe, V79–743, CHO, and CH-III have the cell cycle values shown in TABLE 5. These normally G_1^+ cells were fused with one another in all possible combinations to test whether any of them complement one another with respect to the G_1 period.[14] For example, CH-III ($G_1 = 2.3$ hours) was fused with CHO ($G_1 = 3.0$ hours). In this case all of the hybrids had shorter generation times and were G_1^-. The full set of tests revealed three complementation groups for the four cell lines; DeDe and CHO did not complement each other. The conclusion from this experiment is that the G_1 periods in standard cell lines have different causes. Applying the interpretation of the experiments on the mutant cell lines discussed earlier, it may be hypothesized that these cell lines do not grow rapidly enough to avoid a delay in initiation of DNA synthesis, and the different lines have different bases for a limitation on cell growth. In G_1^- hybrids the limitations are removed by complementation. Why or how growth is limited in these cell lines is not known. It seems unlikely that genes important to cell growth have been mutated. Rather, it may be that the *expressions* of growth-related genes may be partially repressed.

G_1 CAN BE SHORTENED BY LENGTHENING THE S PERIOD

If it is correct that G_1^+ cells have slower growth rates and are therefore delayed in reaching the necessary size to trigger DNA replication, then it should be possible to shorten or even eliminate G_1 by increasing the rate of cell growth. Unfortunately, increasing cell growth rate has not been possible. Alternatively, however, it is possible to slow the rate of DNA synthesis, and this might produce the same final effect on G_1 as increasing the cell growth rate.

Low levels of hydroxyurea (HU) slow DNA synthesis by reducing the rate of synthesis of deoxynucleoside triphosphates. When a low level of HU is added to a culture of G_1^+ cells in the logarithmic phase of cell number increase, all cells undergo an increase in the length of the S period. This delay in completion of S allows more time for growth of the individual cell in each cell cycle. Hence, cells will be larger when they reach mitosis. If DNA synthesis is

TABLE 5

CELL CYCLE VALUES FOR FOUR LINES OF CHINESE HAMSTER CELLS THAT HAVE G_1
PERIODS *

Cell Line	G_1	S	$G_2 + M$	Generation Time
CHO	3.0	9.3	0.75	13.0
DeDe	2.0	8.8	0.75	11.5
V79–743	3.5	9.2	0.75	13.5
CH-III	2.3	8.2	1.0	11.5

* From Liskay et al.[14]

triggered by a critical size in newly divided daughter cells, then the increase in cell size resulting from HU treatment may be sufficient to trigger DNA synthesis immediately, that is, eliminate G_1.

Careful choice of HU concentration increased the length of S without increasing the generation time in two G_1^+ cells, the mutant cell G_1^+-1 (G_1 = 4.25 hours), and in CHO (G_1 = 3.0 hours).[15] The increase in the length of S was accommodated entirely by a shortening in the length of G_1 (TABLE 6). Thus, the result of the experiment was in the direction predicted, supporting once again the thesis that G_1 is caused by a failure of cell growth rate to keep pace with the chromosome cycle. However, even when HU was increased to a concentration that caused the generation time to increase, the G_1 period could not be reduced below approximately 1 hour. Thus, although most of G_1 is eliminated by slowing DNA synthesis, some irreducible portion of G_1 remains that presumably contains events essential for progressing to S.

The results of this experiment are a little puzzling in the face of the existence of the G_1^- cell line. However, the drug HU may have unidentified effects that interfere with reduction of G_1. For example, in the slime mold *Physarum,* HU not only slows DNA synthesis, but also markedly depresses protein and RNA synthesis.[16] On the other hand, G_1^- cells grown in the presence of HU have longer S periods and longer generation times, but no G_1 period is induced by the drug.

TABLE 6

EFFECT OF HYDROXYUREA ON THE CELL CYCLE OF CHO CELLS *

[HU], M	GT	S	G_1
4×10^{-5}	13.6 ± 0.2	11.5 ± 0.2	1.02 ± 0.03
6×10^{-5}	14.6 ± 0.4	12.4 ± 0.4	1.13 ± 0.05
8×10^{-5}	15.9 ± 0.5	13.7 ± 0.4	1.15 ± 0.06

* CHO cells were grown in the indicated concentrations of hydroxyurea and cell cycle analysis was performed. Values (in hours) represent the means of three determinations with the indicated SEM. From Stancel et al.[15]

CONCLUSIONS

The observations described in this paper add to a body of published observations that suggest the following description of the cell cycle in cultured animal cells: The G_1 period is not a part of the cell cycle but rather is the manifestation of a transient interruption in the transit of a cell from mitosis to DNA synthesis. The interruption represents the additional time required by the cell to achieve a size critical for triggering to the "on" position a switch controlling entry into DNA synthesis. Presumably in tissues G_1 periods are not the result of restriction on cell growth rates, but rather are interruptions in transit from mitosis to DNA synthesis caused by specific regulatory signals in the cellular microenvironment that affect an on/off switch for DNA synthesis.

REFERENCES

1. HOLLEY, R. W., P. BÖHLEN, R. FAVA, J. H. BALDWIN, G. KLEEMAN & R. ARMOUR. 1980. Purification of kidney epithelial cell growth inhibitors. Proc. Natl. Acad. Sci. USA **77:** 5989–5992.
2. MCMAHON, J. B., J. G. FARRELLY & P. T. IYPE. 1982. Purification and properties of a rat liver protein that specifically inhibits the proliferation of nonmalignant epithelial cells from rat liver. Proc. Natl. Acad. Sci. USA **79:** 456–460.
3. FORD, D. K. & G. YERGANIAN. 1958. Observations of chromosomes of Chinese hamster cells in tissue culture. J. Natl. Cancer Inst. **21:** 393–425.
4. ROBBINS, E. & M. D. SCHARFF. 1967. The absence of a detectable G_1 phase in a cultured strain of Chinese hamster lung cell. J. Cell Biol. **34:** 684–688.
5. LISKAY, R. M. 1977. Absence of a measurable G_2 phase in two Chinese hamster cell lines. Proc. Natl. Acad. Sci. USA **74:** 1622–1625.
6. LISKAY, R. M. & D. M. PRESCOTT. 1978. Genetic analysis of the G_1 period: Isolation of mutants (or variants) with a G_1 period from a Chinese hamster cell line lacking G_1. Proc. Natl. Acad. Sci. USA **75:** 2873–2877.
7. RAO, P. N. & R. T. JOHNSON. 1970. Mammalian cell fusion. I. Studies on the regulation of DNA synthesis and mitosis. Nature **225:** 159–164.
8. JOHNSON, R. T. & P. N. RAO. 1970. Mammalian cell fusion: Induction of premature chromosome condensation in interphase nuclei. Nature **226:** 717–722.
9. RAO, P. N., B. A. WILSON & P. S. SUNKARA. 1978. Inducers of DNA synthesis present during mitosis of mammalian cells lacking G_1 and G_2 phases. Proc. Natl. Acad. Sci. USA **75:** 5043–5047.
10. YANISHEVSKY, R. M. & D. M. PRESCOTT. 1978. Late S phase cells (Chinese hamster ovary) induce early S phase DNA labeling patterns in G_1 phase nuclei. Proc. Natl. Acad. Sci. USA **75:** 3307–3311.
11. LISKAY, R. M. & D. M. PRESCOTT. 1978. Genetic analysis of the cell life cycle. *In* Cell Reproduction (ICN-UCLA Symposia on Molecular and Cellular Biology). E. R. Dirksen, D. M. Prescott & C. F. Fox, Eds. Vol. **12:** 115–125. Academic Press. New York, NY.
12. KILLANDER, D. & A. ZETTERBERG. 1965. A quantitative cytochemical investigation of the relationship between cell mass and initiation of DNA synthesis in mouse fibroblasts *in vitro*. Exp. Cell Res. **40:** 12–20.
13. LISKAY, R. M., B. KORNFELD, P. FULLERTON & R. EVANS. 1980. Protein synthesis and the presence or absence of a measurable G_1 in cultured Chinese hamster cells. J. Cell. Physiol. **104:** 461–467.

14. LISKAY, R. M., K. E. LEONARD & D. M. PRESCOTT. 1979. Different Chinese hamster cell lines express a G_1 period for different reasons. Som. Cell Genet. **5:** 615–623.
15. STANCEL, G. M., D. M. PRESCOTT & R. M. LISKAY. 1981. Most of the G_1 period in hamster cells is eliminated by lengthening the S period. Proc. Natl. Acad. Sci. USA **78:** 6295–6298.
16. PIERRON, G. & H. W. SAUER. 1980. More evidence for replication-transcription-coupling in *Physarum polycephalum*. J. Cell Sci. **41:** 105–113.
17. LISKAY, R. M. Unpublished results.
18. LISKAY, R. M. & D. M. PRESCOTT. Unpublished results.

MOLECULAR BIOLOGY OF CELL DIVISION *

Renato Baserga, Dieter E. Waechter,† Kenneth J. Soprano,‡
and Norbel Galanti §

*Department of Pathology and Fels Research Institute
Temple University Medical School
Philadelphia, Pennsylvania 19140*

While the extent of cell proliferation in a cell population must be regulated by signals in the environment, the process of cell division must ultimately depend on the genes and gene products through which the cell responds to these signals. Thus, regardless of one's view of the cell cycle, mathematical models and semantic discussions, the key to our understanding of cell division rests essentially on the identification of growth factors and inhibitory factors, and of genes and gene products that regulate the orderly process of cell division.

In terms of genes regulating cell proliferation, one must distinguish between two problems: (1) the identification of those genes; and (2) the mechanism by which these genes are activated or repressed. The latter is just as important as the former since the same genes are clearly present in both resting and proliferating cells, and thus cell division will depend on whether these genes are expressed or not.

In this paper we will summarize our investigations on these two different aspects of cell proliferation. The discussion in this paper will cover the following three things: (1) evidence that unique-copy gene transcription is necessary for the transition of cells from a resting to a growing stage; (2) identification of domains within a single gene that encode the sequences critical for growth in size and for cell DNA replication; and (3) a mechanism by which these genes may be activated or repressed.

NECESSITY OF UNIQUE-COPY GENE TRANSCRIPTION FOR THE TRANSITION OF CELLS FROM A RESTING STATE TO A GROWING STATE

The first suggestion that unique-copy gene transcription was necessary for the transition of cells from a resting to a growing stage came from the pioneer experiments of Lieberman et al.,[1] who showed that low concentrations of actinomycin D inhibited the entry of quiescent cells into the cell cycle, both in cells in culture [1] and in the regenerating liver after partial hepatectomy.[2] The reports of Lieberman and coworkers [1, 2] were repeatedly confirmed in subsequent years (for a review of the effects of actinomycin D on cell proliferation

* This work was supported by Grant CA 12923 from the National Cancer Institute and Grant GM 22359 from the Institute of General Medical Sciences.

† Present address: Friedrich-Miescher-Institut, P.O. Box 273, CH-4002 Basel, Switzerland.

‡ Present address: Department of Microbiology, Temple University Medical School, Philadelphia, Pennsylvania 19140.

§ Present address: Departamento de Biología Celular y Genetica, Universidad de Chile, Santiago 7, Chile.

110

see Baserga [3]), but the question was left unresolved because of the ambiguity of experiments using actinomycin D.[4] Only recently has it been possible to demonstrate rigorously that unique-copy gene transcription is necessary for the transition of cells from either G_0 or mitosis to the S phase of the cell cycle. Two lines of evidence have clearly indicated that RNA polymerase II (the enzyme that transcribes unique-copy genes) is required for cell cycle progression:

(1) tsAF8 cells, a mutant of RNA polymerase II, are incapable of entering S phase at the nonpermissive temperature;

(2) α-amanitin, a drug that is specific for RNA polymerase II, also inhibits the entry of cells into the S phase.

A Temperature-Sensitive Mutant of RNA Polymerase II Arrests in G_1 at the Nonpermissive Temperature

tsAF8 cells were originally isolated from BHK cells by Meiss and Basilico.[5] These cells are bona fide G_1 mutants since (1) when collected by mitotic detachment and plated at the nonpermissive temperature, the cells do not enter S phase; (2) when made quiescent by serum restriction, and subsequently stimulated at the nonpermissive temperature, the cells do not enter S phase; (3) the cells enter S phase at the permissive temperature whether plated after mitotic detachment or stimulated after nutritional deprivation; and (4) the cells arrest in G_1, even when they are shifted up at the nonpermissive temperature in other phases of the cell cycle, that is, if shifted up during S, M, or G_2, they complete the mitotic cycle until they again reach a G_1 point.[6, 7]

These tsAF8 cells have now been identified as a mutant of RNA polymerase II by biochemical [8, 9] and genetic [10] evidence. The final, and rigorous, demonstration that these cells are a mutant of RNA polymerase II came when we microinjected into tsAF8 cells a highly purified preparation of RNA polymerase II. When tsAF8 cells in G_0 were microinjected with RNA polymerase II and then shifted up to the nonpermissive temperature, 45% of the cells were capable of entering the S phase of the cell cycle (TABLE 1). In these experiments only ~10% of the control cells on the same cover slip as microinjected cells, and subjected to exactly the same treatment, entered S phase. These results therefore complete the demonstration suggested by previous reports that tsAF8 cells have a defective RNA polymerase II. These experiments also indicate that a functional RNA polymerase II is required for the entry of cells into S, whether from G_0 or from mitosis.

Microinjected α-Amanitin Inhibits the Entry of Cells into S Phase

The requirement for RNA polymerase II, for entry into S, can also be demonstrated by using the drug α-amanitin, which is specific for the α-amanitin binding subunit of RNA polymerase II. A point mutation in the α-amanitin binding subunit of RNA polymerase II renders mammalian cells completely insensitive to the toxic effect of α-amanitin.[11] Therefore, any effect of α-amanitin on cell cycle progression has to be attributed to its effect on RNA polymerase II.

In previous experiments Wells *et al.*[12] had shown that addition of α-amanitin to the medium of cells in culture inhibited the entry of cells into the S phase of

TABLE 1

EFFECT OF MICROINJECTED RNA POLYMERASE II ON THE ENTRY OF tsAF8 CELLS
INTO THE CELL CYCLE

Treatment	Temperature	Percentage of Labeled Cells
None	34°	7.2
None	39.6°	3.1
10% serum	34°	63.1
	39.6°	13.9
10% serum + buffer *	34°	58.9
10% serum + RNA polymerase II *	39.6°	45.0
10% serum + IgG *	39.6	8.4

NOTE: tsAF8 cells were made quiescent in 0.5% serum and then stimulated with 10% serum or left untreated (first 2 rows).

* Cells were microinjected with either buffer or RNA polymerase II or IgG. The cells were labeled with [³H]-thymidine for 24 hr. The RNA polymerase II preparation was prepared from human placenta by Peter M. McGuire, Erwin Freund, and C. Mark Riggenbach, Department of Biochemistry, University of Florida, Gainesville, Florida.

the cell cycle. We confirmed their results more rigorously by microinjecting α-amanitin directly into the nuclei of cells, using the glass capillary technique of Graessmann and Graessmann.[13] The results are shown in FIGURE 1. When cells are microinjected with α-amanitin, entry into S is inhibited, although α-amanitin does not have a direct effect on ongoing DNA synthesis. In fact, it can be estimated from FIGURE 1 that once the cell has passed a point located roughly 8 hours before S, it becomes insensitive to α-amanitin and the cell enters the S phase of the cell cycle. Interestingly enough this 8-hr point coincides with the execution point of the temperature-sensitive mutation in tsAF8 cells.[14]

The demonstration that a functional RNA polymerase II is necessary for cell cycle progression, and that microinjected α-amanitin inhibits the entry of cells into S, constitutes a rigorous demonstration that unique-copy gene transcription is necessary for the transition of cells from the resting to the growing stage.

GROWTH IN SIZE AND CELL DNA REPLICATION ARE SEPARATE PROCESSES

Although tsAF8 cells, at the nonpermissive temperature, are incapable of entering the S phase of the cell cycle, RNA polymerase I activity is not affected. Indeed, it was shown that even at the nonpermissive temperature tsAF8 cells accumulate RNA just as effectively as at the permissive temperature.[7] The findings indicate that a functional RNA polymerase II is required for entry into S, but not for the growth in size of the cells. They also suggest that the requirements for cell DNA replication may be different from those for growth in size.

This is important because although cell DNA replication and mitosis are the most striking events in the cell division cycle, it is self-evident that the size of the cell must also be carefully regulated. Clearly, if cell size were not to double from early G_1 to mitosis, at each cell cycle the cells would become increasingly smaller and eventually vanish. During balanced growth, under ordinary conditions "the two daughter cells produced at each division are identical to the parent at the same time in the preceding cycle. This requires that all cell components are doubled during each course of the cell cycle." [15] This is true of bacteria, yeasts, and mammalian cells. It says that cell size must be regulated for, in the words of Mitchison,[16] "size control is likely to be an important element in cell cycle mechanisms". In the experiments described below we have demonstrated that it is indeed possible to identify genes that stimulate only cell DNA replication and genes that instead stimulate only the growth in size of the cells.

Adenovirus 2 Infection Stimulates Cell DNA Replication, but Not Growth in Size

Adenovirus 2 stimulates DNA synthesis in infected hamster cells,[17, 18] but does not cause an increase in either the synthesis or the accumulation of ribosomal RNA.[19-21] These experiments indicate that the adenovirus genome contains the necessary information for the stimulation of cell DNA replication, but lacks the necessary information for inducing growth in size of the cells.

Different Domains of the SV40 A Gene Regulate Cell DNA Replication and Growth in Size of Cells

SV40 infection can stimulate cell DNA replication and mitosis in quiescent mammalian cells.[22, 23] Indeed, it has been formally demonstrated that the SV40 T antigen stimulates cellular DNA synthesis.[24] We have investigated whether the capacity to stimulate growth in size can be dissociated from the capacity to stimulate cell DNA replication when cells are induced to proliferate by SV40. Two different sets of experiments were carried out. In one set of experiments we investigated the ability of the SV40 genome to reactivate silent ribosomal

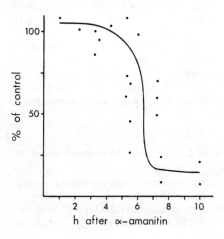

FIGURE 1. Determination of the last α-amanitin-sensitive point in the G_1 period of AF8 cells. Quiescent AF8 cells were stimulated with 10% serum. After 24 hr, when most of the cells were in S phase or near it, they were microinjected into the nucleus with α-amanitin at a concentration of 50 μg/ml. The cells were then incubated for the times indicated on the abscissa, pulse-labeled for 30 min with 1 μCi/ml [³H]-thymidine, and fixed. The percentage of labeled cells was determined by autoradiography and compared with that of cells that were not microinjected ($= 100\%$).

RNA genes, on the reasonable assumption that ribosomal RNA genes constitute a target for any signal that will induce growth in size of the cells. This is not an unreasonable assumption. Nucleic acids and proteins constitute about 50% of the dry weight of cells and ribosomal RNA constitutes about 70% of the total nucleic acids of the cell. In addition, ribosomes are the structure on which proteins are synthesized, and therefore it seems quite reasonable that the ribosomal RNA genes may be one of the primary targets of any signal for the growth in size of the cells. An alternative would be to determine the cellular content of proteins, as done by Rønning et al.,[25] who showed that the doubling time of cells in culture is a function of the doubling of the protein amount. Either proteins or ribosomal RNA are a reasonable measure of cell size. To determine the effect of growth signals on rRNA genes we have used the system of reactivation of silent ribosomal RNA genes.[26] This is a physiologic system since in cells in culture not all the ribosomal RNA genes are active,[27] although they are turned on if an appropriate stimulus is applied.[28] The reactivation of silent ribosomal RNA genes constitutes, therefore, the method of choice for determining whether a gene product has the property of stimulating growth in size of cells.

We have investigated the ability of the SV40 genome to reactivate the ribosomal RNA genes of 55–54 hybrid cells (where reactivation of silent rRNA genes can be more easily studied), using adeno-SV40 hybrid viruses and the microinjection of cloned deletion mutants of SV40. These experiments have been described in detail in the papers by Soprano et al.,[20, 29, 30] as well as in the paper by Galanti et al.[31] The results are summarized in TABLE 2, in which the map coordinates of the SV40 DNA sequences that were tested are given together with the outcome of the test. It should be remembered at this point that the SV40 A gene, which codes for both the large T and the small t, maps from 0.67 to 0.17 map units counterclockwise. From TABLE 2 it is apparent that the large T antigen is sufficient for the stimulation of ribosomal RNA genes. The small t is not required (dl 2005 makes a regular T but no small t). It is also apparent from TABLE 2 that the sequences from 0.67 to 0.39 of the SV40 A gene are not necessary for the reactivation of rRNA genes, and neither are the sequences from 0.33 to 0.17. Therefore, the conclusion is that in the SV40 A gene the sequences that are critical for the reactivation of rRNA genes are those mapping between 0.39 and 0.33 map units of the SV40 genome. These results should be interpreted with caution. They do not mean that the 100 or so amino acids, coded by those 300 nucleotides between 0.39 and 0.33 map units, are sufficient for the reactivation of ribosomal RNA genes. Obviously, tertiary structure of proteins is important for protein function, but what these data convey is that the critical sequences for reactivation of ribosomal RNA genes are indeed specified by this nucleotide sequence. An analogy should be made with the active site of an enzyme or with the antigen binding site of an antibody.

Ability of SV40 Deletion Mutants to Induce Cell DNA Replication

All of these experiments were done by microinjection of cloned deletion mutants of SV40 into quiescent mammalian cells. The experiments consisted of microinjecting cloned SV40 fragments into quiescent ts13 and 3T3 cells, and determining their ability to stimulate cell DNA replication. The results are summarized in TABLE 3, which gives the map coordinates of the SV40 clones microinjected into cells, as well as their ability to stimulate cell DNA replication. From TABLE 3 it is apparent that a fragment of the SV40 A gene extending from 0.67 to 0.42 is sufficient for the induction of cell DNA replication. The sequences downstream from 0.42 map units therefore are not critical for the stimulation of cell DNA replication. A mutant of this kind will code for a protein not larger than 30,000 daltons, and yet it has all the necessary capacity for stimulating cell DNA replication, although this mutant is incapable of reactivating ribosomal RNA genes. Therefore, the information for the stimulation of cell DNA replication is clearly separate from the information for the reactivation of ribosomal RNA genes.

By looking at TABLE 3 one can see that the sequences of the SV40 A gene mapping between 0.67 and 0.49 map units are not critical for the stimulation

TABLE 2

SEQUENCES OF SV40 GENOME REQUIRED FOR THE REACTIVATION OF RIBOSOMAL RNA GENES

Virus or Plasmid	SV40 Sequences (map units)	Reactivation of rRNA Genes
SV40	1.00/0	+
pSV2G	1.00/0.144	+
Hpa II/Pst I A fragment	0.73/0.27	+
Pvu II A fragment	0.70/0.33	+
Hpa I B fragment	0.75/0.37	—
pVR200	0.71/0.42	—
dl 2005	Δ0.59/0.54	+
Adenovirus 2	—	—
Ad2 + ND$_3$	0.18/0.11	—
Ad2 + ND$_1$	0.28/0.11	—
Ad2 + ND$_5$	0.39/0.11	+
Ad2 + ND$_2$	0.44/0.11	+

NOTE: The plasmids or fragments were manually microinjected into the nuclei of 55–54 cells. The effect of viruses was determined by infection of 55–54 cultures. The SV40 sequences are given counterclockwise. Δ = deletion. Details are given in the three papers by Soprano *et al.*[20, 29, 30]

of cell DNA replication. Therefore, the critical sequences for the induction of cell DNA replication seem to lie between 0.49 and 0.42 map units, that is, a total of 360 nucleotides that code for 120 of the 708 amino acids of the SV40 T antigen.

It is too early to say whether the control of cell DNA replication and of ribosomal RNA gene reactivation are also separate in the genome of mammalian cells, but it is clear from the experiments with adenovirus 2, and with SV40, and their hybrids, that the two processes are regulated by different domains on both the SV40 A gene and the adenovirus 2 genome. The prediction of this model is that we should be able to identify among the growth factors those that induce cell DNA replication from those that stimulate growth in size of the cell. Our prediction, though, is that in ordinary physiological conditions the

TABLE 3

STIMULATION OF CELL DNA REPLICATION BY RECOMBINANT SV40-PLASMIDS

Plasmid	SV40 Sequences (map units)	Stimulation of Cell DNA Synthesis
pSVB3	1.00/0	+
pSV2G	1.00/0.144	+
pSV1137	Terminates at 0.51	−
pSV1138	Terminates at 0.49	−
pSV1046	Δ0.46–0.42	−
pVR200	0.71/0.42	+
pSVHpa I	0.70/0.375	+
pSV Pst	1.00/0.272	+
pSV3D	Δ0.63–0.49	+

NOTE: Cell DNA synthesis was determined by labeling with [^{3}H]-thymidine and autoradiography. All plasmids were microinjected manually into nucleic 3T3 and ts13 cells. Map units are given counterclockwise. Δ = deletion. Terminates = point of termination of the A gene which normally extends from 0.67 to 0.17 map units. (Adapted from Galanti et al.[31] and unpublished results from our laboratory.) Some of the recombinant plasmids were constructed by Jim Pipas (University of Pittsburgh) in the laboratory of Daniel Nathans (Johns Hopkins Medical School).

cell would not accept a signal for cell DNA replication unless a signal for growth in size has first been acknowledged. It should be noted, however, that, although there is a strict correlation between amount of proteins and mitosis, cells can enter S phase even with subnormal amounts of proteins.[25]

REGULATION OF GENE EXPRESSION BY DNA METHYLATION

As mentioned in the introduction, it would be interesting to know how genes that are present in both proliferating and resting cells are expressed, and thus to determine whether a cell should grow or not. We have approached this problem by investigating two genes that are involved in cell cycle progression, and asked the question whether the methylation of these genes would affect their expression.

In recent years a number of investigators have suggested that DNA methylation may be responsible for the control of gene expression. The evidence for this hypothesis has been marshalled in a very thorough review by Razin and Riggs.[32] Apart from the fact that certain specific methylation sites in expressed genes are less methylated than in nonexpressed genes,[33, 34] other evidence has been accumulating implicating methylation as a way of regulating gene expression. Among the most convincing experiments were the ones by Doerfler and coworkers using cells transformed by adenovirus. Doerfler and coworkers [35, 36] studied the degree of methylation of adenovirus DNA integrated into chromosomal DNA. Under these conditions some of the adenovirus genes are expressed, whereas others are not. Doerfler's group found that the integrated adenovirus genes that were expressed were unmethylated, whereas the integrated adenovirus genes that were not expressed were highly methylated. In subsequent experiments Doerfler and collaborators [37] methylated adenovirus

DNA and then microinjected it into Xenopus oocytes. Whereas the adenovirus DNA was fully expressed when microinjected into *Xenopus* oocytes, its expression was markedly inhibited when the DNA was methylated before microinjection.

In our laboratory we have also shown that methylation can alter the expression of microinjected genes, although in our case we microinjected the methylated genes into mammalian cells.[38] In these experiments the cloned genes for the simian virus 40 T antigen and the herpes simplex virus thymidine kinase (two genes that are both involved in cell cycle progression) were methylated with ECoRl methylase. The genes were then microinjected into the nuclei of tk⁻ cells, and the expression of the genes was determined by immunofluorescence staining for the SV40 T antigen and by the [³H]-thymidine incorporation, followed by autoradiography, for the HSV-tk. We found that methylation of the SV40 A gene under ECoRl* conditions, resulting in methylation within the gene and the surrounding sequences, has no effect on the expression of T antigen when the gene is manually microinjected into mammalian nuclei. However methylation of the HSV-tk gene at the two ECoRl sites markedly reduces, or abolishes, the expression of this gene. Some new results obtained with this system are presented in TABLE 4. Notice that in these experiments the two genes, the SV40 A gene and the HSV-tk, were inserted into the same pBR322 plasmid. Therefore, these two genes were treated exactly alike and microinjected into the same cell, yet methylation affected the expression of the HSV-tk gene, but had very little effect on the expression of the SV40 A gene.

One of the ECoRl sites on the HSV-tk gene is about 1.1 kilobases downstream from the 3′ end of the gene, and it can be deleted without affecting the expression of the tk gene. The other ECoRl site is 79 basepairs upstream from the 5′ end of the gene and has considerable homology to a regulatory sequence proposed by Benoist *et al.*,[39] a sequence being considered important in gene expression, and as part of the prelude region described by Grosschedl and

TABLE 4

EFFECT OF METHYLATION ON THE EXPRESSION OF MICROINJECTED GENES

DNA Microinjected	Percentage of Cells Expressing T Antigen	Percentage of Cells Incorporating [³H]-Tdr
pC6 unmethylated	169 ± 1%	327 ± 11%
pC6 unmethylated and cut with ECoRl	101 ± 22%	18 ± 11%
pC6 ECoRl * methylated	130 ± 42%	135 ± 59%
pC6 ECoRl * methylated and cut with ECoRl	128 ± 30%	108 ± 30%

NOTE: pC6 is a plasmid containing in pBR322 the SV40 genome and the thymidine kinase gene of herpes simplex virus (HSV-tk). The plasmid was microinjected into tk⁻ts 13 cells. T antigen was determined by immunofluorescence, HSV-tk activity by the ability of cells to incorporate [³H]-thymidine. In each case, 100 cells were microinjected, but they proliferated during the experimental period (24 hr). ECoRl * methylated means the plasmid was methylated under ECoRl * conditions. Details are given in the paper by Waechter and Baserga.[38]

Birnstiel,[40] and which includes other elements, such as the TATAA box. There-fore, modification of a single site, about 70 basepairs upstream from HSV-tk gene, decreases its transcription. On the other hand extensive methylation of the SV40 A gene at various places in the coding region, and in the 5' flanking sequences, but excluding this site, has no effect on its transcription when the gene is microinjected into mammalian cells. Generalized conclusions cannot be drawn from experiments in which only two genes were examined. Further-more, the genes were microinjected as naked DNA, whereas in the cell genes are largely covered with proteins. However, the results make two important points: they clearly show (1) that methylation has different effects on different genes, and (2) that methylation has different effects, depending on the sites in the genes that are methylated.

CONCLUSIONS

We hope that we have been able to reach the goals stated in the introduction to this paper, namely, of demonstrating that: (1) unique-copy gene transcrip-tion is necessary for the transition of cells from a resting to a growing stage; (2) different domains on a single gene encode the critical sequences for growth in size and for cell DNA replication; and (3) the expression of genes that are involved in cell cycle progression can be modified by appropriate modifications of the 5' flanking sequences. The implications of these findings are numerous, but we would like to mention, at this point, the following: (i) The evidence that unique-copy gene transcription is necessary for the transition of cells from a resting to a growing stage justifies the search for mRNAs that are present in G_1, or S phase cells, and are not at present in G_0. Among these mRNAs may be some that are critical, while others are necessary but not sufficient. This is a very urgent problem in the field of cell proliferation and we are actively investigating the possibility of identifying some of these mRNAs. Even if we were not able to identify the mRNA that controls cell proliferation, the estab-lishment of a catalogue, even though incomplete, of gene products that are involved in cell cycle progression, will constitute enormous progress in the area of the control of cell division. (ii) The separation of cell DNA replication from growth in size also opens up new avenues of investigation not only for those interested, as we in our laboratory have been, in the genes and gene products that control cell proliferation, but also for those investigators who are interested in the identification of growth factors. Clearly growth factors that stimulate cell DNA replication and growth factors that stimulate growth in size must be present in the environment and they should be identified. (iii) Finally, it is clear that the expression of genes can be regulated by simply modifying them, especially when the modification occurs in the 5' flanking sequences. This also opens up new avenues for determining how some of these genes can be regulated by signals in the environment.

SUMMARY

Different domains of the SV40 A gene have different functions, such as viral DNA replication, cell DNA replication, and stimulation of cellular RNA synthesis. The sequences in the SV40 A gene that are critical for the induction of cell DNA synthesis lie on the map between nucleotide 4360 and nucleotide 4001, a stretch of 360 nucleotides coding for 120 of the 708 amino acids of the large T antigen. The sequences critical for stimulation of rRNA synthesis lie on the map further downstream, between nucleotides 3827 and 3506, thus indicating that the signals for growth in size and for cell DNA replication can be dissociated. Methylation of the SV40 A gene at multiple ECoRl* sites has no effect on its expression. However, methylation of the HSV-TK gene at one single ECoRl site 70 base pairs upstream from the cap site inhibits its expression. The results indicate that methylation of genes affects their expression, but only when methylation occurs at specific sites.

REFERENCES

1. LIEBERMAN, I., R. ABRAMS & P. OVE. 1963. J. Biol. Chem. **238:** 2141–2149.
2. TSUKADA, K. & I. LIEBERMAN. 1964. J. Biol. Chem. **239:** 2952–2956.
3. BASERGA, R. 1976. Multiplication and Division in Mammalian Cells. Marcel Dekker. New York, NY.
4. CLARK, J. L. & S. GREENSPAN. 1979. Exp. Cell Res. **118:** 253–260.
5. MEISS, H. K. & C. BASILICO. 1972. Nature New Biol. **239:** 66–68.
6. BURSTIN, S. J., H. K. MEISS & C. BASILICO. 1974. J. Cell. Physiol. **84:** 397–408.
7. ASHIHARA, T., F. TRAGANOS, R. BASERGA & Z. DARZYNKIEWICZ. 1978. Cancer Res. **38:** 2514–2518.
8. ROSSINI, M. & R. BASERGA. 1978. Biochemistry **17:** 858–863.
9. ROSSINI, M., S. BASERGA, C. H. HUANG, C. J. INGLES & R. BASERGA. 1980. J. Cell. Physiol. **103:** 97–103.
10. SHALES, M., J. BERGSAGEL & C. J. INGLES. 1980. J. Cell. Physiol. **105:** 527–532.
11. INGLES, C. J. 1978. Proc. Natl. Acad. Sci. USA **75:** 405–409.
12. WELLS, D. J., L. S. STODDARD, M. J. GETZ & H. L. MOSES. 1979. J. Cell Physiol. **100:** 199–214.
13. GRAESSMANN, M. & A. GRAESSMANN. 1976. Proc. Natl. Acad. Sci. USA **73:** 366–370.
14. ASHIHARA, T., S. D. CHANG & R. BASERGA. 1978. J. Cell. Physiol. **96:** 15–22.
15. FRASER, R. S. S. & P. NURSE. 1978. Nature **271:** 726–730.
16. MITCHISON, J. M. 1977. *In* Growth Kinetics and Biochemical Regulation of Normal and Malignant Cells. B. Drewinko & R. M. Humphrey, Eds.: 23–33. Williams & Wilkins. Baltimore, MD.
17. LAUGHLIN, C. & W. A. STROHL. 1976. Virology **75:** 44–56.
18. ROSSINI, M., R. WEINMANN & R. BASERGA. 1979. Proc. Natl. Acad. Sci. USA **76:** 4441–4445.
19. ELICEIRI, G. L. 1973. Virology **56:** 604–607.
20. SOPRANO, K. J., M. ROSSINI, C. M. CROCE & R. BASERGA. 1980. Virology **102:** 317–326.
21. POCHRON, S., M. ROSSINI, Z. DARZYNKIEWICZ, F. TRAGANOS & R. BASERGA. 1980. J. Biol. Chem. **255:** 4411–4413.
22. WEIL, R. 1978. Biochim. Biophys. Acta **516:** 301–388.
23. LEBOWITZ, P. & S. M. WEISSMAN. 1979. Curr. Topics Microbiol. Immunol. **87:** 44–172.
24. TJIAN, R., G. FEY & A. GRAESSMANN. 1978. Proc. Natl. Acad. Sci. USA **75:** 1279–1283.
25. RØNNING, Ø. W., T. LINDMO, E. O. PETTERSEN & P. O. SEGLEN. 1981. J. Cell. Physiol. **109:** 411–418.

26. CROCE, C. M., A. TALAVERA, C. BASILICO & O. J. MILLER. 1977. Proc. Natl. Acad. Sci. USA **74:** 694–697.
27. JHANWAR, S. C., W. PRENCKY & R. S. K. CHAGANTI. 1981. Cytogenet. Cell Genet. **30:** 39–46.
28. SCHMIADY, H., M. MÜNKE & K. SPERLING. 1979. Exp. Cell Res. **121:** 425–428.
29. SOPRANO, K. J., V. G. DEV, C. M. CROCE & R. BASERGA. 1979. Proc. Natl. Acad. Sci. USA **76:** 3885–3889.
30. SOPRANO, K. J., G. J. JONAK, N. GALANTI, J. FLOROS & R. BASERGA. 1981. Virology **109:** 127–136.
31. GALANTI, N., G. J. JONAK, K. J. SOPRANO, J. FLOROS, L. KACZMAREK, S. WEISSMAN, V. B. REDDY, S. TILGHMAN & R. BASERGA. 1981. J. Biol. Chem. **256:** 6469–6474.
32. RAZIN, A. & A. D. RIGGS. 1980. Science **210:** 604–610.
33. MANDEL, J. L. & P. CHAMBON. 1979. Nucleic Acids Res. **7:** 2081–2103.
34. SHEN, C. K. J. & T. MANIATIS. 1980. Proc. Natl. Acad. Sci. USA **77:** 6634–6638.
35. SUTTER, D. & W. DOERFLER. 1980. Proc. Natl. Acad. Sci. USA **77:** 253–256.
36. VARDIMON, L., R. NEUMANN, I. KUHLMAN, D. SUTTER & W. DOERFLER. 1980. Nucleic Acids Res. **8:** 2461–2473.
37. VARDIMON, L., A. KRESSMANN, H. CEDAR, M. MAECHLER & W. DOERFLER. 1982. Proc. Natl. Acad. Sci. USA. **79:** 1073–1077.
38. WAECHTER, D. E. & R. BASERGA. 1982. Proc. Natl. Acad. Sci. USA. **79:** 1106–1110.
39. BENOIST, C., K. O'HARE, R. BREATHNACH & P. CHAMBON. 1980. Nucleic Acids Res. **8:** 127–142.
40. GROSSCHEDL, R. & M. L. BIRNSTIEL. 1980. Proc. Natl. Acad. Sci. USA **77:** 7102–7106.

DIFFERENCES IN GROWTH REGULATION
OF NORMAL AND TUMOR CELLS *

Arthur B. Pardee,† Judith Campisi, and Robert G. Croy

Department of Pharmacology
Harvard Medical School, and
Sidney Farber Cancer Institute
Boston, Massachusetts 02115

A great deal has been learned during the past few years about growth control of mammalian cells in culture,[1] as illustrated by many of the papers in this volume. Comparisons of growth of normal and tumor cells in culture have been very useful, since the neoplastic properties of tumor cells *in vivo* are reflected in their defective growth control in culture. A second subject on which great progress has been made is the molecular genetic nature of the tumorigenic transformation process. This work also is represented in the present symposium. Connections between these two areas—cell biology of growth regulation and molecular biology of neoplastic transformation—are still tenuous. A principal purpose of this paper is to suggest some relations between our efforts in the former area and the findings of molecular geneticists.

ON THE CELL BIOLOGY OF GROWTH CONTROL

Our view of the growth control problem is summarized in the following statements:

1. The growth of nontumorigenic cells is dependent on external conditions, such as the availability of growth factors and nutrients in the medium, and, depending upon the cell type, a substratum and the density of nearby cells.

2. Depending on these conditions, normal cells can either be growing and proceeding through the cell cycle, or alternatively they can be quiescent. These quiescent cells do not divide or make DNA over long periods.

3. A growing cell either proceeds through another cycle or moves into a quiescent state after it reaches a point R in the cell cycle that is a few hours prior to the beginning of DNA synthesis. Growth control can best be considered as a switching mechanism dependent upon external factors that act at this R point (the restriction[2] point). In general, restriction of growth occurs shortly before S, in the G_1 part of the cell cycle.

4. Quiescent (G_0) cells either remain quiescent or enter the cell cycle depending upon external conditions. Re-entry is a two-step process of competence and progression,[3] as discussed elsewhere in this symposium. These events are probably very similar to ones through which cells go in each cycle.

5. Normal cells can be transformed by a variety of agents, such as chemicals, RNA or DNA viruses, radiation, and most recently by transfer of DNA from tumor cells: In some cases introduction of a single viral gene is sufficient for

* This work was aided by Grant GM 24571 from the U.S. Public Health Service.
† Address for correspondence: Sidney Farber Cancer Institute, 44 Binney Street, Boston, Massachusetts 02115.

121

transformation, and this gene may produce only a single protein. These proteins appear to be very similar, or even identical, to normal cell components, but in transformed cells they are present in larger amounts.[4]

6. Transformed cells' growth controls are in general relaxed but not absent: that is, they can grow under some conditions that block the growth of non-transformed cells. They are not as readily arrested at the restriction point as are nontransformed cells.[5]

On the Biochemistry of Cell Growth Control

Both the molecular genetic and the cell biological approaches suggest that specific proteins are at the heart of the growth control problem. Cells transformed by various RNA tumor viruses often overproduce normal cellular proteins, each relatively specifically determined by its virus. The best known example is transformation by Rous sarcoma virus, and production of a 60-K sarc protein.[4] Sarc is a protein kinase and presumably has its main action through phosphorylation of other proteins.[6] Transformation with SV40, a DNA tumor virus, causes appearance of the viral T antigens, one of which (T) forms a complex with a cell-derived protein of about 53-K daltons. T antigen has a number of properties, one being stabilization of this otherwise highly unstable 53-K host-coded protein.[7] The proteins sarc and T are coded by nucleic acid sequences in their respective viruses, and their proteins are thus the primary products of these transforming viruses. They are the beginnings of metabolic chains whose subsequent links are generally unknown. Thus there seems little doubt that transformation by these viruses is primarily dependent upon the appearance in the cell of a protein specific in each case. These proteins can create biochemical changes such as phosphorylations in other specific proteins. Similar changes probably occur in chemically transformed cells. One example of great interest is appearance of the 53-K host-coded protein in a mouse line transformed by methylcholanthrene.[8] It is generally supposed that genetic changes, particularly rearrangements of the chromosome,[9] activate host genes so that they overproduce their products.[10]

Using a completely different approach, we have come to the conclusion that the critical factor in growth control is specific protein production. Our experiments lead to the following conclusions [11, 12]: A few hours before the cells are capable of making DNA, generally during the G_1 period, they start to synthesize a protein that has a half-life of about 2.5 hr. This protein is both being synthesized and degraded during the following hours. Its ability to accumulate in a cell depends upon both its rates of synthesis and of degradation. Therefore its accumulation is highly sensitive to factors that affect both processes. If environmental or intracellular factors are adequately stimulatory, the protein accumulates to a critical level, high enough to start a process which after approximately 2 hours initiates DNA synthesis.

If external conditions are not adequate, for example, when insufficient serum is provided, the synthetic rate does not exceed the degradation rate and the protein cannot accumulate to the critical level. These G_1-arrested cells do not progress into S phase. After a few hours "marking time" in G_1, their various relatively unstable proteins gradually decay, and the cells fall into a G_0 state. They can recover only after conditions are improved. FIGURE 1 caricatures alternative G_1-related states.

We have tested the labile protein model by partly inhibiting the overall rate of protein synthesis, using cycloheximide (CHM) or histidinol as inhibitors of protein synthesis. A moderate inhibition of protein synthesis evidently will change the balance, making degradation predominate over synthesis. Cells thus treated will not be able to synthesize labile proteins sufficiently rapidly relative to their degradation, and will therefore be unable to pass into S phase. Indeed, we found that normal cells exposed to low CHM concentrations are retained specifically in the G_1 phase for long periods.[11] A similar result is seen upon deprivation for essential amino acids; these cells too are arrested with a G_1 DNA content, and eventually they enter a G_0 state.[13, 14]

By varying the CHM concentration, we have obtained quantitative data on the G_1 arrest, and analyzed these data to determine the half-life of the putative unstable protein. By this method we found a half-life of 2.5 hr for 3T3 cells.[11] This calculation is in good agreement with that obtained by another method we

CELL STATES

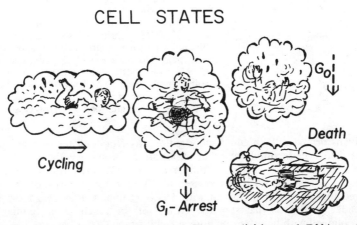

FIGURE 1. Cartoon illustrating G_1 states. Between division and DNA synthesis a cell contains its unduplicated quantity of DNA. It is very different biochemically and kinetically otherwise, depending on extracellular conditions. Like our swimmer, a "G_1" cell can be (i) progressing toward S, (ii) in a dynamic steady state, a true G_1 arrest, (iii) in quiescent (G_0) states from which it can be revived, or (iv) in a terminal, nondividing state.

have used for determining the half-life of this labile protein, which depends upon storing G_1 cells in the presence of a high concentration of CHM for various intervals so that pre-existing unstable protein can decay.[15] In these experiments, 3T3 (A31) cells were synchronized by serum deprivation (48 hr) followed by serum readdition. CHM was added at a time shortly before the earliest cell reached the R point. The inhibitor was removed after periods of 1–6 hr. If the R protein was perfectly stable, the onset of S should be delayed by a period equal to the length of the CHM pulse. Any degradation of the R protein should result in an excess delay equal to the time required for its resynthesis. FIGURE 2 shows that CHM treatment under these conditions resulted in appreciable excess delays (the heavy arrow-headed lines), which increased with longer CHM treatments. From these excess delays, we calculated an R protein half-life of 2.5 hr for A31 cells.[11, 12]

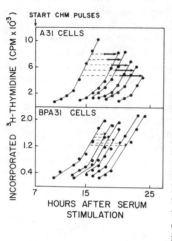

FIGURE 2. The effects of complete protein synthesis blocks on synchronized normal and transformed 3T3 cells. Normal (A31) and transformed (BPA31) 3T3 cells were arrested in G_0 by growth in low serum concentrations (0.5%, 52–56 hours for A31 cells; 0.2%, 78–82 hours for BPA31 cells). At zero time, they were stimulated to grow by the addition of 10% serum. Seven hours later, [³H]-labeled thymidine (0.08 μCi/ml) and CHM (1.5 μg/ml) were added. Control cultures were immediately washed free of the inhibitor; the remaining cultures were washed 2,3,4,5 and 6 hours after CHM addition. After washing, fresh medium containing ³H-thymidine was added to the cultures. At hourly intervals, starting at 10 hours after serum stimulation, incorporation was stopped and the amount of radioactivity in trichloroacetic acid-insoluble material was determined. The left-most line of data points in each panel shows the initiation of DNA synthesis (accumulation of [³H]-thymidine) in the control cultures and the sets of data points to the right of the controls show the initiation of S after CHM pulses of 2,3,4,5 and 6 hours, respectively. The heavy arrow-headed lines illustrate delays in the onset of S which were in excess of the lengths of the CHM pulses.

Transformed cells should respond differently from untransformed cells when exposed to cycloheximide or other inhibitors of protein synthesis, if this labile protein hypothesis is correct. Comparisons of 3T3 cells transformed with a variety of agents—RNA tumor viruses, SV40 DNA tumor virus, or chemicals—showed that a partial inhibition with CHM is unable to arrest these cells in G_1 under conditions that stop the growth of the parent line. Similar results were obtained with hamster and human cell lines.[16]

More recently we have used the complete block technique with CHM or histidinol to demonstrate that transformed cells are far less sensitive than are their untransformed counterparts.[12] FIGURE 2 shows the results of the complete block technique using CHM and BPA31 cells, a benzopyrene-transformed, tumorigenic A31 derivative. These transformed cells show no excess delays, even after long exposures to the inhibitor. We conclude that the protein which is required for transit to S phase is considerably more stable in these transformed cells than it is in untransformed cells.

Serum deprivation rapidly arrests untransformed cells in G_1,[17] but not transformed cells.[2, 5] In recent experiments we have been exploring the effect of serum deprivation upon the stability of the putative regulatory protein. We propose from our other results that low serum either prevents synthesis of the regulatory protein, increases its rate of degradation, or both. 3T3 cells were arrested in G_0 with low serum and then refed to achieve synchrony. After 7 hr, when these cells were about 4 hr from initiation of DNA synthesis, they were put either into medium containing a highly inhibitory CHM concentration, into medium lacking serum, or into medium lacking serum and with high CHM. After 3–5 hr under these conditions the cells were put back into complete medium. It can be seen in FIGURE 3 that exposure to high CHM for 3 or 5 hr caused extra delays of 1.3 and 1.9 hr, respectively. We have calculated that the maximal extra delay of 3T3 cells is approximately 2.8 hr,[12] and therefore a period of even 5 hr in high CHM did not allow total decay of the labile protein. In contrast, exposure to serum-free medium for only 3 hr created essentially the maximal delay, and this was not increased by 5-hr serum deprivation. Therefore, decay in the absence of serum appears to be even faster than decay in the presence of cycloheximide. A combination of the two treatments (high CHM and low serum) was used, and this gave a result very similar to the one observed after serum deprivation alone. Minimally, these experiments show that net R protein synthesis is regulated by serum factors. Barring the possibility that the recovery from serum deprivation is sluggish compared with the recovery from CHM, we may also tentatively conclude that serum factors are very important in stabilizing this regulatory protein.

These experiments immediately suggest a search for the labile regulatory protein, a protein that should be more stable in the transformed cell lines that we have studied. Proteins show highly different half-lives in cells; the average protein has a half-life of several days. Several unstable proteins have been identified, one of the best known being ornithine decarboxylase, which has a half-life of only about 20 min in some cells.[18] These unstable proteins have not been definitely related to growth control. A possible exception is the 53-K protein that is associated with SV40 transformation and is also found in certain other transformed and tumorigenic cell lines.[7, 8, 10] This protein has recently been shown to have a half-life of only about one-half an hour in 3T3 cells. It is also, very interestingly, stable in SV40-transformed 3T3 cells [7] and provides an example of the kind of protein we are seeking. The physical association of p53 with T antigen may be responsible for its greater stability, which results in a 50–100-fold increase in its intracellular concentration in SV40-transformed cells.[7]

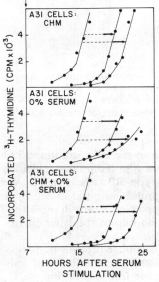

START CHM OR 0% SERUM PULSES

A31 CELLS: CHM

A31 CELLS: 0% SERUM

A31 CELLS: CHM + 0% SERUM

INCORPORATED ³H-THYMIDINE (CPM × 10³)

7   15   25
HOURS AFTER SERUM STIMULATION

FIGURE 3. Effects of complete serum deprivation and protein synthesis blocks on synchronized 3T3 cells. 3T3 (A31) cells were "growth-arrested" in low serum concentrations and stimulated as described in the legend to FIGURE 2. Seven hours later, [³H]-thymidine was added in medium which either contained CHM (1.5 μg/ml), lacked serum (0% serum), or both lacked serum and contained CHM (CHM + 0% serum). Control cultures received 10% serum and [³H]-thymidine. Three or five hours later, the cultures were washed and the medium replaced by 10% serum and [³H]-thymidine. DNA synthesis in the control cultures is shown by the left-most line of data points. Lines of data points to the right of the controls show the initiation of S after 3 or 5 hours of treatment with 0% serum, CHM, or both. The heavy arrow-headed lines show the delays in S which were in excess of the 0% serum or CHM pulses.

We have investigated the rate of turnover of p53 in BP3T3 cells to see if the relaxed growth control in this cell line is correlated with an increased stability of this protein.

Protein p53 was analyzed by immunoprecipitation with monoclonal antibody obtained from hybridoma PAb101 (clone 412).[19] Normal, untransformed Balb/c-3T3 cells (clone A31) and syngenic lines transformed by SV40 or BP were labeled with ^{35}S-labeled methionine. Labeled proteins were subsequently chased for 3 hr with media containing excess unlabeled methionine. Immunoprecipitates were prepared before and after the 3-hr chase period. The results of these experiments are shown in FIGURE 4. We have confirmed that p53 is labile in normal Balb/c-3T3 cells (A31) and stable in the SV40-transformed

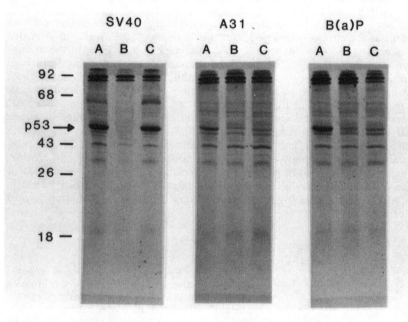

FIGURE 4. Immunoprecipitation of cell extracts with monoclonal antibody against p53. Pulse-chase analysis of the stability of p53 in untransformed Balb/c-3T3 cells (A31) and two Balb/c-3T3 lines transformed with benzo(a)pyrene [B(a)P] or SV40. Lane A, 3-hr pulse, immune media; lane B, 3-hr pulse, control media; Lane C, 3-hr chase, immune media.

line. However we find that p53 is not more stable in the BP-transformed 3T3 cells than in A31 cells. This result is not consistent with the protein inhibition kinetics, which show that the regulatory protein(s) in BP cells is stable. We therefore conclude that p53 is probably not the protein involved in cell cycle regulation at the restriction point. It may still be important in growth regulation, but most likely p53 does not control a rate-limiting step in the latter part of the C_1 phase.

We have been attempting to locate additional candidate proteins using two-dimensional gel electrophoresis to analyze the synthesis and stability of individual proteins in whole cell extracts and in cellular fractions during the G_1

period. These experiments have shown at least a dozen spots in normal cells that have the characteristics we are seeking. Therefore, a class of labile G_1-related proteins exists and we are in the process of studying them further.

EXCESS TRANSFORMATION PROTEINS AND LABILE REGULATORY PROTEINS

While surpluses of specific virus-related proteins are produced in some transformed cells, we nevertheless predict greater stability in other transformed cells of a labile protein whose existence is inferred from cell kinetics. At first glance there seems to be a discrepancy between these two sorts of results (for example, overproduction versus underdegradation). These differences are probably consequences of the various mechanisms by which transformation can be brought about. A protein can accumulate more rapidly in a transformed cell because it is synthesized faster, or because it is degraded more slowly. Either process can lead to excess protein in these cells.

Our prior results with serum starvation and CHM show that various modes of transformation have different effects upon low serum growth arrest in the G_1 phase.[5, 16] The SV40-transformed cells present an extreme; they could not be "growth-arrested" in G_1 under conditions that inhibit progress through G_1 of the normal and other transformed cells.[12, 16, 20]

That transformation can have several different mechanisms has been very elegantly illustrated by cell fusion experiments.[21] When quiescent normal cells were fused with normal G_1 cells, entry into S phase of the G_1 nuclei was inhibited. Similarly, when quiescent cells were fused with a variety of tumorigenic G_1 cells, the entry of these hybrids into S phase was inhibited. These results led to the strong inference that the quiescent cells produce a diffusible internal substance inhibitory to progress towards DNA synthesis. In contrast, fusion of quiescent cells with SV40-transformed cells or HeLa cells caused DNA synthesis to occur in both nuclei. Thus, evidently there are two general classes of transformed cells.

One possible interpretation of these experiments is that quiescent cells have an enzyme that inactivates the regulatory protein, thereby preventing entry into S phase of hybrids made with normal cells and some transformed cells. The SV-3T3 and HeLa cell lines could possess a positive factor which is sufficiently active or in excess to carry even the quiescent cell nuclei into S phase.

Slow, specific R protein degradation could be responsible for diminished growth control in some tumor cells. But the alternative mechanism of more rapid synthesis of a specific stimulatory protein is supported from data with virus-transformed cells. Some of these cells release growth stimulatory factors into the medium, the most extensively studied example being Moloney sarcoma-virus-transformed 3T3 cells which excrete a factor (TGF) that replaces or cooperates with epidermal growth factor.[22] These cells autostimulate their growth in the presence of only traces of serum, in which normal cells that do not produce TGF are incapable of growing. This is clearly an example of overproduction of a positive protein factor, in this case an extracellular one.

Other virus transformants produce intracellular proteins such as sarc. Mechanisms by which the nucleic acid introduced by a virus causes high production of a specific protein have been reviewed elsewhere.[4, 10] The general ideas are derived from microbial control mechanisms. Briefly, the viral gene could have its own highly active promoter. Or, as with leukemia viruses,[23] the genetic element introduced could itself be a highly active promoter which inserts at random, occasionally next to the gene whose product provides potential for growth. It is also possible that extra copies of a normal gene can through their protein production allow a degree of escape from growth control. The chromosome rearrangements often associated with tumorigenicity may create gene amplifications or placement of a critical gene next to a highly active promoter, thereby causing overproduction of this gene's product.

In this brief discussion we have pointed out some relationships between current active research in cell biology and molecular genetics. These studies, it seems to us, are coming together to point towards a possible biochemical model for growth regulation in normal cells and its defects in tumor cells, one that depends upon production of adequate amounts of a protein whose relative stability and rate of synthesis are major factors in determining whether a cell will or will not be neoplastic.

SUMMARY

Normal cells cannot initiate DNA synthesis under inadequate external conditions, yet after growth has started they complete their division cycle under these conditions. The sensitive biochemical event for a growing cell is proposed to be accumulation of a labile protein which in adequate amounts permits entry into S phase, after about 2 hr, and completion of the cycle. Instability of this protein (half-life about 2.5 hr) creates a dynamic state so that its accumulation depends on rates of both synthesis and degradation. Neoplastic cells may show poorly regulated growth either by synthesizing this protein more rapidly or degrading it less rapidly, under conditions that limit normal cells' growth. Known mechanisms of overproduction include: more copies of the protein's structural gene per cell, an adjacent high-activity promoter, or autoproduction of growth factors. Less rapid degradation could result from less protease activity or from stabilizing modifications of the protein. Thus, derangement in the control of a labile growth-regulatory protein acting by any one of these diverse mechanisms could lead to neoplasia.

ACKNOWLEDGMENTS

We thank Gail Morreo and Deborah Ehrenthal for assistance and Marjorie Rider for preparing the manuscript. We are very indebted to the Cell Distribution Center at The Salk Institute for hybridoma Pab101.

REFERENCES

1. HOCHHAUSER, S. J., G. S. STEIN & J. L. STEIN. 1981. Int. Rev. Cytol. 71: 95–243.
2. PARDEE, A. B. 1974. Proc. Natl. Acad. Sci. USA 71: 1286–1290.
3. SCHER, C. D., M. E. STONE & C. D. STILES. 1979. Nature 281: 390–392.
4. BISHOP, J. M. 1981. Cell 23: 5–6.
5. DUBROW, R., V. G. H. RIDDLE & A. B. PARDEE. 1979. Cancer Res. 39: 2718–2726.

6. RUBSAMEN, H., K. SALTENBERGER, R. R. FRIIS & E. EIGENBRODT. 1982. Proc. Natl. Acad. Sci. USA **79:** 228–232.
7. OREN, M., W. MALTZMAN & A. J. LEVINE. 1981. Mol. Cell Biol. **1:** 101–110.
8. DIPPOLD, W. G., G. JAY, A. B. DELEO, G. KHOURY & L. J. OLD. 1981. Proc. Natl. Acad. Sci. USA **78:** 1695–1699.
9. SAGER, R. 1979. Nature **282:** 447–448.
10. KLEIN, G. 1981. Nature **294:** 313–318.
11. ROSSOW, P. W., V. G. H. RIDDLE & A. B. PARDEE. 1979. Proc. Natl. Acad. Sci. USA **76:** 4446–4450.
12. CAMPISI, J., E. E. MEDRANO, G. MORREO & A. B. PARDEE. 1982. Proc. Natl. Acad. Sci. USA **79:** 436–440.
13. STILES, C. D., R. R. ISBERG, W. J. PLEDGER, H. N. ANTONIADES & C. D. SCHER. 1979. J. Cell. Physiol. **99:** 395–405.
14. YEN, A. & A. B. PARDEE. 1978. Exp. Cell Res. **114:** 389–394.
15. SCHNEIDERMAN, M. H., W. C. DEWEY & D. P. HIGHFIELD. 1971. Exp. Cell Res. **67:** 147–155.
16. MEDRANO, E. E. & A. B. PARDEE. 1980. Proc. Natl. Acad. Sci. USA **77:** 4123–4126.
17. MEDRANO, E. E., P. ARANYI & A. B. PARDEE. 1981. *In* Cellular Responses to Biological Modifiers. L. W. Moze, *et al.* Eds.: 49–59. Academic Press. New York, NY.
18. JANNE, J., H. POSO & A. RAINA. 1978. Biochem. Biophys. Acta **473:** 241–293.
19. GURNEY, E. G., R. O. HARRISON & J. FENNO. 1980. J. Virol. **34:** 752–763.
20. KAWASAKI, S., L. DIAMOND & R. BASERGA. 1981. Mol. Cell Biol. **1:** 1038–1047.
21. STEIN, G. H. & R. M. YANISHEVSKY. 1981. Proc. Natl. Acad. Sci. USA **78:** 3025–3029.
22. ROBERTS, A. B., M. A. ANSANO, L. C. LAMB, J. M. SMITH, C. A. FROLIK, H. MARQUARDT, G. J. TODARO & M. B. SPORN. Nature **295:** 417–419.
23. NEEL, B. G., W. S. HAYWARD, H. L. ROBINSON, J. FANG & S. M. ASTRIN. 1981. Cell **23:** 323–334.

GROWTH ACTIVATION OF RESTING CELLS: INDUCTION OF BALANCED AND IMBALANCED GROWTH *

Anders Zetterberg, Wilhelm Engström, and Olle Larsson

Department of Tumor Pathology
Karolinska Hospital
S–104 01 Stockholm 60, Sweden

INTRODUCTION

Nonproliferating, quiescent cells maintained *in vitro* can be stimulated to proliferate by exposure to a large number of various external mitogenic effectors. These effectors include serum,[1] purified growth factors such as epidermal growth factor (EGF),[2] fibroblast growth factor (FGF),[3] or platelet-derived growth factor (PDGF),[4] insulin,[5] somatomedins,[6] proteolytic enzymes in low concentration,[7, 8] calcium pyrophosphate,[9] ions,[10] glutamine,[11] and alkaline pH.[12] When quiescent cells are stimulated to resume proliferation by the addition of mitogenic effectors, a set of distinct metabolic events occurs. Among the earliest detectable events after exposure to stimuli are increased transphosphorylation reactions [13, 14] and increased activity of the enzyme acyl–CoA: lysolecithin–transferase.[14] These immediate events are followed by alterations in membrane permeability for monovalent cations,[15] divalent cations,[16-18] amino acids,[8, 19] sugars,[8, 19, 20] and nucleotides,[8, 19, 20] as well as an increased activity of membrane-bound ATPase[14] and formation of polysomes.[14] It is poorly understood to what extent these events are actually involved in the control of proliferation, and if and how they are interrelated with each other. Most reports concerning control of proliferation have focused on DNA synthesis and cell division, and only in a few studies has attention been drawn to cell size control mechanisms.[21-29]

We have recently found that cells are able to undergo DNA synthesis and cell division in the absence of a concomitant cellular enlargement, indicating that these two sets of processes can be dissociated from one another.[30] This discovery was made by utilizing a recently devised method by which quiescent cells can be irreversibly committed to undergo DNA synthesis and mitosis without growing in size, namely, by a brief exposure to a medium of alkaline pH.[30] However, growth in cell size can be induced by the addition of serum to the culture medium, and the extent to which cells grow in size is found to be dependent on the serum concentration.[31] These results imply that the alkaline treatment is sufficient for the activation of the processes leading to DNA synthesis and mitosis, whereas a macromolecular factor (or factors) in serum is required for growth in cell size. The present study aims to characterize the requirements for the progression towards DNA synthesis and mitosis as well as for growth in cell size.

Our interest has also been focused on developing alternative methods by

* This study was supported by grants from the Swedish National Cancer Society, the Stockholm Cancer Society, the Swedish Society for Medical Sciences, and the Research Funds of the Karolinska Institute.

0077–8923/82/0397–0130 $01.75/0 © 1982, NYAS

which cells can be irreversibly committed to DNA synthesis and mitosis after a brief ($<$ 1 hour) exposure to mitogenic effectors. Two such methods are presented in this paper, the first involving a short (½ hour) exposure to a relative glutamine excess and the second utilizing a short (½ hour) exposure to 10% serum. These two methods as well as the aforementioned short alkaline treatment have been used in this study to characterize the relationship between DNA replication, mitosis, and cellular enlargement after mitogenic stimulation.

PROGRESSION TOWARDS DNA REPLICATION AND MITOSIS

It was recently hypothesized that the addition of serum to quiescent cells initiates a sequence of events that is dependent on the continuous presence of serum.[32] If serum was removed any time during the first 8 hours after addition, the cells failed to respond to the mitogenic stimulation and reentered a state of quiescence. However, if serum was removed after the 8-hour interval, the cells underwent DNA synthesis and mitosis at an unreduced rate, that is, they were irreversibly committed to undergo mitosis. This phenomenon was further characterized by Antoniades, Pledger, and coworkers,[33] who suggested that the process of mitogenic stimulation can be separated into three distinct parts: competence formation, progression and irreversible commitment to DNA synthesis, and mitosis. The term *competence* refers to initial changes in quiescent cells enabling them to respond to critical growth signals. If the required signal(s) is (are) added to competent cells, it (they) must be present for a certain time interval during which the cells proceed towards S phase and mitosis (*progression*). At a certain moment that occurs during this progression the cells become *irreversibly committed* to DNA synthesis and the critical signal(s) can be withdrawn without inhibiting the cellular entrance into S phase. Furthermore, it was suggested that one fraction of serum (platelet-derived growth factor [PDGF]) is responsible for competence formation and another (platelet-poor plasma [PPP]) is responsible for progression and commitment to DNA synthesis and mitosis. The cells become competent after a 5-hour treatment with PDGF, whereas plasma had to be added thereafter for progression into S phase. If plasma was not added within a certain period (13 hours) after competence formation, the cells reentered the state of quiescence. After 12 hours of subsequent incubation in plasma, the cells had become irreversibly committed to DNA synthesis and all macromolecules could be withdrawn without inhibiting the progression towards *mitosis*.

Alkaline Stimulation

It was shown in a recent study [12] that quiescent cells can be irreversibly committed to undergo DNA synthesis and mitosis after only 5 minutes of treatment in alkaline medium (pH 9.5). After this alkaline treatment, the cells could progress towards DNA synthesis and mitosis in the absence of macromolecular factors (that is, they had become irreversibly committed). Kinetic analysis of the stimulatory effects of short alkaline treatment as compared with stimulation by 10% serum (control) revealed an important similarity between these two means of stimulation. The time course for entrance of the cells into the S phase from the state of quiescence was almost identical for both stimulatory situations, suggesting that both types of stimuli acivate an equally long chain of reactions preceding initiation of DNA synthesis.[12, 30] Although the alkaline treatment may be considered a highly unphysiological situation, the method offers one distinct advantage, namely, that both the process of commitment as well as the subsequent progression towards DNA synthesis and mitosis can be studied under chemically defined conditions in serum-free media. Therefore, we aimed to characterize the biochemical requirements as well as to identify specific biochemical events occurring during the alkaline treatment, that is, before the cells have become irreversibly committed to DNA synthesis and mitosis.

TABLE 1

STIMULATORY EFFECT OF A SHORT TREATMENT IN ALKALINE MEDIA OF DIFFERENT COMPOSITIONS

Alkaline Medium Content	Percentage of ^{3}H-Tdr-Labeled Cells
Control 1:	
Continuous exposure to 0.5% serum and DMEM at normal pH (7.3) without alkaline pretreatment	15
0.5% serum and complete DMEM	76
Complete DMEM	73
BSS	69
Calcium- and magnesium-deficient DMEM	72
Calcium-, magnesium-, and phosphate-deficient DMEM	20
0.9% NaCl	14
Control 2:	
Continuous exposure to 10% serum and DMEM at normal pH (7.3) without alkaline pretreatment	99

NOTE: Swiss 3T3 cells were grown in a humidified 6% CO_2–air mixture in Dulbecco's modified Eagle's medium (DMEM) supplemented with 10% serum. Quiescent cells were obtained by washing proliferating cells twice in Earle's balanced salt solution and then exposing them to DMEM supplemented with 0.1% serum for 48 hours. Such cells were exposed to alkalinized (pH 9.5) media with chemical compositions as stated above for 5 minutes. These media were then replaced by a complete DMEM at normal pH (7.3) supplemented with 0.5% serum, which was present for 24 hours. The proportion of cells that had initiated DNA synthesis was determined by autoradiography after continuous labeling during the 24-hour period with 0.5 μCi ^{3}H-thymidine/ml culture medium.

The requirements for low molecular weight compounds during the 5-minute alkaline treatment were studied. TABLE 1 summarizes these findings. If the alkaline medium, to which the cells were exposed during a 5-minute period, was based on 0.9% NaCl only, no stimulatory response was observed. If, however, calcium- and magnesium-deficient balanced salt solution (BSS) was used, there was a significant stimulatory response. This stimulatory response, however, could not be enhanced if calcium, magnesium, or other low molecular weight constituents of Dulbecco's modified Eagle's medium (DMEM) or 0.5% serum were present in the medium during the 5-minute alkaline treatment. It can be concluded, therefore, that calcium, magnesium, glucose, amino acids, vitamins, or serum are not required for the mitogenic activation that takes place during the short alkaline treatment.

The only compound that was found to be required during and immediately after the alkaline treatment was phosphate. If this ion was withdrawn during the 5-minute alkaline treatment, the cells totally failed to initiate DNA synthesis. Although calcium can be removed from the external medium without decreasing the stimulatory response, the possible involvement of calcium in the process of commitment cannot be excluded. Mitogenic stimulation by a short alkaline treatment induces a rapid and persistent change in the cells, which results in a rapid translocation of calcium from an exchangeable to a less exchangeable compartment, possibly located intracellularly.[34] A similar translocation was also observed after mitogenic stimulation of quiescent cells by the addition of 10% serum.[16, 34]

Since it was possible to irreversibly commit quiescent cells to undergo DNA synthesis and cell division by a 5-minute exposure to an alkaline medium only composed of NaCl and phosphate, we aimed to characterize the mechanisms underlying the stimulatory effects achieved by the alkaline pH. Our interest was thereby focused on the processes taking place during the short period of alkaline treatment. Two principally different explanations were hypothesized: The first hypothesis is that an enzymatic process is induced during the short alkaline treatment, for example, an activation of pH-dependent enzymes involved in growth control, either membrane-bound or intracellularly located. Such an enzyme activation could be the initial step in an enzymatic cascade reaction resulting in the irreversible commitment to DNA synthesis. The second is that the alkaline pH could induce a nonenzymatic process (for example, a persistent change in the structure or the composition of the cell membrane or the interior of the cell) responsible for the irreversible commitment. We observed that an alkaline treatment performed at 4° C stimulated quiescent cells to initiate DNA synthesis to the same extent as when performed at 37° C. This indicates that the process of irreversible commitment, taking place during the short period of alkaline treatment, is energy-independent.[35] This finding does not seem to be consistent with the first hypothesis that the stimulatory process taking place during the short exposure to alkaline pH is based on the activation of pH-dependent enzymes, since this process is likely to be energy-dependent. The second suggested alternative, that is, that the stimulatory process is based on a structural change in the cells, therefore seems more likely. Direct evidence in favor of this alternative was provided by the finding that exposure to alkaline pH leads to a detachment of proteins from the cell surface.[35] By exposing the cells to alkaline media with different pHs for various time periods, different stimulatory effects on DNA synthesis could be achieved. Under these different stimulatory conditions it was found that the percentage of cells that had initiated DNA synthesis was closely correlated to the quantity of protein released into the medium during the alkaline treatment.[35]

As previously stated, we have found that the short alkaline treatment by which the cells become irreversibly committed to DNA synthesis is only dependent on the presence of phosphate ions. Furthermore, it has been shown that the subsequent progression towards DNA synthesis can take place in the absence of macromolecular serum factors.[36] It thus became possible to study the requirements for progression in a chemically defined medium. Therefore we devoted ourselves to studying whether the progression depends on an increased influx of any of the low molecular weight constituents of the culture medium. This was studied by determining the effects on DNA synthesis in alkaline-treated cells subsequently incubated in media with altered low molecular weight composition.[36] It was found that if all 13 essential amino acids were withdrawn from the medium, the stimulatory response to an alkaline treatment was significantly inhibited. A similar inhibition was observed if only glutamine was depleted from the medium. However, the other 12 essential amino acids (except glutamine) could be excluded from the medium without inhibiting the stimulatory response to an alkaline treatment on the initiation of DNA synthesis.[36] Nor was the stimulatory effect by the alkaline treatment inhibited by the withdrawal of vitamins or energy sources (glucose and pyruvate) from the medium. It was even found that cells were almost as capable of responding to a short alkaline treatment when they were incubated in a medium consisting of only BSS and glutamine as they were when incubated in a complete DMEM.[36] These results imply that mitogenic signals involved in the progression are not mediated by an increased influx of energy sources, vitamins, or amino acids, except possibly glutamine, since these substances can be excluded from the medium without inhibiting the stimulatory response to the alkaline treatment.

It thereafter became of interest to analyze whether the removal of any of the ionic components in BSS inhibits the stimulatory response to an alkaline treatment. Two principally different results could be expected after the withdrawal of different ions from the medium. Either the cells could remain viable and specifically inhibited in a state of quiescence, or the withdrawal of ions could result in nonspecific toxic effects leading to cellular detachment and cell death. It was found that if calcium or phosphate ions were excluded from the medium after alkaline treatment, the cells failed to initiate DNA synthesis.[36] However, as judged by microscopic examination, the cells appeared to be viable. The ^{3}H-Tdr-labeling percentages were similar ($<15\%$) to those observed when cells were starved to quiescence in low serum concentration (0.1%). It was further shown that alkaline-treated cells detach and die in magnesium-depleted medium. However, if calcium and magnesium together were depleted from the medium, the cells remained quiescent but viable. This result points at an interplay between calcium and magnesium ions within the cell. A normal concentration of calcium ions is toxic to the cells when magnesium is depleted, whereas if both ions are depleted together, the cells remain viable. Since depletion of calcium or phosphate ions from the medium inhibited the mitogenic stimulation of quiescent cells without exerting any observable toxic effects, it is possible that these ions as well as magnesium ions are basically involved in the control of progression towards mitosis. Signals for progression could, for example, be mediated intracellularly via an increased influx of calcium or phosphate ions into the cell. The elimination of other ions in the balanced salt solution (Na^+, K^+, Cl^- or HCO^-_3) from the medium resulted in detachment and death of the alkaline-treated cells.[36] The withdrawal of these ions possibly caused unspecific toxic effects, but it cannot be excluded at this stage that they might be involved in the growth control system. Na^+ and K^+ ions are unlikely mediators of growth signals since the intracellular concentration of these ions can be varied five-fold without any observable inhibitory effects on DNA synthesis.[37] This variation is much larger than the change in the intracellular concentrations of monovalent cations that follows calcium or magnesium depletion or addition.

FIGURE 1 shows the proportion of cells that initiated DNA synthesis after a short alkaline treatment as a function of the serum concentration in the culture medium. An almost complete stimulatory response (>80% labeled cells) could be obtained if the serum concentration was 0.5% or higher. However, when the serum concentration was reduced below 0.5%, the stimulatory response in alkaline-treated cells decreased with decreasing serum concentration. If serum was omitted, the percentage of labeled cells was reduced to 40%, which is still a significantly higher labeling index than that for quiescent cells. In the whole interval from 0–1% serum, the alkaline treatment exerted a significant stimulatory effect on DNA synthesis. However, it appears as if a small amount of serum enhances the stimulatory effect of the alkaline treatment.

It then became of interest to elucidate whether this enhancement effect could also be obtained by the addition of some specific growth factor to the medium. TABLE 2 shows the proportion of alkaline-treated cells that has initiated DNA synthesis after 24 hours of incubation in DMEM supplemented with various growth factors. It was found that addition of albumin, EGF, or

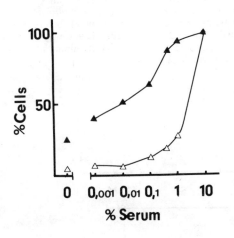

FIGURE 1. Stimulation of DNA synthesis by alkaline treatment in the presence of different serum concentrations in the culture medium. Swiss 3T3 cells, cultured and starved to quiescence as described in TABLE 1, were exposed to an alkaline (pH 9.5) medium for 5 minutes, which was thereafter replaced by a DMEM with different serum concentrations for 24 hours at normal pH (7.3) (▲—▲). Cells continuously exposed to DMEM at normal pH (7.3) with different serum concentration were used as controls (△—△). The proportion of cells synthesizing DNA was determined by autoradiography after continuous exposure during the 24-hour experimental period to 0.5 μCi ^{3}H-thymidine/ml culture medium.

transferrin does not significantly increase the stimulatory response to the alkaline treatment above that obtained in serum-free medium. In contrast addition of insulin in supraphysiological concentrations to alkaline-treated cells results in an almost complete (82% lebeled cells) stimulatory response.

In summary, it was found that alkaline-treated cells are dependent on the presence of glutamine, calcium, and phosphate for progression towards DNA synthesis and mitosis. If any one of these substances is removed, the cells fail to initiate DNA synthesis and return to quiescence. Furthermore, the stimulatory response could be significantly enhanced by adding 0.5% serum to the cells. In order to determine whether the cells require these compounds during any critical moment(s) of the progression, we analyzed the temporal requirements for glutamine, calcium, and phosphate and 0.5% serum. It was found that phosphate was required immediately after the alkaline treatment and could not be withdrawn from the medium until after 15 hours without inhibiting the response to the alkaline treatment (FIG. 2). In contrast, calcium and glutamine

TABLE 2

EFFECTS OF GROWTH FACTORS ON THE INITIATION OF DNA SYNTHESIS

Factors Added to DMEM	Percentage of ³H-Tdr-Labeled Cells	
	No Pretreatment	Short Alkaline Pretreatment
None	5	40
Fetal calf serum (0.5%)	16	95
Fetal calf serum (10%)	99	99
Albumin (1 mg/ml)	15	44
Epidermal growth factor (10 ng/r..)	33	48
Insulin (100 µg/ml)	15	82
Transferrin (10 µg/ml)	18	42
Epidermal growth factor +insulin+transferrin	60	89

NOTE: Swiss 3T3 cells were cultured and starved to quiescence as described in TABLE 1. These quiescent cells were exposed to DMEM supplemented with growth factors for 24 hours as described above. In half of the cultures (*right column*) the cells were exposed to a short alkaline treatment (pH 9.5, 5 minutes) before the growth factors were added. The proportion of cells synthesizing DNA was determined by autoradiography after continous exposure to 0.5 µCi ³H-thymidine per ml culture medium during the entire 24-hour experimental period.

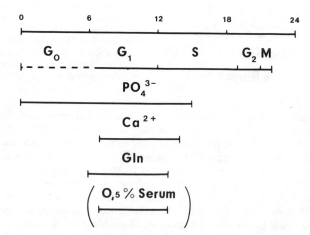

FIGURE 2. Temporal requirements for calcium, phosphate, glutamine, and serum after alkaline stimulation. Swiss 3T3 cells cultured and starved to quiescence, as described in TABLE 1, were exposed for 5 minutes in alkaline DMEM at time 0. These cells were subsequently exposed to DMEM which had been made deficient of one of the indicated constituents. The lacking component was then returned for a limited period of time. The effects on DNA synthesis were determined by autoradiography after continuous labeling with 0.5 µCi ³H-thymidine/ml medium.

were only required during a 6–7-hour interval between the 6th and 13th hours after alkaline stimulation. The small amount of serum (0.5%) that enhances the response to the alkaline treatment was only required between the 7th and 12th hours after onset of stimulation.

These results imply that the set of processes and events that follow after onset of stimulation are dependent on the presence of phosphate ions. This period includes the lag phase preceding the initiation of DNA synthesis as well as a part of the S phase. In contrast, calcium, glutamine and 0.5% serum are required during a discrete 6–7-hour interval which appears to coincide with the transition from G_1 to S phase. It may thus be concluded that these latter factors may be required for the initiation of DNA replication, but less necessary for the preceding events.

Stimulation by a Relative Glutamine Excess

It has been known for some time that an altered balance between the amino acids in the culture medium has a marked impact on cell proliferation.[38–40] We have shown in a previous study [11] that 3T3 cells are sensitive to alterations in the balance between glutamine and the other 12 essential amino acids in the culture medium. Sparse 3T3 cells starved to quiescence in low serum concentration (0.1%) could be stimulated to undergo DNA replication and mitosis by a continuous exposure to a serum-depleted (0.1%) medium containing a relative excess of glutamine.[11] This excess was achieved by keeping glutamine in normal concentration (4 mM) and reducing that of the other 12 amino acids 100- or 1000-fold. We report here that a brief exposure (½ hour) to a relative glutamine excess, as described earlier, followed by a 23.5-hour exposure to complete DMEM (that is, all amino acids including glutamine in normal concentration) is sufficient to irreversibly commit a substantial portion (53%) of the cells to DNA synthesis and mitosis in the absence of serum (TABLE 3). This figure is comparable to the previously reported effect [11] seen after a 24-hour exposure to a relative glutamine excess (51%). In both these two stimulatory situations, glutamine was the only essential amino acid for which this effect was observed.

Stimulation by a Short Exposure to Serum

Quiescent serum-starved cells can be stimulated by a continuous exposure to serum to initiate DNA replication in a semisynchronous fashion after a well-defined lag period.[32, 41] It was originally shown by Brooks [32] that serum has to be present for several (≥8) hours to irreversibly commit the cells to DNA replication and mitosis since otherwise the cells remain in a quiescent state. It is shown in FIGURE 3 that when quiescent cells are exposed to 10% serum for a shorter period than 8 hours (that is, 1–6 hours) and then subsequently exposed to a serum-depleted (0.1%) medium, the stimulatory effect on DNA synthesis decreases with decreasing exposure time. However, if the exposure to 10% serum is limited to a very short period (that is, ½ hour), a substantial portion of the cells (46%) are induced to initiate DNA synthesis and undergo mitosis (FIG. 3). This stimulatory effect of a ½-hour exposure to 10% serum could be significantly enhanced (80% labeled cells) if the cells were subsequently exposed to a serum-depleted (0.1%) medium supplemented with cholesterol. In contrast, no additional stimulatory effect of cholesterol could be achieved if the initial exposure to 10% serum was 2 hours or more.

Table 3

Effect of Different Mitogenic Stimuli on DNA Synthesis in Quiescent Cells

Mitogenic Stimulus	Percentage of ³H-Tdr-Labeled Cells
24-hour exposure to 0.1% serum in complete DMEM (control 1)	7
24-hour exposure to 10% serum in complete DMEM (control 2)	99
Short alkaline treatment (pH 9.5; 5 minutes) followed by 24-hour exposure to 0.1% serum in complete DMEM at pH 7.3	81
24-hour exposure to a relative glutamine excess *	54
Short exposure (0.5-hour) to a relative glutamine excess * followed by 23.5-hour exposure to 0% serum in complete DMEM	53
Short exposure (0.5-hour) to 10% serum followed by 23.5-hour exposure to 0.1% serum in complete DMEM	46
Short exposure (0.5-hour) to 10% serum followed by 23.5-hour exposure to 0.1% serum and 10 μg/ml cholesterol in complete DMEM	80

Note: Swiss 3T3-cells were grown in a humidified 6% CO_2–air mixture in Dulbecco's modified Eagle's medium (DMEM) supplemented with 10% serum. Quiescent cells were obtained by washing proliferating cells twice in Earle's balanced salt solution and then exposing them to DMEM supplemented with 0.1% serum for 48 hours. The quiescent cells were then exposed to different stimulatory media as described above. The proportion of cells synthesizing DNA was determined by autoradiography after continuous exposure to 0.5 μCi ³H-thymidine per ml culture medium during the whole 24-hour experimental period.

* The relative glutamine excess was achieved by keeping the glutamine concentration normal and reducing the concentration of the other 12 amino acids to 1/100 of that in DMEM.

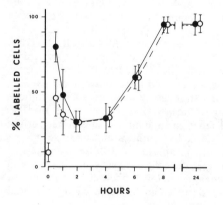

Figure 3. The effect of short exposure to 10% serum on initiation of DNA synthesis in quiescent cells. Swiss 3T3 cells cultured and starved to quiescence, as described in Table 1, were exposed to 10% serum. This medium was replaced up to 8 hours later by a serum-depleted DMEM (0.1% serum) (O—O). In one set of experiments the serum-depleted medium was supplemented with 100 ng cholesterol/ml medium (●—●). The proportion of cells synthesizing DNA was determined by autoradiography after continuous exposure for 24 hours to 0.5 μCi ³H-thymidine/ml medium.

CELLULAR ENLARGEMENT

Most reports concerning control of cellular proliferation have focused on DNA synthesis and cell division, and only in a limited number of studies has attention been drawn to cell size control mechanisms.[21-29] The role of cell size for control of proliferation was discussed by Prescott [21] in a classic study in which he showed that division in amoeba could be stopped for many days by periodic amputation of the cytoplasm. He concluded that the cells did not provide because they were never allowed to reach a critical size. It was later shown that cytoplasmic growth during G_1 is somehow involved in the control of initiation of DNA synthesis in mammalian cells.[22, 23] Cells entering the interphase with a relatively small mass synthesize more protein during the G_1 period and thus spend a longer time in G_1 than do cells entering the interphase with a larger mass.[24] Since the major quantity of the proteins synthesized in the cell during G_1 accumulated in the cytoplasm, it was suggested that DNA synthesis is not initiated until the cell nucleus is surrounded by a certain amount of cytoplasmic protein.[24, 25] Furthermore, direct evidence for a size control for initiation of DNA synthesis in *E. coli* was given by Donachie,[26] who showed that DNA synthesis is initiated at a fixed cell size which is independent of the growth rate. He therefore concluded that there is a "critical" size which controls entrance into S phase in *E. coli*. Initiation of DNA synthesis and mitosis thus appears to be dependent on cellular enlargement, indicating the existence of a cell size control mechanism.[25]

The present study has aimed to characterize the growth in cell size during the progression towards mitosis after mitogenic stimulation. For this purpose we utilized the three principally different methods by which cells can be irreversibly committed to undergo DNA replication and mitosis after a brief exposure (≤ 1 hour) to mitogenic effectors, namely, (*a*) a short alkaline treatment, (*b*) a short exposure to a relative glutamine excess, and (*c*) a short exposure to 10% serum in a fashion just described.

The effects of stimulation by continuous exposure to 10% serum (B) or by a short exposure to a medium of alkaline pH (C) are shown in FIGURE 4. In both stimulatory situations, the proportion of cells with S-phase and G_2-phase DNA values had increased after 12 hours. When continuous exposure to 10% serum was used as a mitogenic stimulus, the protein contents of the S- and G_2-phase cells were substantially increased (B). However, this concomitant increase in cellular protein content was not observed in the cells stimulated in low serum concentration by a short alkaline treatment (C). In the latter stimulatory situation, the protein contents of the S- and G_2-phase cells had not increased above that seen in quiescent cells (A). In order to investigate whether the inability of alkaline-treated cells to grow in size was either due to toxic effects, caused by the elevated pH per se, or to a consequence of the subsequent exposure to a serum-depleted medium, not containing sufficient amount of specific macromolecular factors required for cell size, alkaline-treated cells were subsequently incubated in high serum concentration (10% instead of 0.1%) (D). Such cells (D) grow in size to the same extent as control cells exposed only to 10% serum without an alkaline pretreatment (B). Thus, the capability to grow in size before mitosis was not affected by the alkaline treatment per se but was rather due to the lack of serum factors.

In order to study the extent to which growth in cell size is dependent on macromolecular factors in serum, alkaline-treated cells were exposed to different serum concentrations ranging from 0.1% to 10%. Mitotic cells were sampled from each of the experimental situations and the size of these cells was determined, as described in TABLE 4. Cells incubated in 0.1% serum did not grow in size at all. Cells grown in 0.5% serum increased in size by approximately 30% before mitosis, whereas a 100% increase in cell size, that is, a complete balanced growth, was achieved at 2% serum. These findings clearly indicate that the alkaline treatment mainly activates the cell cycle events responsible for the progression towards DNA synthesis and mitosis, whereas macromolecular factors in serum seem to be required for growth in cell size. These data were found by measuring the dry mass and protein content of individual mitotic post-telophase cells obtained by the procedure of mitotic selection.[31] This approach allows an accurate quantitation of the extent to which cells grow

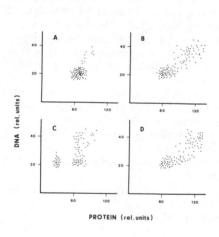

PROTEIN (rel. units)

FIGURE 4. The DNA and protein contents of individual 3T3 cells. These cells were cultivated and starved to quiescence as described in TABLE 1. The cells were then stimulated to proliferation by continuous exposure to 10% serum at pH 7.3 (**B**) or by a short treatment in medium of alkaline pH, as described in FIGURE 1. The alkaline-treated cells were subsequently exposed to 0.1% serum (**C**) or to 10% serum (**D**). Control cells were starved to quiescence in 0.1% serum for 48 hours (**A**). The cells—grown on glass slides in petri dishes—were fixed 24 hours after onset of stimulation in 10% neutral formalin and stained by means of a combined Feulgen–naphtol yellow S procedure as described elsewhere.[42] The cells were then analyzed in a rapid scanning and integrating microspectrophotometer equipped with a field-limiting device.[43] The total extinction at 435 nm was used as a measure of the total amount of cellular protein (naphtol yellow S bound in the cells) and the total extinction at 546 nm was used as a measure of the total amount of DNA (Feulgen-positive material) in the cells.

in size before mitosis. This approach is also of particular value when the proportion of nondividing cells is large and the small proportion of dividing cells can be enriched by mitotic selection. Therefore, this method could be used to study whether a dependency on serum for growth in cell size is only observed in alkaline-treated cells or whether it is a general property of 3T3 cells. Mitotic cells were enriched from unstimulated cultures maintained in different serum concentrations, that is, cultures in which only a limited number of cells undergo spontaneous cell division. Such cells, as shown in TABLE 4, are dependent on the serum concentration to the same extent as alkaline-treated cells for growth in cell size, indicating that the dependency on serum factors is a general characteristic of 3T3 cells rather than an artifact induced by the alkaline

TABLE 4

EFFECTS OF DIFFERENT MITOGENIC STIMULI ON CELLULAR PROTEIN CONTENT AND DRY MASS OF INDIVIDUAL MITOTIC POST-TELOPHASE CELLS

Medium	No Alkaline Treatment			Short Alkaline Pretreatment (pH 9.5 for 5 min)		
	Cellular Protein* Content (rel. units, mean ± 1 SD)	Dry Mass † (pg)	Percentage of ^{3}H-Tdr-Labeled Cells ‡	Cellular Protein* Content (rel. units, mean ± 1 SD)	Dry Mass † (pg)	Percentage of ^{3}H-Tdr-Labeled Cells ‡
10% calf serum and complete DMEM	180.8 ± 6.6	47 ± 8.9	99 ± 0.6	183.1 ± 7.1	47 ± 8.5	99 ± 0.7
2% calf serum and complete DMEM	175.4 ± 6.9	44 ± 3.6	72 ± 4.5	177.0 ± 10.0	45 ± 3.8	99 ± 0.7
0.5% calf serum and complete DMEM	115.5 ± 11.8	31 ± 5.2	20 ± 4.1	121.3 ± 9.2	33 ± 7.8	95 ± 2.1
0.1% calf serum and complete DMEM	94.9 ± 4.6	23 ± 3.7	16 ± 3.1	97.6 ± 5.5	24 ± 4.4	88 ± 4.6

NOTE: 3T3 cells were cultured, starved to quiescence and stimulated to undergo DNA synthesis and mitosis in 50-ml plastic bottles by using three methods, as described in FIGURE 1. The protein and dry mass measurements were performed on individual mitotic post-telophase cells obtained by a mitotic selection procedure as follows: 40 ml of the medium was discarded from the bottle, after which the bottle was shaken for 90 seconds in order to preferentially detach mitotic cells. The remaining 10-ml medium enriched with mitotic cells was poured into a plastic petri dish which contained a glass coverslip on the bottom. The cells were allowed to attach during 30 minutes and then the slides were fixed, either in ethanol or in 10% neutral buffered formalin. The post-telophase cells could easily be identified as 8-shaped cells by microscopic examination.

* Cellular protein content as measured by cytophotometric determination after naphtol yellow S staining at 435 nm of individual mitotic (post-telophase) cells after 24-hour incubation in media as described above.

† Dry mass as measured by microinterferometric determination of individual mitotic (post-telophase) cells after 24-hour incubation in media as described above. The cells were mounted in 4% aqueous formaldehyde for the interferometric measurements. Dry mass was determined in a rapid scanning and integrating microinterferometer.

‡ The percentage of ^{3}H-Tdr labeled cells after 24-hour incubation in media as described above. These media were supplemented with 0.5 μCi ^{3}H-thymidine/ml and the proportion of labeled cells was determined by autoradiography.

treatment. In order to investigate the macromolecular factor requirements for cellular enlargement, we exposed alkaline-treated cells to serum-free media supplemented with different growth factors, as shown in TABLE 5. We found that the addition of albumin, EGF, or transferrin exerted no stimulatory influence on the cellular enlargement. Alkaline-treated cells subsequently exposed to any of these three substances underwent imbalanced growth in the sense that they underwent DNA replication and mitosis without growing in size. However, addition of supraphysiological concentrations of insulin to alkaline-treated cells resulted in a complete balanced growth, that is, an approximate doubling in cell size before mitosis (TABLE 4, FIG. 5B). In contrast it was found that addition of insulin in physiological concentrations resulted in an imbalanced growth, that is, cells underwent DNA replication and mitosis without growing in size (not shown). It thereafter became of interest to test whether the dependency on supraphysiological concentrations of insulin for growth in size was unique for alkaline-treated cells or a general property of cells committed to DNA synthesis but maintained in low serum concentration. It is shown in FIGURE 5 that cells stimulated by a ½-hour exposure to relative glutamine excess (FIG. 5C) or to 10% serum (FIG. 5E) and subsequently exposed to a serum-free medium do not increase in size before mitosis, that is, undergo imbalanced growth. No difference in this respect was observed between cells briefly exposed to 10% serum and subsequently incubated in DMEM and in DMEM supplemented with cholesterol. However, if 100 μg insulin/ml is added after a short exposure to a relative glutamine excess (FIG. 5D) or to 10% serum (FIG. 5F), the cells undergo balanced growth in the sense that they approximately double in size before mitosis. Thus, there is an important similarity between these two mitogenic effectors and the short alkaline treatment in the sense that all three methods require a continuous exposure to high concentration of insulin for balanced growth.

TABLE 5

EFFECTS OF GROWTH FACTORS ON CELLULAR ENLARGEMENT AFTER MITOGENIC STIMULATION BY ALKALINE pH

Factors Added	Balanced Growth	Imbalanced Growth
Albumin (1 mg/ml)		X
Epidermal growth factor (10 ng/ml)		X
Insulin (10 ng/ml)		X
Insulin (100 μg/ml)	X	
Somatomedin C (100 ng/ml)	X	
Transferrin (10 μg/ml)		X

NOTE: Swiss 3T3 cells were cultured and starved to quiescence as described in TABLE 1. These cells were exposed to a short alkaline treatment (pH 9.5, 5 minutes) and then exposed for 24 hours to serum-free DMEM supplemented with growth factors, as listed above. The DNA and protein contents of 100 individual cells in each experimental situation were determined as described in FIGURE 3 in order to decide whether a balanced growth (an approximate two-fold increase in cellular protein content before mitosis) or an imbalanced growth (no [or little] increase in cellular protein content before mitosis) was achieved.

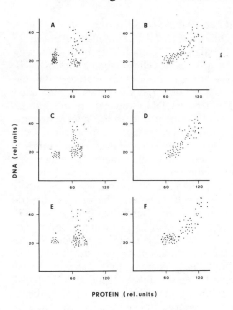

FIGURE 5. The effect of insulin on DNA synthesis and cellular protein content 24 hours after onset of stimulation. Swiss 3T3 cells, cultured and starved to quiescence, as described in TABLE 1, were exposed for 5 minutes to alkaline medium (pH 9.5) **(A, B)** for 30 minutes to a relative glutamine excess **(C, D)** or for 30 minutes to 10% serum **(E, F)**. These cells were subsequently exposed to serum-free DMEM supplemented with 100 μg insulin/ml medium **(A, C, E)** or nothing at all **(B, D, F)** for 24 hours. The cells were fixed and stained and the cellular contents of DNA and total protein were determined.

Since a balanced growth, which is normally obtained only if the serum concentration is above 2%, can be achieved in serum-free medium only if supraphysiological concentrations of insulin are added, it is not likely that insulin per se is responsible for the increase in cell size. Rather, the results suggest that some other macromolecular factor, with a mode of action related to that of insulin, is required for the cellular enlargement after alkaline stimulation. It therefore became of interest to test whether the addition of somatomedin C, which has been suggested to mediate most of the insulin effects,[6] had any effect on the growth in cell size. It was found that addition of somatomedin C in physiological concentrations to alkaline-treated cells resulted in an approximate doubling in cell size, that is, in a balanced growth (TABLE 5).

CONCLUSIONS

Quiescent serum-starved 3T3 cells normally require addition of 5–10% serum to resume proliferation. Little is known about how serum factors generate growth regulatory signals and how these are mediated within the cell. Three alternative means of mitogenic stimulation are presented in this paper. Quiescent 3T3 cells can be irreversibly committed to undergo DNA replication and mitosis in a virtually serum-free medium after an initial exposure of short duration ($\leq$½ hour) to (*a*) a medium of alkaline pH, (*b*) a relative glutamine excess, or (*c*) 10% serum (with or without a subsequent exposure to cholesterol). A kinetic analysis of these stimulatory methods, as compared to stimulation by a continuous exposure to 10% serum, revealed an important similarity between all four means of stimulation; the time period required for entrance of the cells into the S phase from the state of quiescence was almost identical (12 hours) for all four stimulatory situations. This suggests that all these stimuli activate an equally long chain of reactions preceding initiation of DNA synthesis.

A great difference in the coordinate cellular response to the different types of mitogenic stimuli was observed. Quiescent cells continuously exposed to 10% serum underwent a completely "balanced" growth response, including DNA replication and mitosis as well as growth in cell size before mitosis. In contrast, cells stimulated by a short exposure ($\leq \frac{1}{2}$ hour) to a relative glutamine excess, medium of alkaline pH, or to 10% serum, and subsequently incubated for 23.5 hours in serum-free medium, underwent DNA replication and mitosis in the absence of concomitant cellular enlargement and thus underwent "imbalanced" growth. Thus, these three stimulatory means (a, b, and c) seem sufficient for the activation of processes leading to DNA synthesis and mitosis, whereas the continuous presence of a macromolecular factor or factors is required for growth in cell size. Other studies have shown that growth in cell size can be dissociated from progression through the cell cycle towards mitosis under certain experimental conditions. In such situations the cell cycle progression can be blocked in early S phase by chemical inhibitors [44] or in late G_2 by X-radiation.[45] However, synthesis and accumulation of protein continue in both of these two situations. Thus, imbalanced growth can be induced in the sense that DNA synthesis and mitosis are inhibited, but an increase in cell size is allowed to continue. The present study clearly demonstrates that imbalanced growth can also be induced in the reverse sense. DNA replication and cell division can be selectively stimulated in the absence of cellular enlargement. This result is in line with a recent finding by Baserga and coworkers, who showed that by using small oncogenic DNA viruses and manual microinjection of viral DNA fragments it was possible to dissociate DNA synthesis from synthesis of ribosomal RNA in AF8-cells.[46]

The three stimulatory methods (a, b, and c) were then used for studies of the specific requirements for DNA synthesis and mitosis as well as of those for cellular enlargement. In order to determine the requirements for DNA synthesis and mitosis, quiescent serum-starved cells were briefly exposed to media of alkaline pH and subsequently exposed to media with altered chemical composition. It was found that each of the low molecular weight constituents of the DMEM could be excluded without influencing the stimulatory response to the alkaline treatment, with the exception of glutamine and calcium and phosphate ions.

The temporal requirements for these compounds were then studied from the onset of stimulation to the subsequent mitosis. Phosphate ions were found to be required during the alkaline treatment as well as during a period of at least 15 hours after the alkaline treatment. Phosphate ions could not be withdrawn until a few hours prior to mitosis without inhibiting the response to the alkaline treatment. The phosphate-dependent period thus includes the lag phase preceding the initiation of DNA replication as well as a part of the S phase. This result implies that the set of processes that follow after onset of stimulation is dependent on the presence of phosphate ions. In contrast, calcium and glutamine were only required during a 6–7-hour interval between the 6th and 13th hours after the alkaline treatment. It has previously been shown that addition of a small amount of serum (0.5%) enhances the stimulatory response to the alkaline treatment. However, this effect of serum was also limited to a 6–7-hour interval between the 6th and 13th hours after the alkaline treatment. This period coincides with the late parts of G and the early parts of the S phase. It may thus be concluded that these latter factors (that is, calcium, glutamine, and 0.5% serum) are not required during the first part of the lag period after onset of stimulation.

The three recently devised methods (*a*, *b*, and *c*) by which DNA synthesis and mitosis can be selectively stimulated were then utilized to study the specific macromolecular requirements for cellular enlargement. Cells that had been committed to growth by the methods (*a*, *b*, and *c*) were subsequently exposed to growth factors in various concentrations—either one by one or in combination. These experiments revealed an important similarity between these three means of mitogenic stimulation; cellular enlargement could be induced in all three stimulatory situations if the cells were subsequently incubated in supraphysiological concentrations of insulin. A similar effect could be achieved if mitogenically stimulated cells were exposed to physiological concentrations of somatomedin C. This latter result is consistent with the notion that several of the biological effects of insulin are mediated by somatomedin.[6] It might therefore be suggested that the extent to which cells grow in size before mitosis depends on the amount of insulin-like micromolecules in the culture medium, either supplied separately or supplied to the medium by its serum content.

SUMMARY

Little is known about how mitogenic factors generate growth regulatory signals and how these are mediated within the cell. We have developed three different types of mitogenic stimuli in order to identify the possible existence of common denominators in a complex and perhaps pleiotypic signal–response system. 3T3 cells, starved to quiescence by reducing the serum content of the culture medium 100-fold, can be irreversibly committed to undergo DNA replication and mitosis in a serum-free medium after an initial exposure of short duration to (*a*) serum factors and cholesterol, (*b*) a relative excess of glutamine, or (*c*) alkaline pH. Cells stimulated by any of these procedures, and subsequently incubated in serum-free Dulbecco's modified Eagle's medium (DMEM) undergo DNA replication and mitosis in the absence of concomitant cellular enlargement (imbalanced growth). However, cellular enlargement is induced after the initial mitogenic stimuli (*a*, *b*, and *c*, as described previously) if the cells are subsequently incubated in DMEM containing $\geq 0.5\%$ serum, supraphysiological concentrations of insulin, or normal concentrations of somatomedin C.

REFERENCES

1. HOLLEY, R. W. 1974. Serum factors and growth control. *In* Control of Cell Proliferation in Animal Cells. B. Clarkson and B. Baserga, Eds.: 13–18. Cold Spring Harbor Laboratory. Cold Spring Harbor, NY.
2. COHEN, S. & J. M. TAYLOR. 1974. Epidermal growth factor: Chemical and biological characterization. Recent Prog. Horm. Res. **30:** 533–550.
3. GOSPODAROWICZ, D. 1975. Purification of a fibroblast growth factor from bovine pituitary. J. Biol. Chem. **250:** 2515–2520.
4. ROSS, R., J. GLOMSET, B. KARIYA & L. HARKER. 1974. A platelet-dependent serum factor that stimulates the proliferation of arterial smooth muscle cells in vitro. Proc. Natl. Acad. Sci. USA **71:** 1207–1210.
5. VAHERI, A., E. RUOSLAHTI & T. HOVI. 1974. Cell surface and growth control of chick embryo fibroblasts in culture. *In* Control of Cell proliferation in Animal Cells. B. Clarkson and R. Baserga, Eds.: 305–311. Cold Spring Harbor Laboratory. Cold Spring Harbor, NY.
6. VAN WYK, J. J., L. E. UNDERWOOD, R. L. HINTZ, D. R. GLEMMONS, S. VOINA

      & R. P. WEABER. 1974. The somatomedins. A family of insulin-like hormones under growth hormone control. Recent Prog. Horm. Res. **30:** 259–318.

7. BURGER, M. M. 1970. Proteolytic enzymes initiate cell division and escape from contact inhibition of growth. Nature **227:** 170–171.

8. SEFTON, B. M. & H. RUBIN. 1970. Release from density dependent growth inhibition by proteolytic enzymes. Nature **227:** 843–845.

9. RUBIN, H. & H. SANUI. 1977. Complexes of inorganic pyrophosphate, orthophosphate and calcium as stimulants of 3T3 cell multiplication. Proc. Natl. Acad. Sci. USA **74:** 5026–5030.

10. RUBIN, H. 1973. pH, serum and zinc in the regulation of DNA synthesis in cultured chick embryo cells. J. Cell Physiol. **82:** 231–238.

11. ZETTERBERG, A. & W. ENGSTRÖM. 1981. Glutamine and the regulation of DNA replication and cell multiplication in fibroblasts. J. Cell Physiol. **108:** 365–373.

12. ZETTERBERG, A. & W. ENGSTRÖM. 1981. Mitogenic effect of alkaline pH on quiescent serum-starved cells. Proc. Natl. Acad. Sci. USA **78:** 4334–4338.

13. RESCH, K. & E. PERBEN. 1975. The role of phospholipid in lymphocyte activation. Ninth Leukocyte Culture Conference: Immunorecognition.: 281–300. Academic Press. New York, NY.

14. BASERGA, R. 1976. Division and Multiplication of Mammalian Cells. Marcel Dekker. New York, NY.

15. ROZENGURT, E. & L. HEPPEL. 1975. Serum rapidly stimulates ouabain-sensitive ^{86}Rb$^+$ influx in quiescent 3T3 cells. Proc. Natl. Acad. Sci. USA **72:** 4492–4495.

16. TUPPER, J. & F. ZORGNIOTTI. 1977. Calcium content and distribution as a function of growth and transformation in the 3T3 cell. J. Cell Biol. **75:** 12–22.

17. WHITNEY, R. B. & R. M. SUTHERLAND. 1972. Enhanced uptake of Ca^{++} by transformed lymphocytes. Cell. Immunol. **5:** 137–147.

18. PETERS, J. H. & P. HANSEN. 1971. Effect of PHA on lymphocyte membrane transport. Eur. J. Biochem. **19:** 502–511.

19. CUNNINGHAM, D. D. & A. B. PARDEE. 1969. Transport changes rapidly initiated by serum addition to "contact inhibited" 3T3 cells. Proc. Natl. Acad. Sci. USA **69:** 1049–1056.

20. HERSHKO, A., P. MAMONT, R. SHIELDS & G. TOMKINS. 1971. Pleiotypic response. Nature New Biol. **232:** 205–211.

21. PRESCOTT, D. M. 1956. Changes in nuclear volume and growth rate and prevention of cell division in amoeba proteus resulting from cytoplasmic amputations. Exp. Cell Res. **11:** 94–98.

22. KILLANDER, D. & A. ZETTERBERG. 1965. Quantitative cytochemical studies of interphase growth. I. Determination of DNA, RNA and mass content of age-determined mouse fibroblasts in vitro and of intercellular variation in generation time. Exp. Cell Res. **38:** 272–284.

23. ZETTERBERG, A. 1966. Nuclear and Cytoplasmic Growth during Interphase. Almqvist & Wiksell. Uppsala, Sweden.

24. KILLANDER, D. & A. ZETTERBERG. 1965. A quantitative cytochemical investigation of the relationship between cell mass and initiation of DNA synthesis in mouse fibroblasts in vitro. Exp. Cell Res. **40:** 12–20.

25. ZETTERBERG, A. 1970. Nuclear and cytoplasmic growth during interphase in mammalian cells. *In* Advances in Cell Biology. D. Prescott *et al.*, Eds. Vol. **1:** 211–232, Appleton-Century-Crofts. New York, NY.

26. DONACHIE, W. D. 1968. Relationship between cell size and time of initiation of DNA replication. Nature **219:** 1077–1079.

27. BREWER, E. N. & H. P. RUSCH. 1968. Effect of elevated temperature shocks

on mitosis and on the initiation of DNA replication in Physarum polycephalum. Exp. Cell Res. **49:** 79–86.

28. MITCHISON, J. M. 1971. The Biology of the Cell Cycle. Cambridge University Press.

29. ZEUTHEN, E. & L. RASMUSSEN. 1972. Synchronized cell division in protozoa. *In* Research in Protozoology. T. T. Chen, Ed. Vol. 4: 11–145. Pergamon Press. Oxford.

30. ZETTERBERG, A. & W. ENGSTRÖM. 1981. Effects of alkaline pH and glutamine on cell growth and cell multiplication. *In* The Biology of Normal Human Growth. M. Ritzén *et al.* Ed.: 47–57. Raven Press. New York, NY.

31. ZETTERBERG, A. & W. ENGSTRÖM. 1982. Initiation of DNA synthesis and mitosis in the absence of cellular enlargement. Exp. Cell Res. In press.

32. BROOKS, R. F. 1976. Regulation of the fibroblast cell cycle by serum. Nature **260:** 248–250.

33. PLEDGER, W. J., C. D. STILES, H. N. ANTONIADES & C. D. SCHER. 1978. An ordered sequence of events is required before BALB/c 3T3 cells become committed to DNA synthesis. Proc. Natl. Acad. Sci. USA, **75:** 2839–2843.

34. ENGSTRÖM, W. & U. ROSENQVIST. 1981. Effects of mitogenic stimulation in the exchangeable pool of calcium in 3T3 cells. Cell Biol. Intern. Rep. **5:** 501–508.

35. ENGSTRÖM, W. & A. ZETTERBERG. 1981. Membrane protein detachment and mitogenic stimulation induced by alkaline pH. Cell Biol. Int. Rep. **5:** 517–523.

36. ENGSTRÖM, W. 1981. Requirements for commitment and competence to initiate DNA synthesis after growth stimulation in low serum concentration. Exp. Cell Res. **133:** 115–125.

37. RUBIN, H. & H. SANUI. 1979. The coordinate response of cells to hormones and its mediation by the intracellular availability of magnesium. *In* Hormones and Cell Culture, G. Sato and R. Ross, Eds.: 741–750. Cold Spring Harbor Laboratory. Cold Spring Harbor, NY.

38. EAGLE, H. 1955. The specific amino acid requirements of a mammalian cell in the tissue culture. J. Biol. Chem. **214:** 839–853.

39. EAGLE, H. 1955. Nutrition needs of mammalian cells in the tissue culture. Sci. New York **122:** 501–504.

40. HAM, R. 1974. Nutritional requirements of primary cultures. A neglected problem of modern biology. In Vitro **10:** 119–129.

41. BROOKS, R., D. C. BENNETT & J. A. SMITH. 1980. Mammalian cells need two random transitions. Cell **19:** 493–504.

42. GAUB, J., G. AUER & A. ZETTERBERG. 1975. Quantitative cytochemical aspects of a combined Feulgen-naphtol yellow-S staining procedure for the simultaneous determination of nuclear and cytoplasmic proteins and DNA in mammalian cell. Exp. Cell Res. **92:** 323–332.

43. CASPERSSON, T. & G. LOMAKKA. 1970. Introduction to quantitative cytochemistry. G. Bahr and G. Wied, Eds. Vol. 2. Academic Press. New York, NY.

44. AUER, G., A. ZETTERBERG & G. E. FOLEY. 1970. The relationship of DNA synthesis to protein accumulation in the cell nucleus. J. Cell Phys. **76:** 357–363.

45. KILLANDER, D., C. RIBBING, N. R. RINGERTZ & B. M. RICHARDS. 1962. The effect of X-radiation on nuclear synthesis of protein and DNA. Exp. Cell Res. **27:** 63–69.

46. PACHRON, S., M. ROSSIINI, Z. DARZYNKIEWICZ, F. TRAGANOS & R. BASERGA. 1980. Failure of accumulation of cellular RNA in hamster cells stimulated to synthesize DNA by infection with adenovirus 2. J. Biol. Chem. **255:** 4411–4413.

ORGANIZATION AND CELL CYCLE REGULATION OF HUMAN HISTONE GENES *

G. S. Stein, J. L. Stein,† L. Baumbach, A. Leza,†
A. Lichtler, F. Marashi, M. Plumb, R. Rickles,
F. Sierra, and T. Van Dyke

*Department of Biochemistry and Molecular Biology, and
† Department of Immunology and Medical Microbiology
University of Florida
Gainesville, Florida 32610*

Histone genes represent a moderately repeated set of genes in human cells. To study the organization and regulation of human histone genes, we have characterized a series of recombinant lambda Charon 4A phage containing genomic human histone sequences (designated λHHG). Our analyses indicate that human histone genes are clustered, but are not organized in a simple tandem repeat pattern, as is observed for several lower eukaryotes. For example, several of the human genomic fragments we have isolated contain two each of segments coding for H3 and H4 histones. Of particular interest with respect to organization and expression of the human histone genes is the presence of at least seven different H4 histone mRNAs associated with polysomes of S-phase HeLa cells. At least three of the HeLa H4 histone mRNAs are products of distinct genes and two H4 histone genes in the same genomic fragment code for different H4 mRNAs.

We have used our cloned human histone genes to examine the regulation of histone gene expression in human cells. Although it is generally agreed that histone protein synthesis in HeLa cells is restricted to the S-phase of the cell cycle, and therefore parallels DNA replication, both transcriptional and post-transcriptional levels of control have been postulated. By probing electrophoretically fractionated, filter-immobilized RNAs with several cloned genomic human histone sequences representing different histone gene clusters, we have assessed the steady-state levels of histone RNAs in the nucleus and cytoplasm of G_1- and S-phase HeLa S3 cells. The representation of histone mRNA sequences in G_1 compared with S-phase cells was less than 1% in the cytoplasm and approximately 1% in the nucleus. These data are consistent with control occurring primarily at the transcriptional level, but we cannot dismiss the possibility that regulation of histone gene expression is to some extent, and/or under some biological circumstances, mediated post-transcriptionally. If histone gene transcription does occurs in G_1, the RNAs must either be rapidly degraded or be transcribed to a limited extent compared with those of the S phase.

An unexpected result was obtained when a northern gel blot of cytoplasmic RNA from G_1- and S-phase cells was hybridized with λHHG41 DNA (containing H3 and H4 genomic human histone sequences). This clone hybridizes with histone mRNAs present in S-phase cytoplasmic RNA, but also hybridizes with a G_1 cytoplasmic RNA approximately 330 nucleotides in length. This RNA,

* This work was supported by Grant PCM 80–18075 from the National Science Foundation and by Basil O'Connor Starter Research Grant 5–217 from the March of Dimes Birth Defects Foundation.

0077–8923/82/0397–0148 $01.75/0 © 1982, NYAS

present in the cytoplasm of HeLa cells predominantly in the G_1 phase of the cell cycle, is not similar in size or sequence homology to known histone RNAs.

The possibility of prokaryote-like organization and regulation of human histone genes is discussed.

INTRODUCTION

In this paper we will summarize the progress made in our laboratory during the past several years toward understanding the structure, organization, and regulation of human histone genes. By way of introduction, we would like to share our two-fold rationale for pursuing this problem: First, we believe that understanding the molecular mechanisms by which specific genetic sequences are differentially expressed during the cell cycle can provide insight into regulation of the complex and highly interdependent biochemical events required for execution of the proliferative process. Second, and at least equally important, is study of the pivotal role of histone proteins in DNA packaging and their involvement with DNA replication and RNA transcription. So it has been essentially within the context of these reasons that in our laboratory we have been directing our efforts towards examining the human histone genes and their control. This article will focus on two points: (1) The structure and organization of human histone genes will be discussed, primarily because of the functional interrelationship among structure, organization, and regulation, and also because of the utilization of specific regions of genomic histone sequences as probes for analysis of human histone gene organization and regulation of expression. (2) Approaches to assessing levels of control of histone gene expression will be considered, and, here, variations in levels of control under different biological circumstances and the possibility of prokaryotic type of organization and regulation of human histone genes will be evaluated.

STRUCTURE AND ORGANIZATION OF HUMAN HISTONE GENES

We have isolated a series of fifteen genomic clones containing human histone coding sequences, their flanking sequences and noncoding sequences from a λ Charon 4A human gene library constructed by Maniatis and collaborators.[1] These clones were analyzed by hybridization with heterologous probes as well as by hybrid selection–translation (FIG. 1A), nucleotide sequencing (FIG. 1B), and restriction enzyme mapping.[39] While the moderately repeated human histone genes are clustered, they are not arranged in the form of a tandem repeat such as has been observed in sea urchin and *Drosophila*. Rather, human histone genes exhibit at least three types of arrangements with respect to restriction sites and the order of coding sequences; each of these arrangements is clearly distinguishable from the others. The organization of human histone genes is further complicated by the association of Alu family DNA sequences with some but not all of the histone coding regions.[40] Additionally, sequences coding for nonhistone RNA species, some of which are expressed throughout the cell cycle and others of which are expressed during specific periods of the cell cycle, are interspersed among the human histone genes. *In situ* hybridization studies [2, 3] and restriction analysis data from human–rodent hybrids [4] suggest that in humans the histone genes may be clustered on the distal end of the long

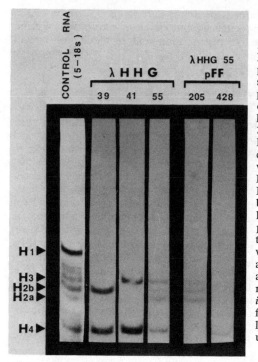

FIGURE 1A. Hybrid selection–
in vitro translation analysis of
DNAs from λHHG recombinant
phage containing human histone
sequences and of recombinant
pBR322 plasmids containing specific regions of the genomic human
histone sequences subcloned from
λHHG phage. Phage or plasmid
DNA was immobilized on nitrocellulose filters and hybridized
with HeLa S-phase polysomal
RNA containing H2A, H2B, H3,
H4 and H1 histone mRNAs. Hybridized RNAs were eluted, translated in a wheat germ cell-free
protein-synthesizing system, and
the in vitro-translated polypeptides
were fractionated electrophoretically in acetic acid–urea polyacrylamide gels. Analysis was by autoradiography. The left lane shows
in vitro translation products (all
five histone polypeptides) translated from the RNA preparation
used for hybrid selection.

arm of chromosome 7 in the G-negative band q34. Partial restriction maps of
each of the three types of arrangements of histone genes, representing information from seven individual genomic clones, are shown in FIGURES 1C and 1D.

Of particular interest with respect to the structure, organization, and expression of human histone genes is an observation we made several years ago of
multiple forms of human H4 and H3 histone mRNAs.[5-7] In our initial studies
we demonstrated that two different mRNA species coding for H4 histones can
be isolated from polysomes of S-phase HeLa cells. The two variants were
separated by polyacrylamide gel electrophoresis of 5–18S polysomal RNA
extracted from synchronized cells. Upon elution from the gel both species were
assayed for template activity in vitro using the wheat germ cell-free protein-
synthesizing system. Both RNAs were translated into H4 histone. Using several

Chicken		GCG	CGT	ACG	AAG	CAG	ACG	GCG	CGT	AAG	TCG	ACG	GGC	GGG	AAG	GCG	CCC	CGC	AAG	CAG	CTG	GCC	ACC	AAG		
Chicken(2.6)	ATG	GCG	CGT	ACG	AAG	CAG	ACG	GCG	CGT	AAG	TCG	ACG	GGT	GGG	AAG	GCG	CCA	CGT	AAG	CAG	CTG	GCC	ACT	AAG		
Sea Urchin		GCA	CGC	ACC	AAG	CAG	ACC	GCT	CGC	AAA	TCT	ACA	GGA	GGG	AAG	GCT	CCC	CGC	AAG	CAG	CTG	GCA	ACC	AAA	GCT	GCC
Mouse	ATG	GCT	CAT	ACA	AAG	CAG	ACT	GCC	CGC	AAA	TCC	ACC	TGT	GGT	AAA	GCA	CCT	AGG	AAA	CAA	CTA	GCT	ACA	AAA	GCT	GCT
Human	ATG	GCT	CGT	ACT	AAA	CAG	ACA	GCT	CGG	AAA	TCC	ACC	GGC	GGT	AAA	GCG	CCA	CGC	AAG	CAG	CTG	GCT	ACC	AAG	GCT	GCC
		ala	arg	thr	lys	gln	thr	ala	arg	lys	ser	thr	gly	gly	lys	ala	pro	arg	lys	gln	leu	ala	thr	lys	ala	ala

FIGURE 1B. Partial nucleotide sequence analysis of the human H3 histone gene in
the 3.1-Kb EcoRI fragment of λHHG17. Shown for comparison are the nucleotide
sequences of several other H3 genes. The asterisk (*) indicates a codon that would
result in an amino acid substitution.

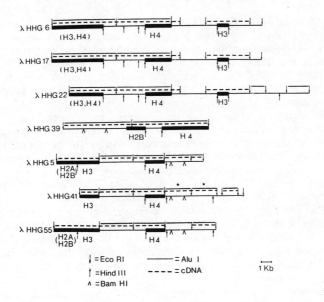

FIGURE 1C. Partial restriction maps of seven recombinant λ phages containing genomic human histone sequences. Also designated are regions of the phage that contain Alu family DNA sequences and nonhistone coding regions that hybridized with cDNA complementary to S-phase polysomal RNAs.

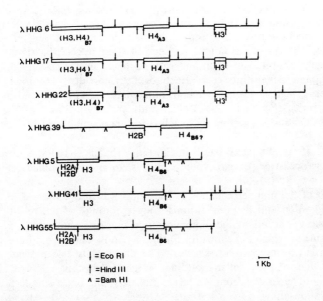

FIGURE 1D. Partial restriction maps of the λHHG phage in which the variant H4 histone mRNA coding sequences are designated.

types of denaturing gels (98% formamide–acrylamide, glyoxal–acrylamide and methyl mercury–agarose), the two H4 mRNAs were found to retain their distinct mobilities, indicating that the two are different in molecular weight. Characterization of the 3' terminus of each H4 mRNA by oligo dT-cellulose chromatography revealed no significant polyA region in either molecule. After treatment of the RNAs with T1, T2 and pancreatic nucleases followed by electrophoresis on DEAE paper, it was shown that both species had a capped 5' terminus.[8] Sequence organization was analyzed by digesting the two RNA species with T1 ribonuclease and subsequently performing two-dimensional fractionation of the resulting oligonucleotides. Although the majority of the oligonucleotides from the two H4 mRNAs migrated similarly, a few variations were noted, suggesting some sequence heterogeneity. This is similar to Grunstein's findings for the C1 and C3 fractions of H4 histone mRNA from sea urchin.[9] Electrophoresis of the *in vitro* translation products of the H4 histone mRNAs in an acetic acid urea system could not separate the independently synthesized products, which comigrate with marker H4. One-dimensional tryptic peptide mapping of the translation products labeled with several different radioactive amino acids revealed no differences between the molecules. Two-dimensional tryptic peptide mapping has also been carried out, and again no differences were detected.[5–7]

More recently, using higher-resolution fractionation procedures, we have observed at least seven different H4 histone mRNA species associated with polysomes of S-phase HeLa S3 cells.[41]

● Electrophoretic fractionation under denaturing conditions of *in vivo*-synthesized, ^{32}P-labeled S-phase HeLa cell histone mRNAs revealed three major H4 histone mRNAs (FIG. 2).

● Subsequent fractionation of the three H4 histone mRNA species under nondenaturing conditions, where advantage was taken of possible variations in secondary structure, resulted in separation of each band into several additional H4 histone mRNA species (FIG. 3). Each of these mRNA bands was excised from the gel, denatured in urea, and refractionated electrophoretically in nondenaturing and denaturing gels. Each of the individual H4 mRNA bands migrated as a single species under both nondenaturing (FIG. 4) and denaturing conditions, indicating that these RNA bands are not artifacts of the electrophoresis system and suggesting that each is in fact a unique H4 histone mRNA species.

● Each of the numbered bands in FIGURE 3 (bands 1–10) was translated in a wheat germ cell-free protein-synthesizing system and each coded for only H4 histone.

● Each of the numbered bands in FIGURE 3 was also subjected to T1 ribonuclease digestion and two-dimensional "fingerprinting" of the resulting oligonucleotides. Variations in the oligonucleotide maps of bands 1, 2, 5, 7, 8, 9, and 10 (some of which are shown in FIGURE 5) show sequence differences in at least seven H4 histone mRNA species. The fingerprints also indicate that the oligonucleotides of the smaller molecular weight H4 histone mRNAs are not a subset of those generated from the larger RNAs, ruling out a simple precursor–product relationship.

● The identity of the H4 histone species was confirmed by hybrid selection with cloned H4 histone gene sequences of *in vivo* labeled S-phase HeLa cell

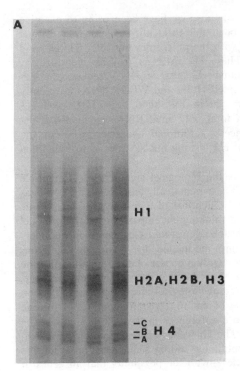

FIGURE 2. Electrophoretic fractionation of 5–18S polysomal RNAs under denaturing conditions. S-phase HeLa cells were ^{32}P-labeled *in vivo* and polysomal RNA was isolated in the presence of vanadyl ribonucleoside complex.[33] The RNA was fractionated on a sucrose gradient and the region between 5S and 18S was pooled. The RNA was ethanol-precipitated and then dissolved in 8.3 M urea–5 mM EDTA (pH 8.0), heated to 100° C and quick-cooled before loading on a 6% (w/v) polyacrylamide—8.3 M urea gel buffered with 50 mM Tris–borate–1 mM EDTA (TBE). The gel was run at 20 watts, which gave a surface temperature of 50–60° C. These conditions are sufficient to denature most RNA molecules.[34] After autoradiography, the bands labeled A, B and C were excised and the RNA was eluted electrophoretically into dialysis tubing.

polysomal RNA and subsequent electrophoretic fractionation under denaturing conditions of the selected RNAs (FIG. 6).

• Variations were observed in the representation of H4 histone mRNA species when polysomal RNAs from HeLa cells and WI–38 human diploid fibroblasts were fractionated electrophoretically, immobilized covalently on diazotized cellulose, and identified by hybridization to ^{32}P-labeled, cloned H4 histone DNA sequences (FIG. 7). At least one H4 histone mRNA species that is observed in WI–38 cells is not represented in the polysomal RNA of HeLa cells, suggesting a possible difference in expression of H4 histone mRNA species in different human cell types.

• We have begun to assign H4 histone mRNA species to individual H4 histone genes using a modification of the Berk and Sharp procedure.[10] As shown in FIGURE 8, when H4 histone mRNA species collectively were annealed with cloned genomic H4 histone sequences, each H4 histone gene formed an S1-nuclease-resistant hybrid with only one H4 mRNA. These results provide convincing evidence that the various H4 histone mRNA species do not represent post-transcriptional processing. It is interesting that where H4 histone mRNA sequences are represented in the genome in close proximity, as in clones λHHG6, λHHG17, and λHHG22, different H4 histone mRNA sequences are encoded in the adjacent H4 genes (FIG. 1C).

We have recently initiated studies directed towards identification, isolation, and characterization of multiple forms of human H3 histone mRNAs. The approaches being pursued are similar to those we have been using to examine H4 histone mRNA species. We have been able to identify at least four distinct H3 histone mRNA species associated with the polysomes of HeLa S3 cells and WI–38 human diploid fibroblasts. These H3 mRNAs can be identified by hybridization of cloned human genomic H3 histone DNA sequences (^{32}P-labeled) to electrophoretically fractionated HeLa and WI–38 RNAs covalently bound to diazotized cellulose. As shown in FIGURE 6, four HeLa cell H3 histone mRNAs can be isolated from total polysomal RNAs by hybrid selection with cloned H3 histone sequences. Additional characterization of the H3 histone mRNAs and assignment of H3 histone mRNA species to individual H3 histone genes are being pursued.

The obvious question that arises is the biological significance of multiple forms of H4 histone mRNAs, which are genetically encoded and serve as templates for the synthesis of apparently identical histone polypeptides. While here we can only speculate, our current thinking encompasses a working model with the following components: All histone genes in a cluster are coordinately controlled, with their expression being modulated by common regulatory sequences and/or regulatory molecules. Only a subset of the reiterated histone genes are expressed, with variations in those histone genes (gene clusters) expressed in different cells and/or in different biological circumstances. Selection of clusters to be transcribed would be based on a requirement for a histone H2A, H2B, H3, or H1 subspecies where differences in the mRNAs and in the histone proteins have been observed. The H4 genes expressed would be predicated on location within a cluster containing coding sequences for a specific H2A, H2B, H3 or H1 histone subspecies—with the possibility that all genes in such a cluster contain similar regulatory sequences.

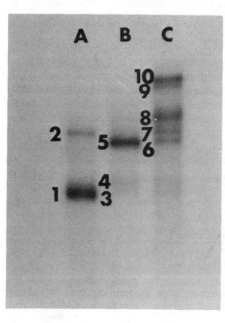

FIGURE 3. Electrophoretic fractionation under nondenaturing conditions of three molecular weight species of human H4 histone mRNAs. RNAs from the gel shown in FIGURE 2 were ethanol-precipitated, dried, and resuspended in 4 M urea–2.5 mM EDTA (pH 8.0). The RNAs were then heated to 100° C and loaded onto a 6% (w/v) polyacrylamide–TBE gel with no urea for fractionation under nondenaturing conditions. The numbered bands were excised and the RNAs eluted electrophoretically.

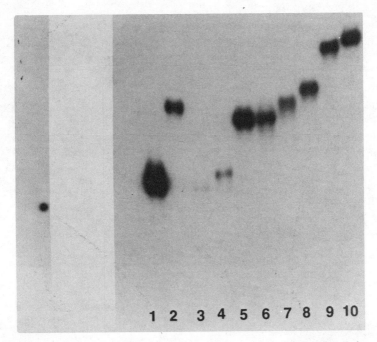

FIGURE 4. Analysis of fractionated H4 mRNA species. RNAs eluted from the numbered gel bands of FIGURE 3 were denatured by boiling in 4-*M* urea (as described in the legend to FIGURE 3) and re-electrophoresed in the same gel system. Each RNA migrated as a single band with the same relative mobility exhibited in the first gel (FIG. 3), eliminating the possibility that the multiple bands in FIGURE 3 are due to conformational isomers of single RNA species.

LEVEL OF CONTROL OF HUMAN HISTONE GENE EXPRESSION

To understand the level at which regulation of histone gene expression resides, it is necessary to establish whether or not histone proteins and histone mRNAs are synthesized in a cell-cycle-stage-specific manner. Equally important is an understanding of the relationship between histone protein synthesis, histone gene transcription, and the histone mRNA sequences in the cell nucleus and cytoplasm.

Histone Protein Synthesis during the Cell Cycle

It has been well documented that in most higher eukaryotic cells the synthesis of histone proteins, with the exceptions of H1 synthesis under certain circumstances [37] and "basal synthesis" of histones in several mammalian cell lines,[38] is primarily if not exclusively restricted to the S phase of the cell cycle in continuously dividing cells and in quiescent cells stimluated to proliferate.[11-21] And, while histone protein synthesis has been reported to occur at a constant rate throughout the cell cycle in S49 mouse lymphoma cells, this appears to be a

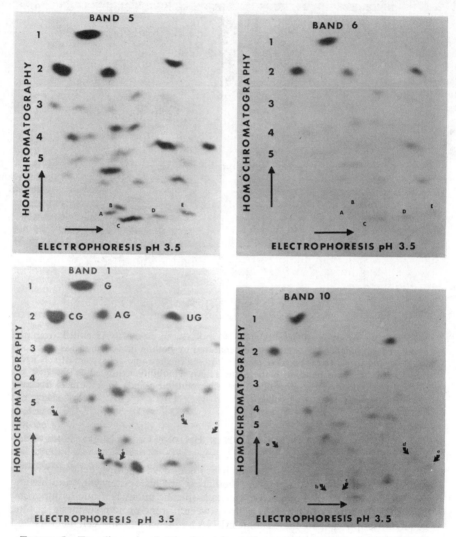

FIGURE 5. Two-dimensional T1 ribonuclease fingerprint analysis of selected H4 histone mRNA species. RNAs eluted from the gel shown in FIGURE 3 were digested with T1 ribonuclease and the resulting oligonucleotides were fractionated on cellulose acetate at pH 3.5 in 7-M urea in the first dimension, followed by homochromatography on PEI–cellulose thin-layer plates in the second dimension. The band numbers correspond to those in FIGURE 3. Bands 5 (*top left*) and 6 (*top right*) are identical, as is shown by the correspondence between the lettered oligonucleotide spots. Bands 1 (*bottom left*) and 10 (*bottom right*) are different, as shown by spots a, b and c in 1, which are not found in 10, and spots d and e from 10, which are not found in 1. Also note that both 1 and 10 differ from 5 and 6.

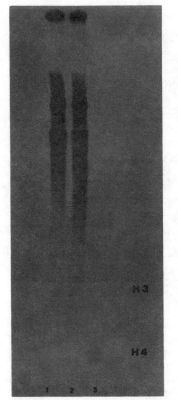

FIGURE 6. Hybrid selection of *in vivo* synthesized histone mRNAs. Fifty µg of plasmid DNA (containing H3 and H4 histone genes) were linearized with *Eco*RI, treated with proteinase K in 2% (w/v) SDS, and extracted with phenol–chloroform–isoamyl alcohol (25:24:1). The DNA was denatured with 0.5 *M* NaOH, neutralized with NaCl–Tris–HCl, and passed through 13-mm Sartorius nitrocellulose filters. The filters were based at 80° C *in vacuo* for 2 hr and then hybridized with ^{32}P-labeled total cytoplasmic RNA from S-phase HeLa cells in 1.5 ml Eppendorf tubes in 50% (w/v) formamide–0.5 *M* NaCl–10 m*M* HEPES (pH 7.3)–1 m*M* EDTA–0.2% (w/v) SDS at 47° for 40 hr. The filters were washed 10 times with 1 ml of 1×SSC–0.5% (w/v) SDS at 68° C and 3 times with 1 ml of 2 m*M* EDTA (pH 7.0) at 68° C. The hybridized RNA was eluted with two 300-µl aliquots of distilled water at 100° for 2 min, ethanol-precipitated, and electrophoresed on an 8.3-*M* urea denaturing gel (as in FIGURE 2) (lane 3) along with total cytoplasmic RNA (lane 1) and RNA from the hybridization mix that did not bind to the filter (Lane 2).

"special situation."[22] Early evidence for S-phase-specific histone synthesis in human cells, both continuously dividing HeLa cells and nondividing human diploid fibroblasts stimulated to proliferate, comes from studies in which cells were pulse-labeled with ^{3}H- or ^{14}C-labeled amino acids and the specific activities of nuclear and/or chromosomal histones were determined.[11–21] To eliminate the possibility that histones are synthesized throughout the cell cycle and become associated with the genome only during S phase, we recently pulse-labeled G_1- and S-phase HeLa cells with ^{35}S-methionine and analyzed unfractionated total cellular proteins (FIG. 9A) or dilute mineral-acid-extractable total cellular proteins (FIG. 9B) for the presence of newly synthesized histone polypeptides. Our ability to detect radioactively labeled histones only in S-phase HeLa cells is consistent with S-phase-specific histone protein synthesis or synthesis of histones predominantly when DNA replication occurs.[23] S-phase-specific histone protein synthesis is also supported by the very low levels of histone synthesis and cytoplasmic histone mRNAs at nonpermissive temperatures in temperature-sensitive cell cycle mutants.[27, 43]

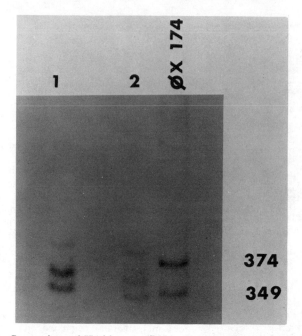

FIGURE 7. Comparison of H4 histone mRNAs from two human cell lines. Seventy-five μg of HeLa (lane 1) and WI-38 (lane 2) cytoplasmic RNAs were preincubated in 50-mM methyl mercury hydroxide and then electrophoretically fractionated on 3% (w/v) low-gelling-temperature agarose gels containing 5-mM methyl mercury. After a neutralization/equilibration step,[35] the nucleic acids within the gel were electrophoretically transferred to diazotized cellulose, as described by Stellwag and Dahlberg.[36] Prehybridization and hybridization solutions were as described[35] except that 5× Denhardt solution (minus BSA), 0.7 mg/ml of carrier nucleic acid, and 0.1% (w/v) SDS were used. The paper was hybridized with a radiolabeled, human H4 DNA fragment (1×10^7 cpm/μg, 1×10^6 cpm/ml) at 50° C for 36 hr. Washing was at 68° C, using decreasing concentrations of SSC. The paper was blotted dry and exposed to Kodak® XAR–5 film at −70° C with a Cronex "Lightning Plus" intensifying screen.

Representation of Histone mRNA Sequences during the Cell Cycle

To gain a more definitive insight into regulation of histone gene expression during the cell cycle, we have used cloned genomic human histone sequences to examine the representation of histone mRNAs in the nucleus and cytoplasm of G_1- and S-phase synchronized HeLa S3 cells.[42] In agreement with our earlier observations from this laboratory and with the findings of others,[6, 24–31] where histone mRNAs were analyzed by RNA excess hybridization with homologous histone cDNAs, histone mRNA sequences are present in significant amounts in the nucleus and cytoplasm of HeLa cells only during S phase, when histone protein synthesis occurs.

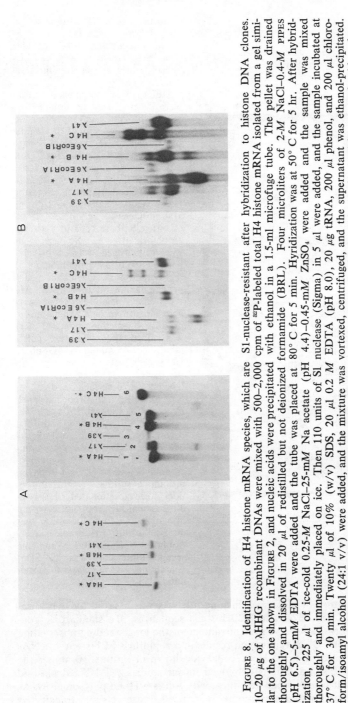

FIGURE 8. Identification of H4 histone mRNA species, which are S1-nuclease-resistant after hybridization to histone DNA clones. 10–20 µg of λHHG recombinant DNAs were mixed with 500–2,000 cpm of ³²P-labeled total H4 histone mRNA isolated from a gel similar to the one shown in FIGURE 2, and nucleic acids were precipitated with ethanol in a 1.5-ml microfuge tube. The pellet was drained thoroughly and dissolved in 20 µl of redistilled but not deionized formamide (BRL). Four microliters of 2-*M* NaCl-0.4-*M* PIPES (pH 6.5)–5-m*M* EDTA were added and the tube was placed at 80° C for 5 min. Hyridization was at 50° C for 5 hr. After hybridization, 225 µl of ice-cold 0.25-*M* NaCl-25-m*M* Na acetate (pH 4.4)–0.45-m*M* ZnSO₄ were added and the sample was mixed thoroughly and immediately placed on ice. Then 110 units of S1 nuclease (Sigma) in 5 µl were added, and the sample incubated at 37° C for 30 min. Twenty µl of 10% (w/v) SDS, 20 µl 0.2 *M* EDTA (pH 8.0), 20 µg tRNA, 200 µl phenol, and 200 µl chloroform/isoamyl alcohol (24:1 v/v) were added, and the mixture was vortexed, centrifuged, and the supernatant was ethanol-precipitated. The dried pellet was dissolved in 8.3-*M* urea–5-m*M* EDTA, heated to 100° C for 2 min, and electrophoresed in an acrylamide gel. S1-resistant samples were electrophoresed in an 8.3-*M* urea gel (**A**) or in a nondenaturing gel (**B**). Results from two different autoradiographic exposure times are shown. Lanes marked H4A, H4B and H4C correspond to marker RNAs.

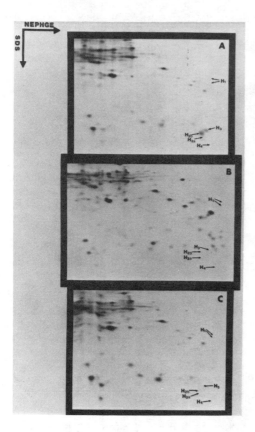

FIGURE 9A. Two-dimensional electrophoretic analysis of ^{35}S-methionine-labeled total cellular proteins. **A** = S phase; **B** = G₁ phase; C = cytosine-arabinoside-treated S phase.

HeLa cells in suspension culture were synchronized by double thymidine block (2 mM). After release from the second thymidine block, cells were maintained at a density of 5 × 10⁵/ml for 1 hr. S-phase cells were incubated for 2 additional hours at 37° C either in the presence or absence of the DNA synthesis inhibitor, cytosine arabinoside (40 μg/ml). Ten ml of either S-phase cells or cytosine-arabinoside-treated S-phase cells were centrifuged, washed in spinner salts solution containing 5 μM methionine (37° C), and resuspended in 2.8 ml of low (5 μM) methionine medium (containing cytosine arabinoside when appropriate). ^{35}S-methionine (140 μCi) was added and cells were pulse-labeled for 45 min at 37°. G₁ phase HeLa cells were obtained by mitotic selective detachment and labeled as described earlier for S-phase cells. Cells were harvested by centrifugation at 1500 × g for 5 min, rinsed with ether, and dried before solubilizing in 9.5 M urea–2% (w/v) NP–40–2% (w/v) ampholine–5% (w/v) mercaptoethanol–0.3-M NaCl–1.0-mg/ml protamine sulfate. ^{35}S-labeled peptides were fractionated in a two-dimensional electrophoretic system in which the first dimension was nonequilibrium pH gradient electrophoresis (NEPHGE) and the second dimension was an SDS-containing, 15% (w/v) acrylamide gel.

The representation of HeLa cell histone mRNAs was assayed by hybridization to cloned H4, H3, H2A and H2B histone sequences. To standardize conditions for the hybridization, we took advantage of the long-standing observation that the inhibition of DNA replication results in a rapid loss of histone mRNAs from the polysomes of S-phase HeLa cells. As shown in FIGURE 10, under the standard hybridization conditions employed in our studies, ^{32}P-labeled plasmid DNAs containing histone sequences anneal with S-phase HeLa polysomal RNAs fractionated electrophoretically in methyl mercury–agarose gels and transferred electrophoretically to diazotized cellulose. Consistent with the anticipated loss of histone mRNA sequences from polysomes after inhibition of DNA synthesis, a greater than 95% inhibition was observed in the hybridization of radiolabeled, cloned histone DNAs to filter-immobilized polysomal RNAs from S-phase HeLa cells when DNA synthesis was blocked by treatment with cytosine arabinoside. The sensitivity of our hybridization assay is such that we can detect less than 500 pg of mRNA.

To find the level at which regulation of histone gene expression occurs during the cell cycle in HeLa S3 cells, we assayed the abilities of ^{32}P-labeled (nick-translated) histone DNAs to hybridize with filter-immobilized RNA from G_1- and S-phase cells. The rationale was that because histone synthesis is confined to S phase, hybridization of the histone DNA probes to RNAs from S-phase cells but not from G_1 cells would be consistent with nuclear and/or transcriptional control. However, hybridization to both G_1- and S-phase RNAs would suggest that regulation of histone gene expression resides at a post-transcriptional step.

As shown in FIGURE 11, hybridization between λHHG55 DNA, a recombinant λ Charon 4A phage containing human genomic H2A, H2B, H3, and H4

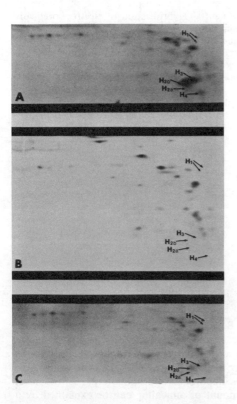

FIGURE 9B. Two dimensional NEPHGE/SDS electrophoresis of acid-extracted nuclear proteins of **(A)** S-phase, **(B)** G_1, and **(C)** cytosine-arabinoside-treated S-phase cells. ^{35}S-methionine-labeled cells were lysed in 10-mM KCl–10-mM Tris–1.3 mM MgCl$_2$ (pH 7.4) containing 0.65% (v/v) Triton X-100, and nuclei were pelleted by centrifugation at $800 \times g$. Nuclear pellets were extracted with 0.4 M H$_2$SO$_4$ for 30 min and the acid-soluble nuclear proteins were precipitated from the supernatant at $-20°$ overnight after addition of three volumes of 95% ethanol.

histone sequences, and G_1 nuclear or cytoplasmic RNAs was barely detectable, while hybridization of λHHG55 DNA with both nuclear and cytoplasmic RNAs of S-phase HeLa cells was apparent. In these experiments G_1 cells were obtained by mitotic selective detachment, a procedure that yields a G_1 population containing less than 0.5% S-phase cells. 100 μg of both G_1- and S-phase RNA were fractionated electrophoretically. Ethidium bromide staining indicated that similar amounts of 18S and 28S RNAs from G_1- and S-phase cells were fractionated in the gels and transferred to diazotized cellulose (greater than 90%

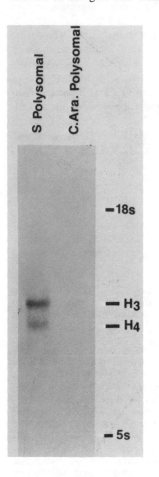

FIGURE 10. Hybridization of electrophoretically fractionated polysomal RNA from S-phase- and cytosine-arabinoside-treated S-phase HeLa cells with ^{32}P-labeled human genomic H3 and H4 histone sequences. One hundred μg of total HeLa cell polysomal RNAs were fractionated in a 2% (w/v) agarose gel containing 5 mM methyl mercury hydroxide, electrophoretically transferred to DBM paper, and hybridized with ^{32}P-labeled (nick-translated) plasmid DNA containing human genomic H3 and H4 histone sequences.

transfer was obtained) in both cases. Because there is an increase in the amount of ribosomal RNA per cell in S phase compared with G_1, the hybridization observed is probably an underestimation of the amount of histone mRNA in S-phase cells. On longer exposure to the "northern blot" some hybridization of the probe with G_1 RNA becomes apparent (approximately 1% the level observed with S-phase RNA); this amount of annealing can be explained by a limited number of S-phase cells in the G_1 population (the biological limits of the system) or by basal level histone synthesis during G_1.[38] When the northern blot of G_1- and S-phase HeLa cell RNAs shown in FIGURE 11 was rehybridized with ^{32}P-labeled plasmid DNA containing different H3 and H4 histone coding sequences, S-phase-specific hybridization was also observed.

An unexpected result was obtained when a northern blot of cytoplasmic RNA from G_1- and S-phase HeLa cells was hybridized with ^{32}P-labeled DNA from λHHG41, a recombinant phage containing H3 and H4 coding sequences derived from another human histone gene unit (FIG. 12). While hybridization with S-phase but not G_1-phase histone mRNAs was observed, intense hybridization was also seen with an RNA of approximately 330 nucleotides present predominantly in G_1 cells.

The increase in the representation of both nuclear and cytoplasmic histone mRNAs in S-phase compared with G_1-phase cells suggests that histone genes are preferentially expressed during the restricted period of the cell cycle when DNA replication occurs. Since synthesis of histone proteins is also confined to the

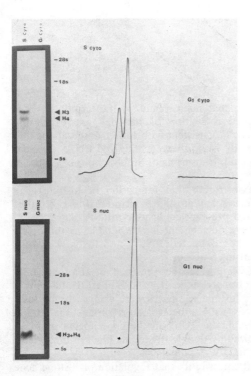

FIGURE 11. Hybridization of human genomic recombinant phage λHHG 55-DNA containing H2A, H2B, H3 and H4 histone sequences with cytoplasmic and nuclear RNA from G_1- and S-phase HeLa cells. S-phase cells were obtained 1 hr after release from two cycles of 2-mM thymidine block, while the G_1 population was obtained by mitotic selective detachment. One hundred μg of total cytoplasmic RNA were fractionated in a 2% (w/v) agarose–5-mM methylmercury hydroxide gel, and equal amounts (100 μg) of nuclear RNA were fractionated in a gel containing 1% (w/v) agarose–5-mM methylmercury hydroxide. The positions of 28S, 18S, and 5S markers were determined optically after staining the gel with ethidium bromide. RNAs were electrophoretically transferred to DBM paper and hybridized with ^{32}P-labeled (nick-translated) λHHG 55 DNA. The blots were analyzed autoradiographically at $-70°$ C using preflashed XAR–5 film (Kodak) with a Cronex "Lightning Plus" intensifying screen. Autoradiograms were scanned with a Joyce-Loebel densitometer and quantitated by planimetric analysis; (*top*) cytoplasmic RNAs, (*bottom*) nuclear RNAs. Note that under these electrophoretic conditions, the mRNAs for H2A, H2B and H3 histones are not resolved.

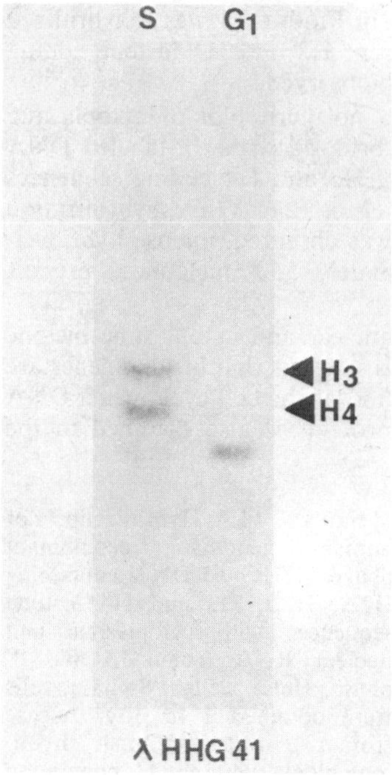

FIGURE 12. Autoradiographic analysis of G_1- and S-phase cytoplasmic RNAs hybridized with DNA from λHHG 41, a recombinant phage containing H3 and H4 human histone sequences. The DBM blot shown in FIGURE 11 (top) was incubated in sterile water at 100° C to remove ^{32}P-labeled λHHG 55 probe. After confirming that the λ55 probe was no longer detectable, the filters containing fractionated cytoplasmic RNAs were annealed with ^{32}P-labeled λHHG 41 DNA.

S phase, it is reasonable to postulate that nuclear and/or transcriptional level control is operative. Transcriptional regulation of histone gene expression during the cell cycle of the HeLa cells is consistent with earlier observations that histone cDNA hybridized preferentially with *in vivo* synthesized RNAs (nuclear and cytoplasmic) and *in vitro* chromatin transcripts of S-phase but not G_1-phase cells.[6, 24–31]

However, an unequivocal demonstration that regulation of histone gene expression during the cell cycle resides solely at the transcriptional level requires establishing that (1) the very limited presence of histone mRNA sequences in G_1 cells obtained by mitotic selective detachment is attributable to those few S-phase cells in the G_1 population (approximately 0.5%) and that (2) histone gene transcription is initiated only during S phase.

Although Melli and coworkers reported the presence of approximately equivalent amounts of histone gene transcripts in G_1- and S-phase HeLa cells,[32] these results are not surprising since histone sequences were assayed by hybridization under nonstringent conditions with a heterologous probe—sea urchin histone DNA sequences cloned in lambda. Also, in the experiments of Melli and coworkers, cells were synchronized by double thymidine block, which yields a G_1 population containing more than 20% S-phase cells.

We cannot completely dismiss the possibility that regulation of histone gene expression during the cell cycle may to some extent be mediated post-transcriptionally. However, the low steady-state level of histone mRNA sequences that we observed in G_1 nuclear RNA would indicate that if histone sequences are transcribed at the same rate throughout the cell cycle, they must be rapidly degraded in G_1 cells. Alternatively, it is possible that histone sequences are transcribed at a much lower level outside of S phase. Such low-level transcription might be functional or might reflect "leaky" transcription of some or all of the histone genes. In this context the persistence of a limited amount of histone transcripts from the previous S phase into the subsequent G_1 phase should be considered.

A definitive explanation for the observed hybridization of ^{32}P-labeled λHHG41 DNA (which contains H3 and H4 human histone genes) with a 330-nucleotide cytoplasmic RNA species present predominantly in G_1 cells is not yet available. However, since the G_1 cytoplasmic RNA species is encoded in a genomic sequence in close proximity to histone coding sequences, a possible regulatory role for the G_1 RNA should not be dismissed. Further analyses of the RNA and the genomic DNA sequences in which it is encoded are under way.

Regulation of Human Histone Gene Expression under Various Biological Circumstances

In agreement with the evidence presented herein for nuclear and/or transcriptional level control of histone gene expression during the cell cycle in continuously dividing HeLa S3 cells, a parallel situation appears to be operative when nondividing WI–38 human diploid fibroblasts are stimulated to proliferate. That is, concomitant with the onset of DNA synthesis, as human fibroblasts make the transition from the prereplicative to the S phase of the cell cycle, there is a comparable stimulation of histone protein synthesis and increased representation of histone mRNA sequences.[29] However, it is unlikely that control of human histone gene expression is mediated at the nuclear level under all biological circumstances. By analogy with the manner in which histone gene expression is regulated during early stages of development in several lower eukaryotes, it is possible that histone gene expression is controlled post-transcriptionally under comparable circumstances in human cells. A very likely possibility, and one which is being pursued experimentally, is that those copies of the human histone genes or those human histone gene clusters expressed concomitantly share similar or identical regulatory sequences, with differences in putative regulatory sequences among those genes whose expression is mediated transcriptionally rather than post-transcriptionally.

Are Human Histone Genes Organized and Regulated in a Prokaryotic Manner?

Several features of human histone gene organization and the expression of these sequences suggest it may be realistic to think in terms of "prokaryote-like" gene organization and control. One striking feature of human histone gene organization that appears to reflect the organization of prokaryotic genes is the apparent absence of intervening sequences. But perhaps the strongest argument for the similarity of human histone genes and prokaryotic genetic sequences comes from the rapid manner in which newly transcribed mRNAs reach the polysomes and become actively engaged in histone protein synthesis— without an extensive amount of post-transcriptional processing and without addition of poly A to the 3′ termini. The "rapid" turnover of human histone mRNAs and the dramatic cell cycle stage-specific variations in the representation of histone mRNA sequences in the nucleus and cytoplasm of HeLa and WI–38 cells provide further support for the prokaryotic analogy, that is, the manner in which histone gene expression parallels the onset of DNA replication is indeed reminiscent of the manner in which *lac* operon expression in *E. coli* reflects the levels of specific sugars in the bacterial growth medium. It will be interesting to determine whether other eukaryotic genes, whose expression is modulated in a cyclic fashion in response to specific yet changing cellular environments (for example, inducible metabolic enzymes), are organized and regulated in a manner similar to that of human histone genes. Such organization and expression are apparently strikingly different from those of other eukaryotic genes such as ovalbumin and globin, but it must be considered that the latter genetic sequences are expressed in conjunction with long-term rather than cyclic cellular commitments, often being permanent commitments of terminally differentiated cells. It remains to be established whether the "simple" or "prokaryotic type" of organization and control reflected by histone genes or the "complex type" as reflected by globin genes is the rule or special situation in eukaryotic cells.

REFERENCES

1. LAWN, R. M., E. F. FRITSCH, R. C. PARKER, G. BLAKE & T. MANIATIS. 1978. Cell **15:** 1157.
2. YU, L. C., P. SZABO, T. W. BORUN & W. PRENSKY. 1978. Cold Spring Harbor Symp. Quant. Biol. **42:** 1101.
3. CHANDLER, M. E., L. H. KEDES, R. H. COHN & J. YUNIS. 1979. J. Science **205:** 908.
4. NAYLOR, S., J. L. STEIN & G. S. STEIN. Unpublished results.
5. STEIN, G. S., J. L. STEIN, P. J. LAIPIS, S. K. CHATTOPADHYAY, A. C. LICHTLER, S. DETKE, J. A. THOMSON, I. R. PHILLIPS & E. A. SHEPHARD. 1978. Miami Winter Symp. **15:** 125. Academic Press. New York, N.Y.
6. STEIN, G. S., J. L. STEIN, W. D. PARK, S. DETKE, A. C. LICHTLER, E. A. SHEPHARD, R. H. JANSING & I. R. PHILLIPS. 1977. Cold Spring Harbor Symp. Quant. Biol. **42:** 1107.
7. LICHTLER, A. C., S. DETKE, I. R. PHILLIPS, G. S. STEIN & J. L. STEIN. 1980. Proc. Natl. Acad. Sci. USA **77:** 1942.
8. STEIN, J. L., G. S. STEIN & P. M. McGUIRE. 1977. Biochemistry **16:** 2207.
9. GRUNSTEIN, M., S. LEVY, P. SCHEDL & L. KEDES. 1973. Cold Spring Harbor Symp. Quant. Biol. **38:** 717.
10. BERK, A. J. & P. A. SHARP. 1978. Proc. Natl. Acad. Sci. USA **75:** 1274.
11. SPALDING, J., K. KAJIWARA & G. MUELLER. 1966. Proc. Natl. Acad. Sci. USA **56:** 1535.
12. ROBBINS, E. & T. W. BORUN. 1967. Proc. Natl. Acad. Sci. USA **57:** 409.
13. STEIN, G. S. & T. W. BORUN. 1972. J. Cell Biol. **52:** 292.
14. STEIN, G. S. & D. L. THRALL. 1973. FEBS Lett. **34:** 35.
15. GALLWITZ, D. & G. C. MUELLER. 1969. J. Biol. Chem. **244:** 5947.
16. BORUN, T. W., M. D. SCHARFF & F. ROBBINS. 1967. Proc. Natl. Acad. Sci. USA **58:** 1977.
17. BUTLER, W. B. & G. C. MUELLER. 1973. Biochim. Biophys. Acta. **294:** 481.
18. BREINDL, M. & D. GALLWITZ. 1974. Eur. J. Biochem. **45:** 91.
19. BORUN, T. W., F. GABRIELLI, K. AJIRA, A. ZWEIDLER & C. BAGLIONI. 1975. Cell **4:** 59.
20. JACOBS-LORENA, M., C. BAGLIONI & T. W. BORUN. 1972. Proc. Natl. Acad. Sci. USA **69:** 2095.

21. GALLWITZ, D. & M. BREINDL. 1972. Biochem. Biophys. Res. Commun. **47:** 1106.
22. GROPPI, V. E. & P. COFFINO. 1980. Cell **21:** 195.
23. MARASHI, F., L. BAUMBACH, R. RICKLES, F. SIERRA, J. L. STEIN & G. S. STEIN. 1982. Science **215:** 683.
24. STEIN, J. L., C. L. THRALL, W. D. PARK, R. J. MANS & G. S. STEIN. 1975. Science **189:** 557.
25. DETKE, S., A. LICHTLER, I. PHILLIPS, J. L. STEIN & G. S. STEIN. 1979. Proc. Natl. Acad. Sci. USA **76:** 1995.
26. STEIN, G. S., W. D. PARK, C. L. THRALL, R. J. MANS & J. L. STEIN. 1975. Nature **257:** 764.
27. DELEGEANE, A. M. & A. S. LEE. 1981. Science **215:** 79.
28. DETKE, S., J. L. STEIN & G. S. STEIN. 1978. Nucl. Acids Res. **5:** 1515.
29. JANSING, R. L., J. L. STEIN & G. S. STEIN. 1977. Proc. Natl. Acad. Sci. **74:** 173.
30. PARKER, I. & W. FITSCHEN. 1980. Cell Diff. **9:** 23.
31. CHIU, I. M., D. COOPER & W. F. MARZLUFF. 1979. Abstracts of the Second Annual meeting of the American Cancer Society (Florida Division). Cancer Res. Sem. Abstr No. 38.
32. MELLI, M., G. SPINELLI & E. ARNOLD. 1977. Cell **12:** 167.
33. BERGER, S. L. & C. S. BIRKENMEIER. 1979. Biochemistry **18:** 5143.
34. PEATTIE, D. A. 1979. Proc. Natl. Acad. Sci. USA **76:** 1760.
35. ALWINE, J. L., D. J. KEMP, B. A. PARKER, J. REISER, J. RENART, G. R. STARK & G. M. WAHL. 1979. Meth. Enzymol. **68:** 220.
36. STELLWAG, E. J. & A. E. DAHLBERG. 1980. Nucl. Acids. Res. **8:** 299.
37. BRADBURY, M. Personal communication.
38. WU, R. S. & W. M. BONNER. 1981. Cell **27:** 321.
39. SIERRA, F., A. LICHTLER, F. MARASHI, R. RICKLES, T. VAN DYKE, S. CLARK, J. WELLS, G. STEIN & J. STEIN. 1982. Proc. Natl. Acad. Sci. USA **79:** 1795.
40. SIERRA, F., A. LEZA, F. MARASHI, M. PLUMB, R. RICKLES, T. VAN DYKE, S. CLARK, J. WELLS, G. S. STEIN & J. L. STEIN. 1982. Biochem. Biophys. Res. Commun. **104:** 785.
41. LICTHLER, A. C., F. SIERRA, S. CLARK, J. R. E. WELLS, J. L. STEIN & G. S. STEIN. 1982. Nature. **298:** 195.
42. RICKLES, R., F. MARASHI, F. SIERRA, S. CLARK, J. WELLS, J. STEIN & G. STEIN. 1982. Proc. Natl. Acad. Sci. USA **79:** 749.
43. VAN DYKE, T., F. MARASHI, R. BASERGA, J. STEIN & G. STEIN. Unpublished results.

CELL KINETICS, CELL STRUCTURE,
AND RADIOTHERAPY *

Anna Goldfeder

Laboratory of Cancer and Radiobiological Research
New York University
New York, New York 10003

Since the appearance of a publication from this laboratory demonstrating that two analogous mouse mammary adenocarcinomas differed in their rate of growth, metabolic activity, and radiosensitivity,[1] investigations are continuously being carried out to reveal the structural and biological factors that may be involved in these vital processes. Soon after the classic publication appeared defining the four phases of the proliferating cell cycle [2] and after the successful synthesis of labeled thymidine (^{3}H-TdR),[3] studies in this laboratory were initiated to determine the life cycle of experimental mouse tumors propagated in syngeneic hosts.[4] It was then observed that the time of DNA synthesis (T_s) differed significantly between the two types of tumors, a sarcoma (DBAG) and carcinoma (DBAH). This finding was contrary to the opinion at the time that the T_s is a constant characteristic of all cell types.[5] The fact that both types of tumors were maintained by serial transplants in syngeneic hosts excluded the possibility of host influence on the cell cycle parameters of these two types of tumors. Two postulates were offered concerning that which may have influenced the difference in T_s of these tumors: (1) efficiency in DNA synthesis and (2) ploidy. These two postulates were based on the following observations: (1) The hyperploidy of the sarcoma cells consisted of a high percentage of tetra- and octaploids, whereas the carcinoma consisted mainly of diploid cells. I suggested that for a cell to produce DNA for tetra- or octaploid cells, more time was needed as compared with that of a cell producing DNA for two daughter cells. (2) Some of the metabolic events that are involved in DNA synthesis may be slower in the sarcoma cells. This inference was based on previous studies showing the inferior qualities and smaller quantities in this tumor of the cytoplasmic components that are known to be operative in DNA synthesis.[6] These tentative hypotheses called for further extensive experiments to shed light on the proposed postulates. The five types of tumors that are available in this laboratory offered suitable experimental systems to pursue such studies. Furthermore, to my knowledge, no correlative studies of cellular ultrastructural integrity and kinetic properties of tumor cells as reported herein are available in the literature.

* This investigation was supported by the National Cancer Institute and by the American Cancer Society.

0077-8923/82/0397-0168 $01.75/0 © 1982, NYAS

MATERIAL AND METHODS

Tumors

dbrB

dbrB is a mammary carcinoma that had developed spontaneously in a female mouse of the DBA/1J strain.[7] It has been propagated by subcutaneous transplants in syngeneic mice of the DBA/1J strain for the past 10 years in this laboratory. The tumor is rapidly proliferating, having a latent period averaging 4 days, and invades the chest wall and metastasizes to the lungs and liver. The cells are rich in cytoplasmic organelles. The characteristic mammary tumor virus (MTV) has been revealed by electron microscopy in some parenchymal tumor cells (FIGS. 1 and 2).

DBAH

DBAH is a mammary adenocarcinoma that developed spontaneously in a female mouse of the inbred DBA/2J strain [8] and has been continuously propa-

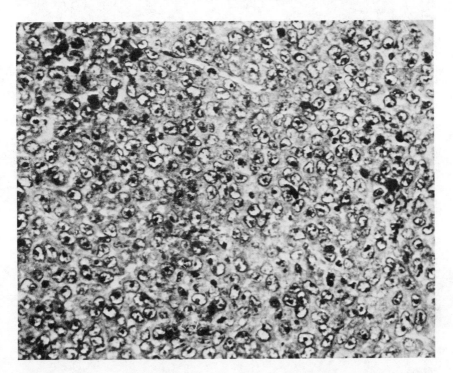

FIGURE 1. Electron micrograph of section from dbrB mammary carcinoma. Sheets of loosely distributed cells are shown; nuclei vary in shape and size, and nucleoli are prominent. (Hematoxylin and eosin stain; original magnification × 350; reduced by 7%.)

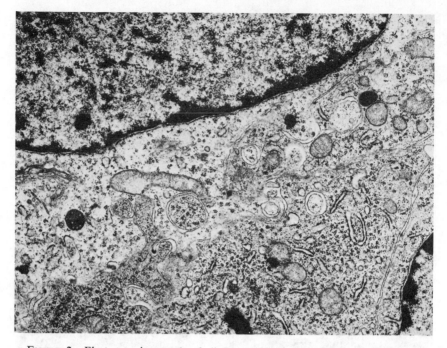

FIGURE 2. Electron micrograph of dbrB mammary carcinoma. Portions of two nuclei are seen showing condensed chromatin along the limiting membrane and chromatin clumps within the nucleoplasm. The cytoplasm is filled with ribosomes, polyribosomes, vesicles of endoplasmic reticulum, and mitochondria filled with cristae. (Original magnification × 18,500; reduced by 15%.)

gated by subcutaneous implants in syngeneic mice. Throughout the years, it has retained its morphologic characteristics, such as bands and nests of closely adjacent tumor cells. Despite its cellular compactness, central necrosis or cystic areas are minimal or none, even in large tumors. The characteristic MTV particles are seen electron microscopically in parenchymal tumor cells (FIGS. 3 and 4).

MT2

This mammary adenocarcinoma has been induced in a female mouse of the inbred X/Gf strain by urethan treatments.[9] It consists of nests of closely adjacent parenchymal tumor cells. The compact cell nests are separated by wide bundles of fibrous stroma. The characteristic MTV particles are occasionally seen electron microscopically in some parenchymal tumor cells (FIGS 5 and 6).

TEC

This tumor was derived from an embryonic cell culture line established from an X/Gf mouse embryo. One of the cultures underwent malignant transformation after 16 consecutive subcultures. This was evident by their ability to produce a tumor upon subcutaneous implantation into syngeneic X/Gf mice. The new subcutaneous tumor was diagnosed microscopically as a spindle-cell type of sarcoma (FIGS. 7 and 8).

DBA/3

This tumor developed spontaneously in a male mouse of the DBA/2J strain. It was diagnosed as a lymphoblastic type of lymphoma. DBA/3 proliferates

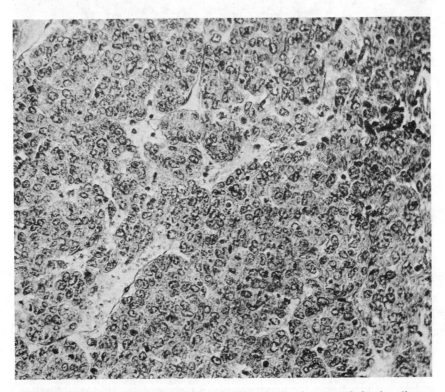

FIGURE 3. Section of DBAH mammary carcinoma showing nest of closely adjacent tumor cells separated by narrow septa of fibrous stroma. (Hematoxylin and eosin stain; original magnification × 350.)

rapidly, metastasizing to the lungs and liver. No apparent virus particles of any type have been revealed electron microscopically in cells of this tumor (FIGS. 9 and 10).

Tumor Growth

For the determination of growth curves, measurements in three dimensions were made with vernier calipers, three times weekly, from the time a palpable

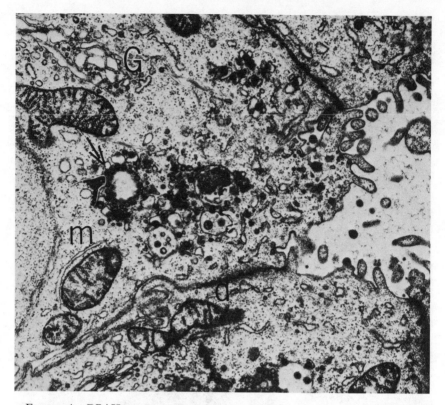

FIGURE 4. DBAH mammary carcinoma. Portions of cells are connected by desmosomes (D) and the following can be seen: surface microvilli extended into the lumen of the acinus; portion of Golgi complex (Gc); cytoplasm filled with ribosomes; polyribosomes; mitochondria (M) of different shape and size containing internal membranes (cristae); type "B" virus particles lying free in the lumen and within the cytoplasmic vacuoles (arrow): The limiting membrane of the cytoplasmic vacuole is lined up with type "A" virus particles (arrow); and a portion of nucleus shows nuclear pores in its limiting membrane. (Original magnification $\times$ 37,500.)

nodule was noted until the tumor reached a large size and started to ulcerate. The tumor volume was calculated by the formula:

$$V = (\pi/6) \times D_1 \times D_2 \times D_3$$

in which D_1 to D_3 are 3 diameters in cm. The mean $\pm$ SD of each tumor is shown in FIGURE 11.

Cell Cycle Determination

Hosts of each tumor line, bearing a tumor of approximately 0.4 cm³ in size, were injected intraperitoneally with 1.0 μCi/gm body weight of methyl-³H-labeled thymidine, specific activity 1.9 μCi/mmol (Schwarz-Mann Radiochemical, Orangeburg, NY). The mice were sacrificed by cervical dislocation at 15 min to 50 hours after the injection of the nucleotide. Tumor tissue was removed, cut into small pieces, fixed in Carnoy's solution, and processed routinely. Paraffin sections, 3 μm thick, were placed on absolutely clean slides. Autoradiography was performed by the dipping technique,[10] using Eastman Kodak® NTB2 nuclear truck emulsion, exposed in black, light-tight plastic boxes (containing silica gel desiccant) at 4° C for 16 to 60 days, depending on the tumor type and labeling intensity, as predetermined by "test" slides. The emulsion was developed with Eastman Kodak D-19 for 6 minutes at 16° C, with slight agitation, rinsed in 1% acetic acid, and fixed in Kodak-fix for 10 minutes; then the fixer was removed by running water for about 1 hour. The tumor sections were stained with hematoxylin and eosin through the emulsion. The labeling of each sample microscopically was evaluated by observing 100 to 200 anaphase or metaphase cells. Autoradiographic background was established by grain counts over mitoses of unlabeled control tumor sections, which were placed at the end of the same slide with labeled tumor. Background was subtracted from the counts and true labeling calculated.[11, 12]

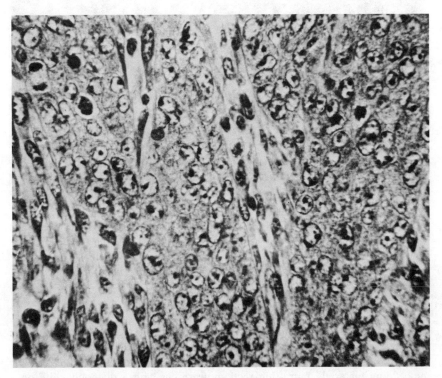

FIGURE 5. Section of MT2 mammary carcinoma. Bands of adjacent tumor cells separated by bundles of fibrous cells can be seen. Nuclei vary in size and shape; mitotic figures are in anaphase and metaphase. (Hematoxylin and eosin stain; original magnification × 400.)

Electron Microscopy

The freshly excised tumor tissue was cut with a sharp razor blade into small cubes of approximately 1 mm³ in one drop of cold 3% glutaraldehyde in phosphate buffer, pH 7.4, and then transferred to a vial containing the same fixative; it was kept in chopped ice for 1 to 2 hours, rinsed three times in cold phosphate buffer sucrose solution and left overnight at 3° C. Then, the tissues

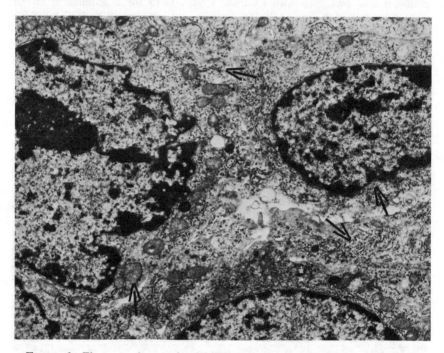

FIGURE 6. Electron micrograph of MT2 mammary carcinoma in which portions of four adjacent cells are seen. The dense cytoplasmic matrix is filled with ribosomes, polysomes, and mitochondria of various sizes (arrow); fibrillar material is seen as well (arrow). There is margination of nuclear material along the nuclear membranes, and chromatin clumps are within the nucleoplasm; invaginations of the nuclear membranes are also shown (arrow).

were rinsed with phosphate buffer sucrose solution, postfixed in 1% osmium tetroxide in phosphate buffer for 1 to 2 hours, dehydrated in graded alcohols, and processed by means of standard procedures. Epon 812 served as the embedding material. Ultra-thin sections were cut with a diamond knife on a Huxley ultramicrotome, stained with uranyl acetate and lead citrate, mounted on bare 300 mesh grids, and viewed and photographed in a 300 Philips electron microscope.

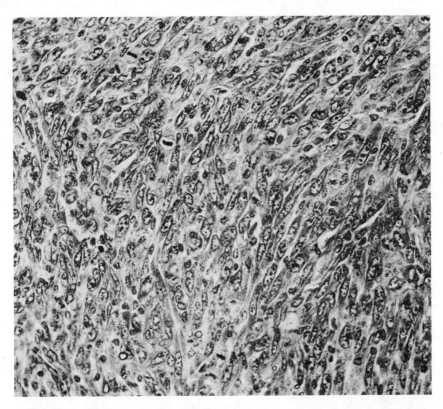

FIGURE 7. Section of spindle-shaped cell sarcoma (TEC). Bundles and whorls of spindle-shaped cells and mitoses in metaphase can be seen. (Hematoxylin and eosin stain; original magnification × 350.)

Computation of Data

A "fraction-labeled mitoses" curve was fitted to a set of percentages of labeled mitoses, and the values of the best fitting parameters of the cell cycle were estimated using a computer program.[13]

RESULTS

Growth of Tumors

The average latent period and the volume-doubling time (VDT) of each type of tumor are recorded in TABLE 1. The average rate of growth of each type of tumor is presented in FIGURE 11. It is apparent that the most rapidly growing tumor is dbrB, which has the shortest latent period (3 days) and a VDT of 0.7 days. The DBA/3, representing a lymphoblastic type of lymphoma, increases rapidly in size after a latent period averaging 4 days and has VDT of

2 days. The MT2 mammary adenocarcinoma shows the most gradual increase in growth. This may be due to its morphologic architecture, which shows bundles of fibrous stroma (FIG. 5), presumably limiting the spread of tumor cells, and also producing hypoxic conditions. The DBAH tumor shows a gradual increase in size after the latent period of 7 days, having a VDT of 1.7 days. The TEC tumor shows a VDT of 2.2 days, and a latent period of 9 days.

Cell Cycle Analysis

Computed labeled mitoses curves are presented in FIGURE 12 and derived cell cycle parameters are listed in TABLE 1. Each data point represents the mean value obtained by three observers on three to four tumors of each type. As mentioned earlier, the data obtained for the five types of tumors were analyzed using a computer program.[13]

Cell Cycle Parameters and Discussion

The cell cycle curves presenting the computed data obtained from auto-radiographic analysis for each type of tumor (dbrB, DBAH, DBA/3, MT2 and TEC) are seen in FIGURE 12. It is apparent that the timing of each phase

TABLE 1

VOLUME-DOUBLING TIME AND CELL CYCLE PHASES (HOURS)*

Tumor Line	Size (cm³)	Days †	VDT ‡ (days)	Emulsion Exposure (days)	T_{G1}	T_S	T_{G2}	T_C
dbrB	0.5 ± 0.1	3	0.7 ± 0.3	20	4.3	5.5	3.2	13.0
	1.3 ± 0.2	8	1.5 ± 0.8		(0.7)§	(0.4)	(0.3)	(0.6)
DBAH	0.5 ± 0.1	7	1.7 ± 0.8	12	2.9	6.4	4.8	14.0
	1.8 ± 0.2	14	2.5 ± 0.5		(0.2)	(0.1)	(0.1)	(0.2)
MT2	0.4 ± 0.1	10	2.2 ± 0.6	16	14.0	11.8	6.5	32.3
	1.8 ± 0.2	21	3.9 ± 0.8		(0.9)	(0.4)	(0.4)	(0.9)
TEC	0.4 ± 0.1	9	2.2 ± 0.5	18	5.8	9.5	4.1	19.5
					(1.1)	(3.8)	(2.3)	(4.1)
DBA/3	0.3 ± 0.1	4	2.2 ± 0.5	60	1.8	5.5	4.7	10.5
					(1.1)	(2.3)	(0.9)	(2.5)

* Cell cycle analysis of the five tumor lines were computerized by Steel and Hanes' method.[13]

† Day 1 = day first nodule of a growing tumor is detectable.

‡ VDT (volume-doubling time), log $(10 \times V) - (\pi/6) \times D_1 \times D_2 \times D_3$; $D_1 - 3$ are three diameters measured by calipers.

§ Standard error is shown in parentheses.

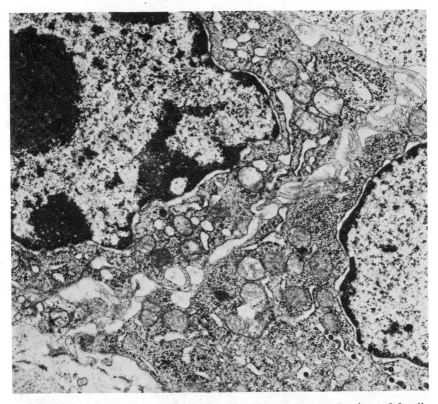

FIGURE 8. Electron micrograph of TEC spindle-cell sarcoma. Portions of 2 cells are seen and the elongated portions of both cells show ribosomes and polyribosomes. Mitochondria are either empty (that is, free of cristae) or show a single membrane; many vacuoles are apparent. Margination of chromatin is seen along the nuclear membranes, and clumps of chromatin appear within the nucleoplasm; there are many vacuoles within the cytoplasmic matrix. (Original magnification × 22,000.)

during the cell cycle time differs with each tumor type. Specifically, the post-synthetic period (T_{G_2}) varies from 3.2 hours for the dbrB tumor, 4.8 hours for the DBAH tumor, 6.5 hours for the MT2 tumor, 4.5 hours for the TEC tumor, and 4.7 hours for the DBA/3 tumor. The frequency of labeled mitoses rises rapidly after the G_2 period and reaches a peak of approximately 98% of labeled mitoses within about 5 hours for the dbrB tumor. The frequency of labeled mitoses after the G_2 period of the two other mammary tumors (DBAH and MT2) reaches peaks at about 88% and 82% of labeled mitoses, respectively. There is, however, a significant difference in the time the waves of labeled mitoses need to reach a peak. This difference is expressed to a greater extent by the MT2 tumor, which reaches its peak of labeled mitoses within 10 hours; whereas about 8 hours is needed by the DBAH tumor for the same process. A still greater difference lies in formation of the second peak by the wave of labeled mitoses for these two mammary tumors. Namely, whereas a second wave of labeled mitoses of the DBAH tumor reaches a peak at about 58% at 24 hours post injection of the labeled precursor, the second wave of labeled mitoses of the MT2 mammary tumor is far away from the descending arm of the first wave, and terminates at 45 hours post injection of the labeled precursor, forming a wide trough, which indicates intermitotic times. The slower growth of the MT2 mammary carcinoma (compared with the mammary carcinomas dbrB and DBAH) may be attributed to the long G_2 phase of 6.5 hours and the long T_c of 32 hours. The waves of labeled mitoses of the DBA/3 lymphoblastic type of lymphoma and that of the TEC spindle-cell sarcoma produced only single peaks at about 65% and 75%, respectively. The descending arms of the curves were short and continued to horizontally form wavy "fading" curves, terminating at about 50 hours after the administration of the labeled nucleotide. The almost complete absence of the second peak of the TEC and DBA/3 tumors may imply that the initial synchrony of the cohort of labeled cells had been lost during one cell cycle. It was possible, however, to make estimates of the cell cycle phases of these tumors (TABLE 1).

According to Steel,[14] "fading" may indicate a progressive loss of labeled proliferating cells or a progressive accumulation of unlabeled proliferating cells. Fade can also be expected in cases of any cell population that has a slowly proliferating stem-cell pool. Another possibility of "fading" may occur if

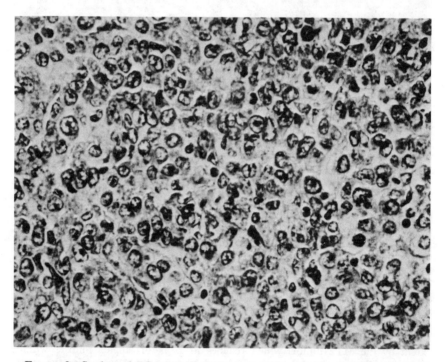

FIGURE 9. Section of DBA/3 lymphoblastic type lymphoma. The nuclei of the tumor cells vary greatly in size; nucleoli are prominent. (Hematoxylin and eosin stain; original magnification × 350.)

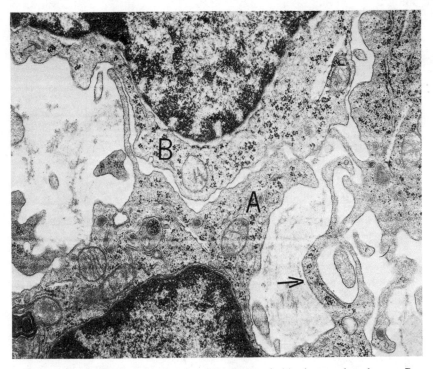

FIGURE 10. Electron micrograph of DBA/3 lymphoblastic type lymphoma. Portions of three cells show projections of plasma membranes (arrow). Cell **A** shows four mitochondria, of which only one has three thin cristae; others are free of cristae, and ribosomes and polyribosomes fill the cytoplasmic matrix. Cell **B** shows a narrow rim of cytoplasm, one empty mitochondrion, polyribosomes, and ribosomes. (Original magnification × 35,200; reduced by 15%.)

primitive cells have a lower ratio of S-phase duration to mean intermitotic time. In such a case, the labeled mitoses curve will progressively decay to the "fading" level.

Electron Microscopic Observations

At the ultrastructural level, each of the five types of tumors show their individual intracellular characteristics (FIGS. 2, 4, 6, 8, and 10). These characteristics are particularly evident from the quality and quantity of the cytoplasmic components, and these in turn are reflected in cellular population kinetics. Specifically, as the electron micrographs illustrate, the portions of the cytoplasm of the dbrB, DBAH, and MT2 mammary carcinomas are rich in ribosomes and polyribosomes (both important in protein biosynthesis), in mitochondria, the carriers of oxidative enzymes, which are important for metabolic processes, including DNA synthesis, thereby controlling the events

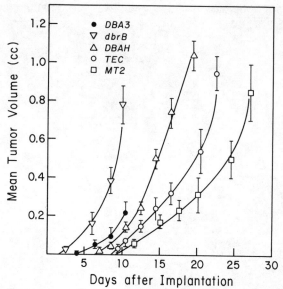

FIGURE 11. Curves presenting the rate of growth of the five types of tumors.

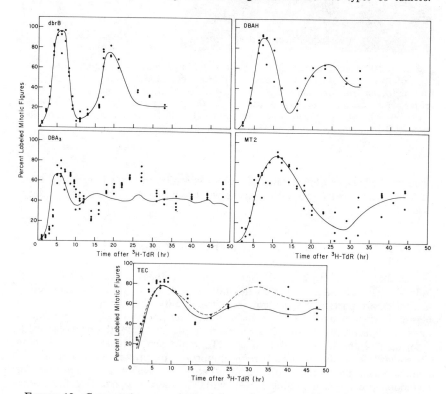

FIGURE 12. Computed curves obtained from the data on cell proliferation kinetics of the five types of tumors.

of the cell cycle proliferation. This is borne out by the labeled mitoses curves of these five types of tumors (FIG. 12). Specifically, the dbrB, DBAH, and MT2 mammary tumor cells, rich in cytoplasmic organelles, resulted in labeled mitoses curves with two well-defined peaks. Conversely, the cytoplasmic matrix of the TEC and DBA/3 tumors, showing paucity of mitochondria and other cytoplasmic components of the tumor cells, failed to produce second waves of labeled mitoses. In other words, the cells of the TEC and DBA/3 tumors were able to traverse only one cycle. Thus, the present study appears to have shown a controlling influence on cell proliferation kinetics by the integrity of cytoplasmic components.

RADIOTHERAPY

Studies on the effects of ionizing irradiation on various types of tumors have been performed in this laboratory for many years. The results from these studies have been published in various scientific journals in this country and in Europe. It would be too lengthy to give an account of this work. Instead, the interested reader is referred to recent publications, which give brief accounts of studies concerning radiation effects on biological systems at tissue, cell, and subcellular levels.[16]

At this time, I am giving a concise account of the current investigations dealing with combined treatments using either ionizing irradiation, such as X-rays, or nonionizing radiation, such as microwaves. A typical example is briefly described: Mice matched for predetermined size of tumors are selected. A number of tumor-bearing mice are assigned to a specific treatment group and an equal number serve as untreated controls. The tumor-bearing mouse is placed in a lead cylinder of 2.4 cm internal diameter and a 0.6-cm-thick wall; the tumor and its enveloping skin are elevated above a longitudinal 0.2-cm-wide opening in the lead wall, obstruction of blood supply being avoided. This device proved to protect the rest of the animal's organs, while the tumor was exposed to radiation treatment.

In recent years there has been an increased interest in using various drugs for therapy of neoplasms (human and animal) in combination with irradiation. Also interest has been renewed in the use of hyperthermia alone or in combination with X-irradiation and drugs in the treatment of tumors. Briefly, an experiment performed in this laboratory resulted in an enhancement factor of 3.9 when treatment was applied to a mammary carcinoma in which triple agents—X-rays, microwave hyperthermia, and a specific drug, misonidazole—were simultaneously administered.[15] Currently, we are obtaining total regressions of tumors in mice by treatments with microwave hyperthermia alone.†

SUMMARY

This study was carried out on five types of experimental tumors maintained by serial subcutaneous transplants in isogeneic mouse hosts. These tumors involved three mammary carcinomas (dbrB, DBAH, MT2), a spindle-cell sarcoma (TEC) and a lymphoblastic type of lymphoma (DBA/3). Growth

† Initial results of this study were presented at the annual meeting of the Radiation Research Society, held in Minneapolis, Minnesota in June 1981 and were published in Abstracts of Papers for the Twenty-Ninth Annual Meeting of the Radiation Research Society (abstract Gbp1): 101.

curves of these tumors are presented. Computed percent labeled mitoses curves for the five types of tumors, the derived cell cycle parameters (T_{G_1}, T_{G_2}, T_s, T_c), and the volume-doubling time (VDT) in days are also presented. The histologic and morphologic appearance of each type of tumor is seen by light microscopy, and the ultrastructural morphology of each type of tumor is seen in electron micrographs. The variation in the kinetic parameters and the autoradiographic exposure time needed to obtain comparable labeling intensity for the five types of tumors is interpreted on the basis of the ultrastructural integrity of the cytoplasmic components of the individual tumor type. The response of these five tumor types to radiotherapy was investigated. The therapy consisted of administering combined treatments of three agents: X-rays, the radiosensitizing drug, misonidazole, and microwave hyperthermia. This treatment resulted in an enhancement factor of 3.9, compared with that of X-rays alone. Total tumor regressions were obtained with microwave hyperthermia alone. The required time of exposure to hyperthermic treatments differed, depending on the response of each type of tumor.

ACKNOWLEDGMENT

I wish to express my appreciation to Dr. Gordon G. Steel of the Imperial Cancer Institute, Surrey, England, for computing the data obtained from the studies on the kinetic characteristics of the tumors.

REFERENCES

1. GOLDFEDER, A. 1950. Further studies on the relationship between radiation effects, cell viability and induced resistance to malignant growth. Radiology **54:** 93–115.
2. HOWARD, A. & S. R. PELC. 1951. Nuclear incorporation of 32P as demonstrated by autoradiography. Exp. Cell Res. **2:** 178–187.
3. HUGHES, W. L., V. P. BOND, G. BRECHER, *et al.* 1958. Cellular proliferation in the mouse as revealed by autoradiography with tritiated thymidine. Proc. Natl. Acad. Sci. USA **44:** 470–483.
4. GOLDFEDER, A. 1965. Biological properties and radiosensitivity of tumors: Demonstration of the cell cycle and time of synthesis of deoxyribonucleic acid using tritiated thymidine and autoradiography. Nature **207:** 612–614.
5. CAMERON, I. L. 1964. Is the duration of DNA synthesis in somatic cells of mammals and birds a constant? J. Cell Biol. **20:** 185–188.
6. GOLDFEDER, A. 1963. Radiosensitivity at the subcellular level. Laval Med. **34:** 12–43.
7. GREEN, E. L. 1966. Biology of the Laboratory Mouse. McGraw-Hill. New York, NY.
8. GOLDFEDER, A. 1954. Studies on radiosensitivity and immunizing ability of mammary tumors of mice. Brit. J. Cancer. **VIII:** 320–335.
9. GOLDFEDER, A. 1972. Urethan and X-ray effects on mice of a tumor resistant strain, X/Gf. Cancer Res. **32:** 2771–2777.
10. ROGERS, A. W. 1967. Technique of Autoradiography. Elsevier. Amsterdam.
11. STILLSTROM, J. 1963. Grain Counts Corrections in Autoradiography. Int. J. Appl. Radiat. Isot. **14:** 113–138.

12. BENASI, M., R. PAOLUZI & F. BRESCIANI. 1973. Computer subtraction of background in autoradiography with tritiated thymidine. Cell Tissue Kinet. 6: 81–85.
13. STEEL, G. G. & S. HANES. 1971. The technique of labeled mitoses: Analysis by automatic curve fitting. Cell Tissue Kinet. 4: 93–105.
14. STEEL, G. G. 1977. Growth Kinetics of Tumors. Clarendon Press. Oxford, England.
15. GOLDFEDER, A. 1979. Enhancement of radioresponse of a mouse mammary carcinoma to combined treatments with hyperthermia and radiosensitizer misonidazole. Cancer Res. 39: 2966–2970.
16. GOLDFEDER, A. 1976. An overview of fifty years in cancer research: Autobiographical essay. Cancer Res. 36: 1–9.

THE SYNTHESIS AND RETENTION OF METHOTREXATE POLYGLUTAMATES IN CULTURED HUMAN BREAST CANCER CELLS

Jacques Jolivet, Richard L. Schilsky, Brenda D. Bailey, and Bruce A. Chabner

Clinical Pharmacology Branch
Division of Cancer Treatment
National Cancer Institute
Bethesda, Maryland 20205

INTRODUCTION

Methotrexate ($4\text{-}NH_2\text{-}10\text{-}CH_3\text{-}PteGlu_1$; MTX) is an antineoplastic agent commonly used in the treatment of acute lymphoblastic leukemia, choriocarcinoma, osteogenic sarcoma, breast cancer, and other tumors. The drug is a potent inhibitor of the enzyme dihydrofolate reductase (DHFR) and thus prevents the reduction of the folate cofactors oxidized during the synthesis of thymidylate from dUMP. This inhibition eventually depletes the intracellular pool of reduced folates and inhibits purine, thymidylate, and DNA synthesis.[1] The cytotoxic effects of MTX appear to depend on the maintenance of intracellular drug concentrations in excess of DHFR's binding capacity for the drug, since its biochemical effects are rapidly reversed by washout of the free drug from the extracellular space.[2]

Like the physiological folate cofactors, MTX is metabolized intracellularly by many human and animal tissues to poly-γ-glutamyl derivatives.[3] These derivatives are synthesized *in vivo* by human red blood cells[4] and liver[5] and *in vitro* by human fibroblasts,[6] bone marrow aspirates,[7] and various murine tissues and tumors.[8-11] The role of these metabolites in MTX's cytotoxic effects, however, is still controversial. Methotrexate polyglutamates are selectively retained intracellularly in human fibroblasts and murine hepatoma cells and continue to inhibit thymidylate synthesis and cell growth after removal of the extracellular parent drug.[10, 12] Conflicting evidence has been forthcoming, however, from other experiments. Poser *et al.* found that the MTX polyglutamates were not retained *in vitro*[13] or *in vivo* by L1210 cells.[11] In addition, they were unable to correlate polyglutamate formation with the drug's cytotoxic effects on L1210 cells and various normal murine tissues. The functional importance of these metabolites might thus vary among different tissues and tumors of different species.

In the present studies, we have examined the formation, intracellular binding, and retention of MTX polyglutamates in the human breast cancer cell line MCF-7. These studies indicate that these metabolites are selectively retained in this human tumor in amounts sufficient to saturate the cell's MTX binding capacity for prolonged periods after removal of extracellular drug. These metabolites might thus play an important role in sustaining MTX's cytotoxic effects.

184

0077–8923/82/0397–0184 $01.75/0 © 1982, NYAS

MATERIALS AND METHODS

Chemicals

[3′,5′,9-^{3}H]MTX (specific activity 20 Ci/mmol) was purchased from Amersham (Arlington Heights, IL). The drug was further purified by DEAE-cellulose chromatography with elution along a linear gradient of 0.1 to 0.4 NH_4HCO_3, pH 8.3.[14] Unlabeled MTX was obtained from the Drug Synthesis and Chemistry Branch, National Cancer Institute (Bethesda, MD) and purified by the same procedure. Purified synthetic 4-NH_2-10-CH_3-PteGlu[2, 3, and 4] were provided by Drs. John Montgomery (Southern Research Institute, Birmingham, AL) and C.M. Baugh (Department of Biochemistry, University of South Alabama, Mobile, AL).[15] Aquassure liquid scintillation counting fluid was purchased from the New England Nuclear Corporation (Boston, MA), L-glutamine from Flow Laboratories (Hamden, CT) and fetal calf serum (FCS) from Biofluids, Inc. (Rockville, MD). Acetonitrile (CH_3CN) and tetrabutyl ammonium phosphate (PicA®) were obtained from Waters Associates (Milford, MA). Sephadex G-75 was purchased from Pharmacia (Uppsala, Sweden). All other chemicals were of reagent grade and purchased either from Fisher Scientific Co. (Pittsburgh, PA) or Sigma Chemical Co. (St. Louis, MO).

Propagation of Cells in Culture

MCF-7 cells, a line of human breast cancer cells in continuous monolayer culture, were provided by Dr. Marc Lippman (National Cancer Institute, Bethesda, MD). The human derivation, hormonal dependency, and growth characteristics of these cells have been previously described.[16] The cells were grown in improved minimal essential medium (IMEM; NIH Media Unit, Bethesda, MD) supplemented with 10% FCS, L-glutamine at 584 μg/ml, penicillin at 124 μg/ml, and streptomycin at 270 μg/ml under 5% CO_2 at 37° C.

Uptake and Binding Capacity for ^{3}H-MTX in MCF-7 Cells

To determine the ability of the MCF-7 cells to transport MTX intracellularly, cells growing in 25-cm[2] culture flasks (Costar, Cambridge, MA) were exposed to 2 μM [^{3}H]-MTX in IMEM (without folic acid) at 37° C for various periods of time up to a maximum of 60 min. At the end of incubation, the cells were processed as described by Schilsky *et al.*[17] The MCF-7 cells' binding capacity for MTX was determined as follows: Following a 24-hr incubation with 2 μM ^{3}H-MTX, the cells were washed in iced phosphate-buffered saline (PBS), disrupted by three cycles of freeze-thawing, and spun at 100,000 × g for 60 min. The supernatant fraction was then applied to a Sephadex G-75 column and the MTX-dihydrofolate reductase complex was eluted as described below. The amount of bound MTX was then determined by liquid scintillation counting. If we assume a binding stoichiometry of 1:1 for enzyme and inhibitor, the DHFR binding capacity of MCF-7 cells was determined to be 5.7 ± 0.85 nmol/g.

Assay of Intracellular MTX Polyglutamates

The intracellular content of MTX and its poly-γ-glutamyl metabolites was determined as follows: At the end of an incubation period with MTX, the medium was aspirated and the cells washed with ice-cold PBS. The cells were scraped off the flask surface with a rubber policeman and lysed by adding 4.5 ml of ice-cold water. The cell lysate was quickly transferred to a test tube containing 0.5 ml of 100% trichloroacetic acid (TCA) so that a final concentration of 10% TCA was achieved. Cellular debris was pelleted by centrifugation at 10,000 $\times$ g for 15 min and the cell extract injected into a Sep-Pak® C_{18} cartridge (Waters Associates) which had been prepared by prior injection with 2 ml 100% CH_3CN followed by 5 ml of water. The cartridge was then washed by injecting 5 ml of water, after which MTX and its metabolites were eluted with 2 ml of 100% CH_3CN. The sample was evaporated to dryness under N_2 and resuspended in the initial HPLC mobile phase. Of the radioactivity present in the TCA extract, 71 $\pm$ 10% was recovered in the resuspended sample. Most of the unrecovered drug was not adsorbed on the cartridge and was lost during the sample injection and water-washing steps. The recovery rates of authentic MTX and 4-NH_2-10-CH_3-PteGlu$_{2-4}$ were tested individually using the Sep-Pak procedure and determined to be identical for each compound. The total amount of intracellular drug was determined in nmol/g as calculated from the radioactivity in the TCA supernatant, the specific activity of [3H]-MTX used, and the amount of protein in the TCA precipitate as measured by a Lowry protein assay.[18] MTX and its polyglutamate derivatives were separated by means of a recently described HPLC assay [19] that has been modified to give faster but equivalent separations: The mobile phase was prepared by a model 660 solvent programmer (Waters Associates) mixing the effluents of two model 6000A pumps (Waters Associates). Pump A's solvent was KH_2PO_4, 10 mM, with PicA, 5 mM, at pH 5.5, while pump B contained 100% CH_3CN. Sample fractions containing about 2000 dpm were injected onto a Radial-Pak C-8 cartridge (Waters Associates) in an RCM-100 Radial Compression Module (Waters Associates) and eluted at 2 ml/min along gradients of 21 to 27% CH_3CN and 3.95 to 3.65 mM PicA for 15 min, followed by 27% CH_3CN and 3.65 mM PicA for the last 10 min of the separation. The retention times of authentic 4-NH_2-10-CH_3-PteGlu$_{1-4}$ were determined by monitoring ultraviolet absorbance at 313 nm. One-min fractions were collected directly into scintillation vials using an LKB 2112 RediRac fraction collector and assayed for radioactivity by liquid scintillation counting.

Characterization of DHFR-Bound and -Free Intracellular MTX

Separation of DHFR-bound drug from free intracellular MTX was achieved by chromatography of cell extracts on Sephadex G75, as previously described.[20] After incubation with 3H-MTX, cells were washed, scraped off the flask surface, and disrupted by three cycles of freeze-thawing. Cytosol, obtained by centrifugation at 100,000 $\times$ g for 60 min in a Beckman L5–50 ultracentrifuge, was then applied to a 1 $\times$ 25-cm Sephadex G75 column equilibrated with 0.5 M KH_2PH_4, pH 5.9, at 4° C. Fractions of 0.5 ml were collected with the same buffer and a portion of each was taken for liquid scintillation counting and for assay of DHFR activity by a spectrophotometric assay.[21] Fractions containing both tritium and enzyme activity were assayed for MTX polyglutamates using gel filtration on Sephadex G15 as described previously.[20] The molecular weight of the protein co-migrating with MTX was estimated by calibration of the Sephadex G75 column with standard proteins of known molecular weight.

RESULTS

Methotrexate Uptake in MCF-7 Cells

FIGURE 1 illustrates the time course of uptake of [³H]-MTX by MCF-7 cells during a 60-min exposure to a drug concentration of 2 μM. Uptake appeared to be linear during the initial 10 min of drug exposure, after which the rate of drug accumulation slowed and approached a steady-state level of 10 nmol/g, which was sufficient to fully saturate the cell's binding capacity of 5.7 nmol/g. As shown previously by Sephadex G15 chromatography,[20] no significant polyglutamate formation occurred in the MCF-7 cells during a 60-min exposure to 2 μM [³H]-MTX.

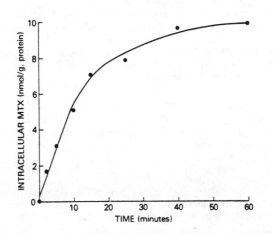

FIGURE 1. Uptake of 2 μM [³H]-MTX by MCF-7 cells.

Methotrexate Polyglutamate Formation in MCF-7 Cells

MCF-7 cells were incubated with 2 μM [³H]-MTX for 24 hours in folate-free IMEM containing 2 mM L-glutamine with 10 μM thymidine (dT) and deoxyinosine (dI) added to prevent cytotoxicity during the incubation period. At the end of incubation, the intracellular distribution of MTX and its γ-glutamyl metabolites was determined by HPLC, and the results of a representative experiment are shown in FIGURE 2 (left upper panel). Five radioactive peaks were identified within the cells: The first four co-chromatographed, respectively, with authentic 4-NH$_2$-10-CH$_3$-PteGlu$_{1-4}$ and made up 46.9, 10.6, 18.2, and 15.2% of the total intracellular drug. The fifth peak, yielding 9.0%

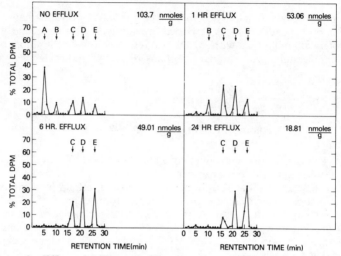

FIGURE 2. Efflux of MTX polyglutamates from MCF-7 cells. After a 24-hr incubation with 2 μM [^{3}H]-MTX, the medium was aspirated, washed once with ice-cold phosphate-buffered saline, and placed in drug-free IMEM. This medium was changed after 1 and 6 hours of efflux. Cell extracts were prepared at the end of incubation and after 1, 6, and 24 hours in drug-free IMEM, and then they were analyzed by HPLC. Peaks A to E represent, respectively, 4-NH$_2$-10-CH$_3$-PteGlu$_1$ (MTX) to 4-NH$_2$-10-CH$_3$PteGlu$_5$. The total amount of intracellular drug in nmol/g of cell protein is given at each time point.

of intracellular drug, eluted with a retention time consistent with 4-NH$_2$-10-CH$_3$-PteGlu$_5$, as shown previously.[19] The cells now contained 103.7 nmol/g of total intracellular MTX, 10 times more than after a 1-hr incubation with the same drug concentration.

TABLE 1

DISTRIBUTION OF INTRACELLULAR MTX AND MTX POLYGLUTAMATES IN MCF-7 CELLS AFTER A 24-HOUR INCUBATION WITH 2-μM MTX [24 (0)] AND AFTER 1 [24 (1)], 6 [24 (6)], AND 24 HOURS [24 (24)] IN DRUG-FREE MEDIUM

	24 (0)	24 (1)	24 (6)	24 (24)
Total Intracellular Drug (nmol/g)	103.7	53.06	49.01	18.81
Amount of Intracellular 4-NH$_2$-10-CH$_3$-PteGlu$_n$ (nmol/g)				
n = 1	48.6	1.8	0.6	0.5
n = 2	11.0	7.5	0.9	0.2
n = 3	18.9	17.6	14.1	2.7
n = 4	15.8	15.3	16.5	6.0
n = 5	9.3	11.0	16.9	9.4

NOTE: After a 24-hr incubation with 2-μM ^{3}H-MTX and after another 1, 6, and 24 hours in drug-free medium, cell extracts of MCF-7 cells were assayed by HPLC for MTX polyglutamates. The total amount of intracellular drug and the respective amounts of 4-NH$_2$-10-CH$_3$-PteGlu$_{1-5}$ are shown from one representative experiment.

Characterization of DHFR-Bound and -Free Intracellular MTX

To determine whether the MTX polyglutamates formed in the MCF-7 cells were bound to DHFR, the fraction of intracellular drug bound to DHFR was examined after a 24-hr incubation with 2 μM ^{3}H-MTX. After the incubation, cell cytosol obtained by disruption of the cells and centrifugation at 100,000 $\times$ g for 60 min was applied to a Sephadex G75 column, as described in the MATERIALS AND METHODS section. Radioactive material eluted at a position that coincided with DHFR activity (FIG. 3A) and that corresponded to a protein of molecular weight 19,800 (FIG. 3B). A late-eluting radioactivity peak was also found and presumed to represent free intracellular MTX. Disruption of the MTX-DHFR complex by boiling followed by Sephadex G15 chromatography [20] demonstrated that greater than 70% of enzyme-bound MTX was in the form of polyglutamates (FIG. 3C).

Retention of MTX Polyglutamates by MCF-7 Cells

The ability of the breast cancer cells to retain MTX and its polyglutamates in drug-free medium after an initial period of drug exposure was next investigated. The amounts of MTX and MTX polyglutamates were determined by

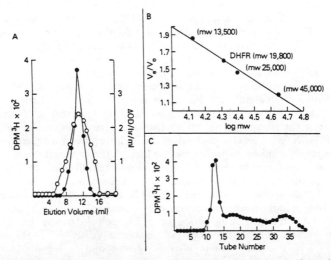

FIGURE 3. Characterization of DHFR-bound MTX. After incubation with 2 μM [^{3}H]-MTX for 24 hours, MCF-7 cells were placed in drug-free medium for a 1-hr efflux period. (A) Cell extracts were chromatographed on Sephadex G75, pH 5.9, at 4° C. Aliquots of each fraction were taken for liquid scintillation counting (●) and for DHFR activity (○). Free intracellular MTX was eluted at 20–30 ml. (B) The M_r of the protein co-migrating with [^{3}H]-MTX was estimated by calibration of the Sephadex G75 column with proteins of known M_r, V_e, elution volume; V_o void volume. (C) Fractions containing both radioactivity and DHFR activity were boiled to dissociate drug from enzyme and rechromatographed on Sephadex G15. The early peak (tubes 10–15) represents 4-NH$_2$-10-CH$_3$-PteGlu$_{2-5}$, while the late peak (tubes 30–35) co-chromatographs with MTX.

HPLC in the MCF-7 cells at the end of a 24-hr incubation with 2 μM ^{3}H-MTX and after 1, 6, and 24 hours in drug-free IMEM following the end of drug incubation; 10 μM dT and dI were added to prevent cytotoxicity during the efflux period. The results of a representative experiment are shown in FIGURE 2 and TABLE 1. Most (60%) of the drug efflux occurred in the first hour in drug-free medium and was almost completely accounted for by the loss of parent drug. Almost all of the 4-NH$_2$-10-CH$_3$-PteGlu$_{2,3}$ left the cells (98 and 86%, respectively), while 38% and 100% of the 4-NH$_2$-10-CH$_3$-PteGlu$_{4,5}$ were retained intracellularly in sufficient amounts (6.0 and 9.4 nmol/g, respectively) to exceed the cells' MTX binding capacity (5.7 nmol/g), even after 24 hours in drug-free medium.

DISCUSSION

Naturally occurring folates undergo a process of polyglutamation in which as many as 7 glutamyl residues are added to the vitamin through γ-peptide linkage.[3] The role of this process in folate metabolism is incompletely understood, although folate polyglutamates are preferentially retained intracellularly and have greatly increased affinity for certain folate-requiring enzymes compared with that of the parent compounds.[3]

The corresponding polyglutamates of the folate analog MTX have been identified in a variety of normal and neoplastic cells.[4-13, 17, 19, 20] In the present experiments, we have used a highly specific HPLC technique [19] to separate and quantify MTX and polyglutamate derivatives containing one to four additional amino acids. This method offers the significant advantage of allowing examination of the formation and retention of each of these derivatives.

MTX polyglutamates are active metabolites of MTX: They not only bind to DHFR but have also been shown in human fibroblasts and murine hepatoma cells to inhibit thymidylate synthesis and cell growth.[10, 12] These metabolites might play an important role in MTX's action if retained for significant periods of time after the disappearance of extracellular drug. Since the biochemical effects of MTX are quickly reversed when its intracellular concentration falls below the cell's binding capacity for the drug,[2] the retained higher polyglutamates could continue to saturate DHFR even after efflux of the parent drug, and consequently prolong drug effects. This phenomenon could help to explain how a cell-cycle-specific agent such as MTX exerts cytotoxic effects against slow-growing tumors such as human breast cancer. Although the selective retention and prolonged drug action of MTX polyglutamates has been confirmed in human fibroblasts [12] and rat hepatoma cells,[10, 22] it did not occur in vitro in L1210 cells [13] and in vivo in various murine tumors and normal tissues.[11] Since the authors of the latter study could not correlate MTX polyglutamate formation with the drug's cytotoxic effects in these tissues,[11] the synthesis of these metabolites could conceivably have a lesser impact on drug action in tissues where they are not selectively retained.

In the MCF-7 human breast cancer cell line, MTX polyglutamate formation occurs progressively during an incubation with 2 μM MTX over a 24-hr period, after which time the metabolites can be identified bound to DHFR.[20] Furthermore, when MTX is removed from the culture medium, 4-NH$_2$-10-CH$_3$PteGlu$_{4 \text{ and } 5}$ are retained intracellularly in sufficient amounts to overwhelm DHFR's binding capacity for MTX and, as determined in experiments not shown here, to persistently inhibit DHFR and cell growth more than 24 hours after drug removal. Consequently, MTX polyglutamate formation and retention probably play an important role in the drug's mechanism of action in the MCF-7 cell line. Many other questions, however, such as the relative binding affinities of MTX and its polyglutamate derivatives to DHFR and the precise characterization by HPLC of the enzyme-bound and -free drug fractions in the cytosol, remain to be elucidated.

The formation of MTX polyglutamates may be an important step in the action of MTX in man. Along with drug transport [23] and target enzyme concentration [24], MTX polyglutamate formation needs to be considered as a possible mechanism of *de novo* or acquired drug resistance.

REFERENCES

1. CHABNER, B. A. 1982. Methotrexate. *In* Pharmacologic Principles of Cancer Treatment. B. A. Chabner, Ed.: 229–255. Saunders. Philadelphia, PA.
2. WHITE, C. J., S. LOTFIELD & I. D. GOLDMAN. 1975. The mechanism of action of methotrexate. III. Requirement of free intracellular methotrexate for maximal suppression of ^{14}C-formate incorporation into nucleic acids and protein. Mol. Pharmacol. **11:** 287–297.
3. COVEY, J. M. 1980. Polyglutamate derivatives of folic acid coenzymes and methotrexate. Life Sci. **26:** 665–678.
4. BAUGH, C. M., C. L. KRUMDIECK & M. G. NAIR. 1973. Polygammaglutamyl metabolites of methotrexate. Biochem. Biophys. Res. Commun. **52:** 27–34.
5. JACOBS, S. A., C. J. DERR & D. G. JOHNS. 1977. Accumulation of methotrexate diglutamate in human liver during methotrexate therapy. Biochem. Pharmacol. **26:** 2310–2313.
6. ROSENBLATT, D. S., V. M. WHITEHEAD, M. M. DUPONT, M. J. VUCHICH & J. VERA. 1978. Synthesis of methotrexate polyglutamates in cultured human cells. Mol. Pharmacol. **14:** 210–214.
7. WITTE, A., V. M. WHITEHEAD, D. S. ROSENBLATT & M. J. VUCHICH. 1980. Synthesis of methotrexate polyglutamates by bone marrow cells from patients with leukemia and lymphoma. Dev. Pharmacol. Ther. **1:** 40–46.
8. WHITEHEAD, V. M., M. M. PERRAULT & S. STELCNER. 1975. Tissue-specific synthesis of methotrexate polyglutamates in the rat. Cancer Res. **35:** 2985–2990.
9. WHITEHEAD, V. M. 1977. Synthesis of methotrexate polyglutamates in L1210 murine leukemia cells. Cancer Res. **37:** 408–412.
10. GALIVAN, J. 1980. Evidence for the cytotoxic activity of polyglutamate derivatives of methotrexate. Mol. Pharmacol. **17:** 105–110.
11. POSER, R. G., F. M. SIROTNAK & P. L. CHELLO. 1981. Differential synthesis of methotrexate polyglutamates in normal proliferative and neoplastic mouse tissues *in vivo*. Cancer Res. **41:** 4441–4446.
12. ROSENBLATT, D. S., V. M. WHITEHEAD, N. VERA, A. POTTIER, M. DUPONT & M. J. VUCHICH. 1978. Prolonged inhibition of DNA synthesis associated with the accumulation of methotrexate polyglutamates by cultured human cells. Mol. Pharmacol. **14:** 1143–1147.
13. POSER, R. G., F. M. SIROTNAK & P. L. CHELLO. 1980. Extracellular recovery of methotrexate polyglutamates following efflux from L1210 leukemia cells. Biochem. Pharmacol. **29:** 2701–2704.
14. GOLDMAN, I. D., N. S. LICHTENSTEIN & V. T. OLIVERIO. 1968. Carrier-mediated transport of the folic acid analogue methotrexate in the L1210 leukemia cell. J. Biol. Chem. **243:** 5007–5017.

15. NAIR, M. G. & C. M. BAUGH. 1973. Synthesis and biological evaluation of poly-gamma-glutamyl derivatives of methotrexate. Biochemistry **12:** 3923–3927.
16. SOULE, H. D., J. VAZQUEZ, A. LONG, S. ALBERT & M. BRENNAN. 1973. A human cell line from a pleural effusion derived from a breast carcinoma. J. Natl. Cancer Inst. **51:** 1409–1416.
17. SCHILSKY, R. L., B. D. BAILEY & B. A. CHABNER. 1981. Characteristics of membrane transport of methotrexate by cultured human breast cancer cells. Biochem. Pharmacol. **30:** 1537–1542.
18. LOWRY, O. H., N. J. ROSENBROUGH, A. I. FARR & R. I. RANDALL. 1951. Protein measurement with the folin phenol reagent. J. Biol. Chem. **193:** 265–275.
19. JOLIVET, J. & R. L. SCHILSKY. 1981. High-pressure liquid chromatography analysis of methotrexate polyglutamates in cultured human breast cancer cells. Biochem. Pharmacol. **30:** 1387–1390.
20. SCHILSKY, R. L., B. D. BAILEY & B. A. CHABNER. 1980. Methotrexate polyglutamate synthesis by cultured human breast cancer cells. Proc. Natl. Acad. Sci. USA **77:** 2919–2922.
21. OSBORN, M. J. & F. M. HUENNEKENS. 1958. Enzymatic reduction of dihydrofolic acid. J. Biol. Chem. **233:** 969–974.
22. BALINSKA, M., J. GALIVAN & J. K. COWARD. 1981. Efflux of methotrexate and its polyglutamate derivatives from hepatic cells *in vitro.* Cancer Res. **41:** 2751–2756.
23. ROSOWSKY, A., H. LAZARUS, G. C. YUAN, W. R. BELTZ, L. MANGIN, H. T. ABELSON, E. J. MODEST & E. FREI, III. 1980. Effect of methotrexate esters and other lipophilic antifolates on methotrexate-resistant human leukemic lymphoblasts. Biochem. Pharmacol. **29:** 648–652.
24. BERTINO, J. R., W. L. SAWICKI, A. R. CASHMORE, E. C. CADMAN & R. T. SKEEL. 1977. Natural resistance to methotrexate in human acute nonlymphocytic leukemia. Cancer Treat. Rep. **61:** 667–673.

ONCOGENIC TRANSFORMATION PRODUCED BY AGENTS AND MODALITIES USED IN CANCER THERAPY AND ITS MODULATION *

Carmia Borek and Eric J. Hall

Radiological Research Laboratory
Department of Radiology and Pathology
Cancer Center/Institute of Cancer Research
Columbia University
College of Physicians and Surgeons
New York, New York 10032

INTRODUCTION

The long-term survival of certain patients after treatment with radiation or chemotherapeutic agents has allowed the realization that agents that effectively control cancer in the human subject may also possess an oncogenic potential, resulting in secondary malignancies in a significant proportion of surviving patients.[1]

A quantitative assessment of the oncogenic effects of these agents at a cellular level is important, as is information on conditions and agents that may effectively alter the development of the neoplastic state.

Cell culture systems where the neoplastic transformation of cells can be scored after exposure to carcinogens offer powerful tools for evaluating the oncogenic potential of radiation and chemotherapeutic agents.

ONCOGENIC TRANSFORMATION BY RADIATION

Hamster Embryo Cells

The initial unequivocal demonstration that mammalian cells can be transformed *in vitro* by radiation utilized freshly cultured hamster embryo cells exposed to X-rays.[2-4] The following conditions were required for an effective transformation of cells into neoplastic cells that ultimately gave rise to tumors in suitable hosts: (1) the exposed cells must replicate soon after treatment in order to fix transformation as a hereditary property of the cells;[3] and (2) several cell replications are required for expression of transformation *in vitro* into cells with a markedly different morphologic pattern from the norm[3, 4] (FIG. 1). While a near-diploid karyotype, as assessed by banding methods, is seen at early stages of transformation,[5] a variety of striking membrane-associated changes are observed soon after transformation in the X-ray-transformed cells as compared with the normal ones.[5-7] These include changed surface features as seen by scanning electron microscopic[6] changes in Na^+ transport enzymes,[7] incomplete synthesis of gangliosides,[5] and increased levels of cellular proteases.[5, 8]

* This investigation was supported by Grant CA 12536–11 to the Radiological Research Laboratory/Department of Radiology.

193

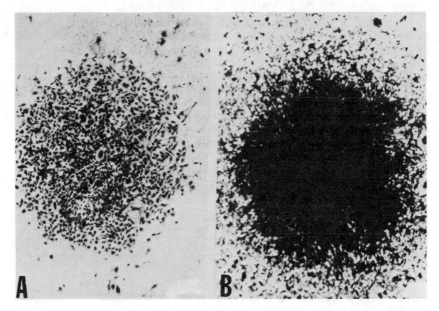

FIGURE 1. (A) a colony of normal hamster embryo cells. (B) a colony of X-ray-transformed hamster embryo cells.

Our early quantitative studies on radiation-induced transformation were carried out utilizing the hamster embryo system described above. These studies include the dose-neoplastic effects of X-rays,[8, 9] neutrons,[8] and argon ions,[8] the transforming potential of split doses of X-rays as compared with the oncogenic effects of the same total dose delivered in a single exposure; [10, 11] and the relative biological effectiveness (RBE) of X-rays versus gamma rays.[12]

The protocol for the utilization of the hamster embryo cell systems as a quantitative assay has been described in detail previously,[8, 9] but the essentials, which are illustrated in FIGURE 2, are as follows: A cell suspension is prepared by mincing and dissociating the tissue of a midterm embryo with trypsin. Cells are plated at low density and treated with radiation or chemical agents after overnight attachment. The cells are incubated for 10 days to allow colony formation before they are fixed and stained, by which time transformed clones can be distinguished by their altered morphologic pattern. The counting of the number of normal and transformed clones in treated versus control dishes allows an assessment of both the surviving fraction and the transformation frequency within the same dishes. FIGURE 3 shows transformation data for hamster embryo cells exposed to X-rays and to 430-KeV monoenergetic neutrons. Many of these data have been published previously,[8] but recent data down to 3 mGy (1 Gy = 100 rad) have been added. The cell-survival data from the same experiments are shown in FIGURE 4.

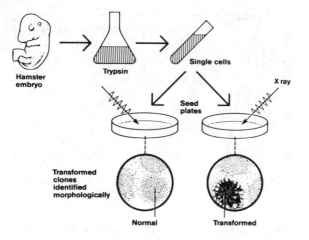

FIGURE 2. *In vitro* assay of hamster embryo cells transformed by radiation.

Several conclusions can be drawn from the hamster embryo data. First, the transformation data for neutrons might be adequately represented by a straight line with a slope of unity on the double logarithmic plot of FIGURE 3. This would imply that the incidence of transformation is proportional to dose. Secondly, the neutron RBE is clearly changing with dose for both cell killing and transformation, and over the limited dose range where both endpoints can be scored, RBE values are similar.

More recent experiments have focused on the RBE for X-rays versus gamma rays, over a range of 1.5 Gy down to 0.03 Gy. While larger doses are utilized in

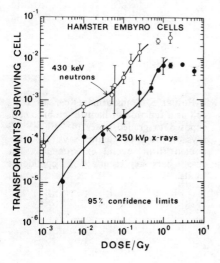

FIGURE 3. Pooled data for the hamster embryo cells of the number of transformants per surviving cell after irradiation with 250-kVp X-rays (*solid circles*) or 430-KeV monoenergetic neutrons (*open circles*) produced at the Radiological Research Accelerator Facility. The error bars indicate 95% confidence intervals for the estimated value. The curves were obtained using B-spline fitting (in the least-squares sense) and with the additional constraint of nontoxicity upward; they will be regarded only as a smooth representation of the shape of the data with a minimum of parametric-related bias.

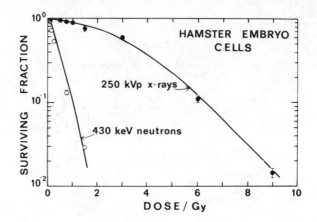

FIGURE 4. Pooled data for the survival of hamster embryo cells irradiated with 250-kVp X-rays (*open circles*) or 430-keV monoenergetic neutrons (*solid circles*). The error bars indicate the estimated standard deviations. The curves are the result of fitting the expression in Equation 1 to the data using the maximum likelihood method.

therapy, clearly the surrounding field of the areas treated are exposed to a range of doses. Our findings, seen in FIGURE 5, indicate that the oncogenic potential of X-rays is twice that of gamma rays at a low dose of 0.3 Gy, while at a higher dose their effectiveness is similar.[12] These results indicate that when the oncogenic effects of these two types of low LET radiation are compared, the extrapolation from high to low doses may be neither conservative nor prudent, depending on the distribution of dose in time.

Another illustration of caution required in extrapolation is illustrated in our studies on the effectiveness of acute versus protracted doses of X-rays.

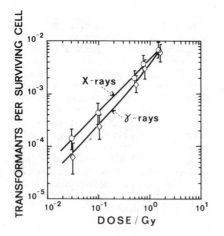

FIGURE 5. Transformants per surviving cell as a function of hamster embryo cells exposed to graded doses of 250-keV X-rays or cobalt-60 gamma rays. Data are pooled from several experiments. The error bars represent 95% confidence limits.

Our findings *in vitro,* illustrated in detail elsewhere,[10, 11] indicate that at doses of 75 and 50 rad (0.75 and 0.50 Gy) the deliverance of the total dose in two fractions separated by 5 hours results in a 70% enhancement of transformation compared with results with the same total amount of radiation absorbed as one single dose. At the higher doses of 150 to 600 rad (1.5 to 6.0 Gy), fractionation leads to a protective effect.[11] Cell survival was enhanced in all cases of fractionated doses, both at low as well as at higher dose levels, suggesting that cellular mechanisms responsible for repair of transformation lesions differ from repair mechanisms responsible for cell survival.[10] Similar results have been obtained using the 10T½ cell line, as described later.

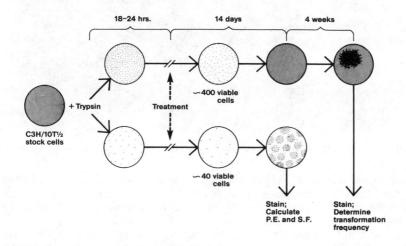

FIGURE 6. Protocol for experiments with 10T½ cells; see text for details.

Experiments with Mouse 10T½ Cells

The advantages of the hamster embryo system lie in the fact that these diploid cells are removed by only a few divisions from growth *in vivo.* Both survival and transformation can be scored in the same plate. Transformants are immortal while the normal cells become senescent. For long-term studies there is a disadvantage in using cell strains, since cloning of normal cell population with a finite life span is a limiting factor. An alternative to the use of cell strains is the utilization of cell lines, although one must be aware of their heteroploid nature. Cell lines enable the continuous experimentation with cells from a common population which possesses an infinite life span. One such line, which is a cloned mouse fibroblast line, is that of the C_3H 10T½ cell system.[13]

We have utilized this cell line in parallel with the hamster embryo cell system, and have found that qualitatively results are similar.[14-18]

The way in which experiments are conducted with this cell line is illustrated in FIGURE 6. Cells are seeded at two concentrations. To assess plating efficiency and surviving fraction, a sufficient number of cells are seeded per dish so that

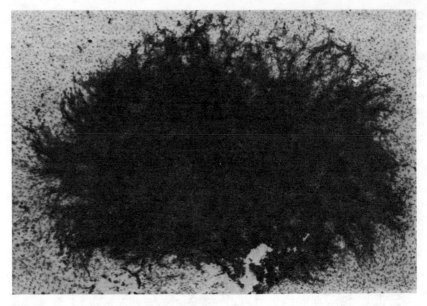

FIGURE 7. A focus of transformed 10T½ cells on a background of normal cells.

about 50 will survive the treatment and grow into colonies that can be counted 14 days later. For the transformation assay, cells are seeded so that about 300 viable cells survive treatment. By two weeks post irradiation, the cells have formed a confluent layer and stop dividing, but a further 4 weeks is needed after confluent incubation before the transformed foci can be identified by their changed morphologic configuration: densely stained piled-up cells with a criss-cross pattern at the periphery of the focus, against a background of lightly stained, contact-inhibited nontransformed cells (FIG. 7).

Pooled data from several experiments relating transformation incidence and cell survival following exposure to single doses of X-rays are shown in FIGURE 8,

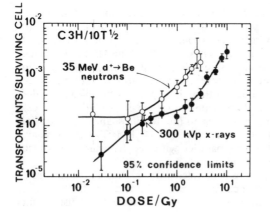

FIGURE 8. Pooled data obtained with 10T½ cells for the fraction of transformants per surviving cell after irradiation with 300-kVp X-rays (*solid circles*) or neutrons produced with 35-MeV d⁺→Be (*open circles*). The error bars indicate 95% confidence intervals for the estimated value of the fraction.

together with the more limited data for high-energy cyclotron-produced neutrons (35 MeV) at the Naval Research Laboratory in Washington. The X-ray data involved the use of more than 30,000 petri dishes with about 1500 transformed foci scored from roughly 12 million cells at risk.

The X-ray dose–response relationship has a complex shape. At doses above 1 Gy the data are consistent with a slope of 2, implying a quadratic transformation dependence on dose. Below 0.3 Gy, the data are consistent with a slope of 1, implying direct proportionality to dose. Between 0.3 and 1 Gy, the curve is very shallow; indeed within the confidence intervals of the data points, the transformation frequency might not vary with dose over this range.

A number of conclusions can be drawn from these data. The RBE values for cell killing and transformation are similar at a given dose. For transformation the RBE increases with decreasing dose. The shape of the neutron dose–response curve at low doses is of interest; the 0.02-Gy data point comes from one single experiment, but if the result is confirmed in future studies, this would imply an absence of proportionality between dose and effect in a dose region where the traversal of no more than one charged particle per cell nucleus would be expected.

Experiments have also been performed with single and split X-ray doses and the data published.[17] The results are simliar to those with the hamster cells. At doses above 1.5 Gy, fractionation leads to a reduction in transformation frequency compared with results with a single exposure. In contrast, between 0.3 and 1 Gy, fractionation enhances the incidence of transformation. This results directly from the changing slope of the dose–response relationship for single exposures if complete recovery between the split doses is assumed.

The similarity in data between those obtained for split doses of hamster embryo cells and those for the 10T½ cells is clearly seen in FIGURE 9. Similar results on enhanced transformation by splitting low doses has been reported in the 3T3 cell line.[19]

ONCOGENIC TRANSFORMATION BY CHEMOTHERAPEUTIC AGENTS

Experiments were undertaken using the 10T½ cells to assess the oncogenic effects of commonly used chemotherapeutic agents and the hypoxic cell radio-

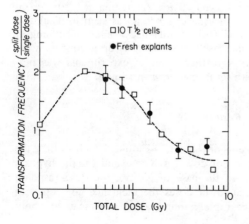

FIGURE 9. Ratio of the transformation incidence for split and single X-ray doses as a function of total X-ray dose. (Data for hamster cells from Borek[11] and for 10T½ cells from Miller and Hall.[17])

sensitizer, misonidazole, and to compare them to the oncogenic potential produced by X-rays.[20] The cells were cultured as described above. Briefly, cells between passage 8 and 13 were grown in Eagle's basal medium, supplemented with 10% heat-activated fetal bovine serum together with penicillin and streptomycin to retard bacterial contamination.

For transformation studies with X-rays or misonidazole, cells were seeded into 50-cm² petri dishes so that approximately 400 reproductively viable cells per dish survived the subsequent treatment. After overnight incubation at 37° C to allow the cells to adhere, they were exposed to X-rays or to misonidazole.

In the case of X-rays, cells were treated at room temperature using a Siemens ortho-voltage X-ray unit operating at 300 kVp and 12 mA, with 0.2 mm Cu added filtration. On the basis of measurements with a Victoreen R-meter the dose rate at the location of the cells was calculated to be 0.36 Gy min⁻¹ (1 Gy = 100 rad). For misonidazole, a 3-day exposure was used in a range of drug concentrations.

Because the quantities of some of the chemotherapeutic agents were limited, a modified experimental technique was used so that cells were treated at high density in a few dishes and subsequently trypsinized and reseeded at low density to assay for transformation. Briefly, cells from stock flasks were seeded at 5×10^5 cells per cm² flask. Three days later the drug was added and remained in contact with exponentially growing cells for 24 hours, after which the drug was removed and the cells trypsinized and replated into 50-cm² petri dishes. To determine the frequency of oncogenic transformation, cells were plated at appropriate cell densities to allow about 400 reproductively viable cells per dish. At the same time dishes were seeded at one-quarter of the cell densities used in the transformation assay and incubated for 12 to 14 days, by which time individual macro-colonies were visible. Colonies were fixed with 10% formalin, stained with Giemsa, and counted to determine plating efficiency and drug-induced cell killing. Cells being tested for drug-induced transformation were refed every 10 days (20 ml of medium per dish) with fresh medium for a total of 5 weeks and then fixed and stained. Transformed foci were scored as described earlier.

All drugs were weighed and then diluted in growth medium to the required concentration. The concentration of the five chemotherapeutic drugs was selected so that cell killing would not exceed 70%. Vincristine at 0.001 µg/ml and melphalan at 0.1 µg/ml resulted in little cell killing, as seen in TABLE 1. Adriamycin (0.001 µg/ml and 5 aza C (0.1 µg/ml) had similar cell killing at about 50%. Cis-platinum showed increased cell killing as drug concentration increased from 0.05 to 0.2 µg/ml. A further series of experiments was performed to compare cis-platinum with its isomer trans-platinum.

Results

Pooled data from many experiments are shown in FIGURE 10, illustrating the transformation incidence as a function of dose for X-rays and for the hypoxic cell radiosensitizer, misonidazole.[21] In the case of X-rays, the dose–response relationship has a complex shape: at lower doses the incidence goes up with dose, slowly at first and then more rapidly, but reaches a plateau at about

TABLE 1

24-HOUR EXPOSURE OF C3H/10T½ CELLS TO CHEMOTHERAPEUTIC DRUGS

	SF(PE)	Number of Dishes	Type II	Type III	Number of Dishes with Transformations	Fraction of Dishes with Transformations	Transformation Frequency $(10^{-4}) \pm 1$ SE (Transformants/ Surviving Cell)
Control	(0.22)	36	0	0	0	0	0
Vincristine, 0.001 µg/ml	0.94	100	0	4	4	0.04	0.66 ± 3.3
Melphalan, 0.1 µg/ml	0.94	59	1	15	15	0.25	4.45 ± 1.1
Adriamycin, 0.001 µg/ml	0.52	35	1	9	10	0.29	8.48 ± 2.7
5 aza C, 0.1 µg/ml	0.46	40	1	19	15	0.38	15.90 ± 3.6
Cis-platinum 0.05 µg/ml	0.66	148	0	4	4	0.027	0.68 ± 3.4
0.1 µg/ml	0.35	156	0	6	6	0.038	0.92 ± 3.8
0.2 µg/ml	0.063	77	0	10	10	0.130	12.90 ± 4.1

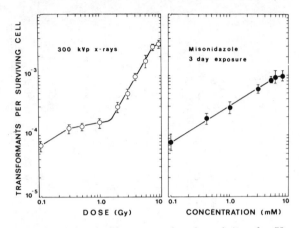

FIGURE 10. Transformation incidence as a function of dose for X-rays (*left*) and for a 3-day exposure to the hypoxic cell radiosensitizer, misonidazole (*right*)

3×10^{-3} for doses of 6 Gy and above. The maximal concentration of misonidazole that can be obtained in the serum of a patient after an oral administration of the drug is about 0.5 mM, which corresponds to an X-ray dose of about 0.5 Gy and produces a transformation incidence of 10^{-4} (0.01%).

FIGURE 11 shows the incidence of transformation obtained for the various chemotherapeutic agents tested; *cis*-platinum produced the highest rate and vincristine the lowest. *Cis*-platinum and *trans*-platinum are compared in FIGURE 12 for their effectiveness in cell killing and their efficiency in producing transformations. These compounds differ only slightly in structure, but produce quite different incidence of oncogenic transformation. The reason for the difference is that *cis*-platinum produces crosslinks between the two strands of DNA. For example, it is suggested that it forms a chelate between two

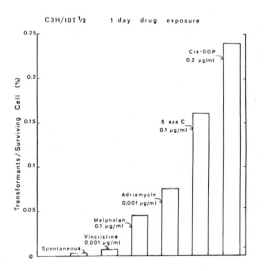

FIGURE 11. Transformation incidence produced by various chemotherapeutic agents.

guanine bases. By contrast, the *trans* isomer tends to bind monofunctionally and is less efficient at producing interstrand crosslinks.[22-25] The concentration scales for *cis*- and *trans*-platinum differ by an order of magnitude, which approximately equalizes their cell survival curves, that is, the concentration of *trans*-platinum must be ten times higher than that of *cis*-platinum to produce equal effect. Even with the difference of cytotoxicity factored out, it is still evident that *cis*-platinum produces transformation at a much higher rate than the *trans* isomer.

The data described above for chemotherapeutic agents, all obtained in the same laboratory, with the same biological system over a relatively short time interval, indicate a big disparity between different compounds in their ability to induce transformations. *Cis*-platinum is far and away the most potent agent

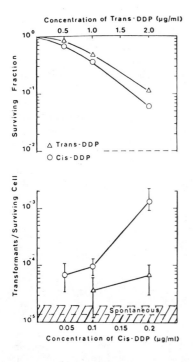

FIGURE 12. Cell survival (*top*) and transformation incidence (*bottom*) or *cis*-platinum and *trans*-platinum. The dose scales for the two drugs differ by a factor of 10.

tested, followed by 5 aza C. On the other hand, vincristine produces a transformation incidence not significantly above the control level. Three reports have been published from different laboratories, involving different assay systems.[26-28] Our own data do not show such high absolute levels of transformation as has been seen in previously published data. However, the relative transformation incidence characteristic of different agents is similar, as is the observation that some agents do not produce transformation at measurable levels. The conclusion is clear that in many cases there is a choice, and that in patients with a good prognosis for long-term survival, combinations of agents should be chosen that are ineffective in producing transformation.

MODULATION OF TRANSFORMATION

Although exposure to agents possessing oncogenic potential may be inevitable in cancer therapy, we can nevertheless seek ways to minimize their oncogenic effects.

One may regard neoplastic development as a sequence of multiple events. Initial processes are associated with initiation and later events are related to expression of neoplastic transformation and its promotion to frank neoplasia *in vivo* or as seen *in vitro*, to a colony of cells with neoplastic potential.[29] While we may influence more readily the later events and slow down the process, we aim at interfering with the early processes and inhibiting initiation.

Retinoids

In recent years retinoids have been found to be effective inhibitors of neoplastic growth *in vivo*,[30] in both experimentally induced tumors as well as clinically, where the course of development of certain cancerous lesions was suppressed.

We have investigated our *in vitro* systems to discern whether retinoids inhibit gamma- and X-ray-induced oncogenic transformation. Utilizing both the hamster embryo cells as well as the 10T½ cells, we have indeed found that exposure of single cells to X-rays or gamma rays in the presence of an analog of retinyl, a wide or *trans* retinoic acid, significantly inhibited the frequency of neoplastic transformation [37] (FIG. 13). The action of retinoids is apparently mediated via its effect on gene expression. This was suggested by the fact that

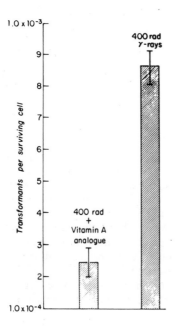

FIGURE 13. The inhibition of γ-ray-induced oncogenic transformation in C3H/10T½ cells by the retinoid, trimethylmethoxyphenyl analog of *n*-ethyl retinamide. (Data derived from Harisiadis *et al.*[37])

the levels of the membrane-associated enzyme Na/K ATPase was reduced in the presence of retinoid.[16, 17, 31] In contrast, when sister chromatid exchanges were used as an indicator of DNA damage, it was found that inhibition of transformation by X-rays was not reflected in changes in SCE.[16, 17, 30]

We also found that retinoids can inhibit the synergistic interaction between chemicals and radiation[31] as well as effectively eliminate the enhancing effect on X-ray transformation exerted by the phorbol-ester-derivative TPA, a tumor-promoter.[16, 17, 31] Thus, exposure to a combination of agents that may act in additive or synergistic fashion to produce oncogenic transformation may possibly be inhibited by dietary factors, such as retinoids, and also by the micronutrient, selenium.[31]

Thyroid Hormones

While retinoids appear to act as inhibitors of late events in neoplastic development we have recently found that a hypothyroid condition *in vitro* renders hamster embryo and mouse 10T½ cells insensitive to the neoplastic transformation induced by X-rays[18, 32] and by chemical agents.[33] Addition of the thyroid hormone triiodothyronine (T_3) at the time of exposure to the oncogenic agent resulted in the appearance of transformation. The frequency of transformation was directly related to the T_3 dose within a physiological dose of 10^{-12}–10^{-9} M (Fig. 14). The T_3 effect appeared to be crucial for the initiation period of transformation and required the metabolically active hormone.[32] The addition of T_3 at 12 hours prior to irradiation resulted in the highest transformation rate, whereas adding it 12 hours after irradiation resulted in no observed transformation. While we do not yet know the mechanisms involved, ongoing experiments raise the possibility that the thyroid hormone induces a host protein that mediates X-ray-induced transformation.[32] This hypothesis is supported by the finding that T_3 modulation of X-ray-induced transformation was suppressed by 50 μg/ml cyclohexamide and eliminated by 100 μg/ml of the same drug.

In many persons the role of thyroid hormones in the etiology of cancer is unclear. Radiotherapy results in a temporary hypothyroid state which, perhaps, if left temporarily unsupplemented, may be protective during further therapy against the development of secondary malignancies.

SUPEROXIDE DISMUTASE AS A PROTECTOR

The generation of reactive oxygen species in living systems exposed to radiation and various chemicals has long been recognized.[34, 35] The use of *in vitro* systems has enabled us to evaluate the inhibitory effects of superoxide dismutase (SOD), a free radical scavenger, on neoplastic transformation by X-rays and bleomycin in the hamster cell system[35] as well as by X-rays and the hypoxic radiosensitizer, metronidazole, in the 10T½ cells.[34] Cells exposed to these agents used in cancer therapy can undergo transformation, but the presence of SOD significantly lowers this transformation rate (TABLE 2; FIGS. 15 and 16). These observations suggest that the oncogenic effects of X-rays, bleomycin, and metronidazole are in part mediated via free radical action; these agents, in their capacity to cause membrane peroxidation and alterations

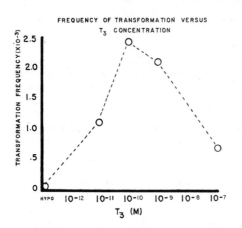

FIGURE 14. The effect of thyroid hormone triiodothyronine (T₃) on radiation-induced transformation in C3H/10T½ cells. No transformation was observed when cells were grown and maintained under hypothyroid condition.

in DNA, may clearly play a role in genetic and epigenetic factors leading to a neoplastic state. The use of radioprotectors, which scavenge these radicals, may serve as a means to reduce the oncogenic effects of the agents used in cancer therapy.

HUMAN CELL TRANSFORMATION

Although *in vitro* systems of animal cells have proved useful for quantitative studies of oncogenesis, the development of a human cell system for assessing radiation-induced cancer risk is desirable.

In recent studies we have transformed human diploid skin fibroblasts by 400 rad of X-rays in cells that were capable of growing in agar and forming tumors in nude mice [36] (FIG. 17). Radiation transformation was potentiated by β-estradiol.

Transformation rate in the human cell system appears lower than that observed in the hamster cells at a dose of 400 rad. In contrast to the hamster cells, where capacity to grow in agar is acquired long after exposure to radiation and upon many subsequent passages, the human transformed cells are able to

TABLE 2

INHIBITING EFFECT OF SUPEROXIDE DISMUTASE ON HAMSTER EMBRYO CELL
TRANSFORMATION BY X-RAYS AND BLEOMYCIN *

Treatment	S.F.	Percentage of Transformation
300 rad	0.75	0.7 ± 0.14
300 rad + SOD	0.91	0.17 ± 0.06
Bleomycin	0.65	1.30 ± 0.09
Bleomycin + SOD	0.75	0.33 ± 0.10

* Data taken in part from Borek and Troll.[35]

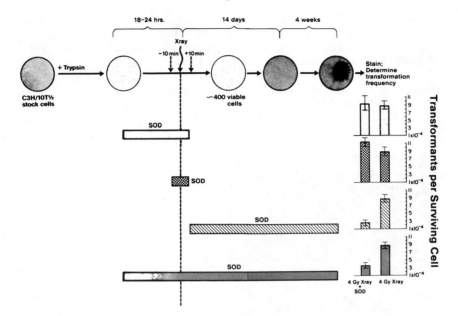

FIGURE 15. The effect of superoxide dismutase (SOD) on the incidence of transformation produced by 4 Gy of X-rays. The SOD at a concentration of 10 units/ml was applied in various protocols, as shown. (From Miller *et al.*[34] Reproduced by permission.)

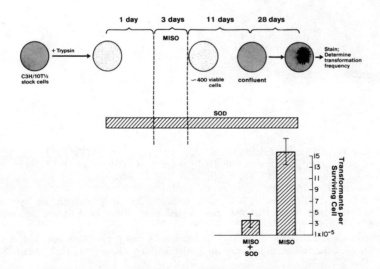

FIGURE 16. The effect of superoxide dismutase (10 units/ml) on the incidence of oncogenic transformation produced by misonidazole (m*M* for 3 days). (From Miller *et al.*[34] Reproduced by permission.)

grow in agar at the same time as they form visible transformed foci in culture (FIG. 17). Both transformed human cells as well as tumor cells derived from the tumors in nude mice exhibited a near-diploid or diploid karyotype. Thus, marked chromosomal change did not reflect the neoplastic state.

Future detailed qualitative and quantitative analysis of X-ray-induced human cell transformation will shed light on similarities and differences between the animal and human cell systems in their progression from a normal to a neoplastic state.

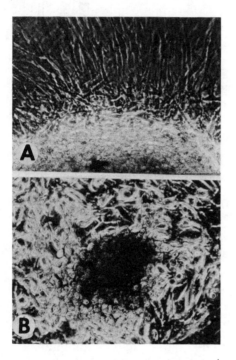

FIGURE 17. Human skin fibro-blasts transformed *in vitro*. (A) focus of transformed cells; (B) similar focus after treatment with low-calcium medium.

REFERENCES

1. ARSENEAU, J., G. P. CANELLAS, R. JOHNSON & V. T. DeVITA. 1977. Risk of new cancer in patients with Hodgkins disease. Cancer **40:** 1912–1916.
2. BOREK, C. & L. SACHS. 1966. *In vitro* cell transformation by x-irradiation. Nature **210:** 276–278.
3. BOREK, C. & L. SACHS. 1967. Cell susceptibility to transformation by x-irradiation and fixation of the transformed state. Proc. Natl. Acad. Sci. USA **57:** 1522–1527.
4. BOREK, C. & L. SACHS. 1968. The number of cell generations required to fix the transformed state in x-ray induced transformation. Proc. Natl. Acad. Sci. USA **59:** 83–85.
5. BOREK, C., C. PAIN & H. MASON. 1976. Transformation of embryo cells x-irradiated *in utero* and assayed *in vitro:* Qualitative and quantitative aspects. Radiat. Res. **67, 68:** 629.

6. BOREK, C. & C. M. FENOGLIO. 1976. A scanning electron microscope study of surface features of hamster embryo cells transformed *in vitro* by x-irradiation. Cancer Res. **36:** 1325–1334.

7. BOREK, C. & D. L. GUERNSEY. 1981. Thyroid hormone modulated neoplastic transformation *in vitro*. J. Supramol. Struct. and Cell. Biochem. Suppl. **5:** 218.

8. BOREK, C., E. J. HALL & H. H. ROSSI. 1978. Malignant transformation in cultured hamster embryo cells produced by x rays, 450 keV monoenergetic neutrons and heavy ions. Cancer Res. **38:** 2997–3005.

9. BOREK, C. & E. J. HALL. 1973. Transformation of mammalian cells *in vitro* by low doses of x-rays. Nature **244:** 450–453.

10. BOREK, C. & E. J. HALL. 1974. Cell transformation *in vitro* by monoenergetic neutrons. J. Cell Biol. **63:** 33a.

11. BOREK, C. 1979. Neoplastic transformation following split doses of x-rays. Brit. J. Radiol. **52:** 845.

12. BOREK, C., E. J. HALL & M. ZAIDER. The oncogenic potential of x-rays and γ-rays *in vitro*. Radiat. Res. In press.

13. REZNIKOFF, C. A., J. S. BERTRAM, D. W. BRANKOW & C. HEIDELBERGER. 1973. Quantitative and qualitative studies of chemical transformations of cloned C3H mouse embryo cells sensitive to postconfluence inhibition of cell division. Cancer Res. **33:** 3239–3249.

14. BOREK, C., R. MILLER, C. PAIN & W. TROLL. 1979. Conditions for the inhibiting and enhancing effect of protease inhibitor Antipain on x-ray induced neoplastic transformation in hamster and mouse cells. Proc. Natl. Acad. Sci. USA **76:** 1800–1803.

15. BOREK, C., R. C. MILLER, C. R. GEARD, D. GUERNSEY, R. S. OSMAK, M. RUTLEDGE-FREEMAN, A. ONG & H. MASON. 1981. Modulating effect of retinoids and tumor promoters on malignant transformation, sister chromatid exchanges and Na/K ATPase. *In* Modulation of Cellular Interaction by Vitamin A and Derivatives (Retinoids). L. M. DeLuca and S. S. Shapiro, eds. Ann. NY Acad. Sci. **359:** 237–238.

16. MILLER, R. C., C. R. GEARD, R. S. OSMAK, M. RUTLEDGE-FREEMAN, A. ONG, H. MASON, A. NAPHOLZ, N. PEREZ, L. HARISIADIS & C. BOREK. 1981. Modification of sister chromatid exchanges and radiation-induced transformation in rodent cells by the tumor promotor 12-0-tetradecanoylphorbol-13-acetate and two retinoids. Cancer Res. **41:** 655–659.

17. MILLER, R. & E. J. HALL. 1978. X-ray dose fractionation and oncogenic transformations in cultured mouse embryo cells. Nature **272:** 58–60.

18. GUERNSEY, D. L., A. ONG & C. BOREK. 1980. Thyroid hormone modulation of x ray-induced *in vitro* neoplastic transformation. Nature **288:** 591–592.

19. LITTLE, J. B. 1979. Quantitative studies of radiation transformation with the A31–11 mouse BALB/3T3 cell line. Cancer Res. **39:** 1474–1480.

20. HALL, E. J., R. C. MILLER, R. OSMAK & M. ZIMMERMAN. 1982. A comparison of the incidence of oncogenic transformation produced by x-rays, misonidazole and chemotherapeutic agents. Radiology. In press.

21. MILLER, R. C. & E. J. HALL. 1978. Oncogenic transformation *in vitro* by the hypoxic cell sensitizer misonidazole. Br. J. Cancer **38:** 411–417.

22. MANSY, S., B. ROSENBERG & A. J. THOMPSON. 1973. Binding of cis and trans dichloramine platinum to nucleosides. J. Am. Chem. Soc. **95:** 1633–1640.

23. PASCOE, J. M. & J. J. ROBERTS. 1974. Interactions between mammalian cell DNA and inorganic platinum compounds. Biochem. Pharmacol. **23:** 1345–1357.

24. ZWELLING, L. A., T. ANDERSON & K. W. KOHN. 1979. DNA-protein and DNA interstrand crosslinking by cis- and trans-platinum (II) diamminedichloride in L1210 mouse leukemia cells, and relation to cytotoxicity. Cancer Res. **39:** 365–369.

25. ZWELLING, L. A., BRADLEY, O. MATTHEWS, N. A. SHARKEY, T. ANDERSON & K. W. KOHN. 1979. Mutagenicity, cytotoxicity and DNA crosslinking in V79 Chinese hamster cells treated with cis- and trans-Pt (II) diamminedichloride. Mutation Res. **67:** 271–280.

26. BENEDICT, W. F., A. BANERJEE, A. GARDNER & P. A. JONES. 1977. Induction of morphological transformation in mouse C3H/10T½ clone 8 cells and chromosomal damage in hamster cells by cancer chemotherapeutic agents. Cancer Res. **37:** 2202–2208.

27. TURNBULL, D., N. C. POPESCU, J. A. DIPAOLO & B. C. MYHR. 1979. Cis-Platinum (II) diamine dichloride causes mutation, transformation, and sister chromatid exchanges in cultured mammalian cells. Mutation Res. **66:** 267–275.

28. MARQUARDT, H., F. S. PHILLIPS & S. S. STERNBERG. 1976. Tumorigenicity *in vivo* and induction of malignant transformation and mutagenesis in cell cultures by adriamycin and daunomycin. Cancer Res. **36:** 2065–2069.

29. HECKER, E. *et al.,* Eds. 1982. Carcinogenesis and Biological Effects of Tumor Promotors. Raven Press. New York, NY.

30. DOLL, R. & R. PETO. 1981. The causes of cancer: Quantitative estimates of avoidable risks of cancer in the United States today. J. Natl. Cancer Inst. **66:** 1193–1308.

31. BOREK, C. 1982. Vitamins and micronutrients modify carcinogenesis and tumor promotion *in vitro. In* Molecular Interrelations of Nutrition and Cancer. M. Arnot *et al.,* Eds.: 337–350. Raven Press. New York, NY.

32. GUERNSEY, D. L., C. BOREK & I. S. EDELMAN. 1981. Crucial role of thyroid hormone in x-ray-induced neoplastic transformation in cell culture. Proc. Natl. Acad. Sci. USA **78:** 5708–5711.

33. BOREK, C., D. L. GUERNSEY, A. ONG & I. S. EDELMAN. Proc. Natl. Acad. Sci. USA In press.

34. MILLER, R. C., R. OSMAK, M. ZIMMERMAN & E. J. HALL. 1982. Sensitizers, protectors and oncogenic transformation *in vitro.* Int. J. Rad. Oncol. Biol. Phys. **8:** 771–775.

35. BOREK, C. & W. TROLL. Modifiers of free radicals inhibit *in vitro* the oncogenic action of x rays, bleomycin and the tumor promotor TPA. Proc. Natl. Acad. Sci. USA. In press.

36. BOREK, C. X-ray-induced transformation of human diploid cells. Nature **283:** 776–778.

37. HARISIDIADIS, L., R. C. MILLER, E. J. HALL & C. BOREK. 1978. Vitamin A analogue inhibits radiation-induced oncogenic transformation. Nature **274:** 486–487.

INDUCTION OF DIFFERENTIATION OF HUMAN MYELOID LEUKEMIAS BY PHORBOL DIESTERS: PHENOTYPIC CHANGES AND MODE OF ACTION *

Giovanni Rovera, Dario Ferrero, Giovanni L. Pagliardi,
Jasmine Vartikar, Silvana Pessano, Lisabianca Bottero,
Sam Abraham, and Deborah Lebman

*The Wistar Institute of Anatomy and Biology
Philadelphia, Pennsylvania 19104*

INTRODUCTION

12-*O*-Tetradecanoyl-phorbol-13-acetate (TPA) induces marked morphologic, biochemical, and functional changes in primary cultures and established cell lines of acute myeloblastic leukemias.[1-6]

When human promyelocytic leukemia HL60 cells [7] are treated with nanomolar amounts of TPA, they differentiate into macrophage-like cells.[1-3] The cells develop a number of mature myelomonocytic markers and monocytic-specific markers, including α-naphthylacetate esterase activity,[1] isozymes of acid phosphatase,[8] the ability to phagocytize to latex beads and IgG-coated erythrocytes,[1] increased levels of lysozyme [1] and of 5'-nucleotidase,[9] and decreased myeloperoxidase activity.[1] TPA-treated cells also become cytotoxic for malignant cells.[11]

Studies by two-dimensional gel electrophoresis of cytoplasmic proteins of HL60 cells treated with TPA show a *de novo* synthesis of at least 58 proteins with a pattern quite similar to that observed in normal monocytes.[12] TPA-treated cells, however, lack the HLA-DR surface antigen and do not secrete complement (C2 or C4).[9] The cells are able to phagocytize nonopsonized yeasts,[13] but are unable to ingest opsonized bacteria.[9] These findings suggest that the process of terminal differentiation induced by TPA is defective.

Among the early functional changes induced by TPA treatment of HL60 cells is an irreversible arrest of cell proliferation. The treated cells rapidly shift from exponential growth to arrest in the G_1 phase of the cell cycle.[14]

Using a number of monoclonal antibodies directed against the surface of myelomonocytic cells,[15-19] we have investigated the changes that occur at the level of the surface membrane of HL60 cells after TPA treatment and their relationship with the arrest of cell proliferation.

MATERIALS AND METHODS

Cell Line

HL60 cells [7] were grown in RPMI 1640 medium supplemented with 15% fetal calf serum and induced to differentiate with 1.7×10^{-8} *M* TPA, as previously described.[1, 12]

* This research was supported by Grants CA 10815, CA 21124, and CA 25875 from the National Cancer Institute and Grant CH 202 from the American Cancer Society. D. F. was supported by Comitato G. Ghirotti and Regione Piemonte (Italy).

211

Monoclonal Antibodies

Myelomonocytic monoclonal antibodies were produced in our laboratory as described,[15, 16] or were obtained from Drs. Z. Steplewski and H. Koprowski.[25] Mon 2 antibody [18] was purchased from Bethesda Research Laboratory (BRL). OKM1 [19] was the gift of Dr. G. Goldstein (Ortho Pharmaceuticals, Raritan, NJ).

Cytofluorimetry

The percentage of fluorescent cells and the mean intensity of fluorescence were determined using a 50HH cytofluorograph cell sorter (Ortho Instruments). Indirect immunofluorescence was performed as described previously.[15, 16]

Binding Experiments

Transferrin and L5.1 monoclonal antibodies labeled with ^{125}I using the chloramine T method [20] were used at a concentration from 0.125 μg/ml to 5 μg/ml. In a typical experiment, 25 μl of labeled proteins was added to 5×10^5 cells in 25 μl of buffer (0.13 M NaCl, 0.005 M KCl, 0.0074 M MgCl$_2$, 0.01 M HEPES, 1 mg/ml bovine serum albumin, pH 7.4). Transferrin binding was measured after incubation for 30 minutes at 37° C. L5.1 binding was measured after incubation for 1 hour at 4° C. Nonspecific binding was determined by incubating parallel cultures with a 500-fold excess of unlabeled transferrin or L5.1 antibody. Bound (pellet) and unbound (supernatant) radioactivity was determined and a Scatchard analysis done.[21]

Acridine Orange and Propidium Iodide Staining

Cells were fixed in 70% ethanol, washed with PBS, and stained with acridine orange, as previously described.[24] Acridine orange at a final concentration of 2.5×10^{-5} M was added to a cell suspension of 5×10^5 cells/ml. A stock solution of acridine orange (8×10^{-2} M) was stored in the dark at 4° C. Alternatively, after indirect immunofluorescence, cells were fixed with 1% paraformaldehyde and stained with propidium iodide.[32]

RESULTS

TABLE 1 summarizes the monoclonal antibodies that were used in this study. They are specific for a given cell lineage when considered within the framework of hematopoietic cell lineages, though most of them are reactive with other cell types (chiefly neuroblastoma cells and colon carcinoma cell lines). These monoclonal antibodies are grouped according to their reactivity as follows: (1) myeloid-specific (reactive only with elements of the myeloid lineage); (2) monocyte-specific (reactive only with monocytes); (3) myelomonocyte-specific (reactive with myeloid cells and monocytes); and (4) reactive with immature myeloid cells and other blast cells. Several of the antigens recognized by these

TABLE 1

MONOCLONAL ANTIBODIES REACTING WITH MYELOID AND MONOCYTIC CELLS

Hybridoma	Isotype	Antigen	Specificity
R1B19	IgM	p150	Myeloid
WGHS-291	IgM	SSEA-1	Myeloid
L12.2	IgG1	p110	Myeloid
L13.1	IgM	ND	Myeloid
S5.25	IgM	ND	Myelomonocyte
B13.4	IgM	ND	Myelomonocyte
B9.8	IgM	ND	Myelomonocyte
OKM1	IgG2b	ND	Myelomonocyte
WCDK-6	IgG2a	ND	Monocyte
Mon 2	IgG1	p200	Monocyte
B44.1	IgM	ND	Monocyte
L5.1	IgG2a	gp 87	Early myeloid + erythroblasts + lymphoblasts
S5.7	IgG1	p20	Stem cells + monocyte subset + T-lymphocytes

antibodies have been biochemically characterized as proteins or glycoproteins, and at least one is a glycolipid. The structure of the other antigens is not known. All these antibodies bind to different surface structures, as is shown by the different patterns of reactivity with cells at different stages of differentiation and with leukemic cells.[10, 15] The reactivity of the monoclonal antibodies with myelomonocytic cells at different stages of differentiation has been identified by flow cytofluorimetry of normal human bone marrow cells as previously described.[10, 15, 16] These results are summarized in TABLE 2. Reactivity with normal myeloblasts could not be identified with certainty using the cell sorter, but could be confirmed by studying the effect of the IgM antibodies in the presence of complement in a CFUc myeloid stem cell assay system.[26] From the data in TABLE 2 it is possible to deduce the phenotype of promyelocytes and monocytes. The phenotype of an exponentially growing population of HL60 cells was determined using these same monoclonal antibodies and was found to be identical to that of normal promyelocytes, that is, R1B19+, WGHS-291+, L13.1±, L12.2−, S5.25±, B13.4−, B9.8−, WCDK-6±, L5.1±, S5.7+, OKM1, Mon 2−, B44.1−.

After TPA treatment, the phenotype of HL60 cells changed, but not drastically. TABLE 3 shows the phenotypic characteristics of HL60 cells at time 0 and at 2 and 5 days after continuous treatment of the cells with 1.7×10^{-8} M TPA. The final phenotype of TPA-treated cells is not that of normal monocytes (R1B19−, WGHS-291−, L13.1−, L12.2−, S5.25+, B13.4+, B9.8+, WCDK-6+, L5.1−, S5.7+, OKM1+, Mon 2+, B44.1+), but rather that of a cell that expresses some monocytic markers but lacks other markers and maintains several that are myeloid-specific (R1B19+, WGHS-291+, L13.1±, L12.2−, S5.25+, WCDK-6−, L5.1−, S5.7±, OKM1+, Mon 2−). Previous

TABLE 2

DIFFERENTIATION STAGE-SPECIFICITY OF MYELOMONOCYTIC ANTIBODIES

Hybridoma	Myeloblast	Promyelo	Myelo	Meta	Granulo	Mono
R1B19 *	+	+	+	+	+	−
WGHS-291	+	+	+	+	+	−
L13.1 †	−	±	±	+	+	−
L12.2 †	−	−	−	+	+	−
S5.25 †	−	±	+	+	+	+
B13.4 *	−	−	+	+	+	+ +
B9.8 *	−	−	−	+	+	+ +
WCDK-6 ‡	−	−	−	−	−	+
B44.1 *	−	−	−	−	−	+ +
L5.1 §	+	+	−	−	−	−
S5.7 ‖	+	+	−	−	−	±

* Perussia et al.[15]
† Pessano et al.[30]
‡ Magnani et al.[29]
§ Lebman et al.[16]
‖ Pessano et al.[31]

studies have indicated that TPA-treated cells are positive for myelomonocyte-specific antibodies B13.4 and B9.8 [17] and negative for monocytic-specific antibody B44.1.[10]

The early changes induced after TPA treatment include the disappearance of the surface antigen recognized by monoclonal antibody L5.1. This antibody

TABLE 3

TPA-INDUCED PHENOTYPIC CHANGES IN HL60 CELLS AS DETECTED BY
MONOCLONAL ANTIBODIES

Hybridoma	Days After Treatment		
	0	2	5
R1B19	87*	70	57
WGHS-291	84	62	52
L13.1	15	25	26
L12.2	1	3	5
S5.25	9	16	48
B13.4	1	44	65
OKM1	14	57	71
WCDK-6	7	6	1
B44.1	1	1	1
Mon 2	2	1	1
L5.1	50	3	1
S5.7	76	45	17

* Percentage of fluorescent cells as determined by cytofluorimetry using an Ortho 50 HH Cytofluorograf.

has been shown to bind to the receptor for transferrin,[16] a molecule that is essential for the growth of HL60 cells in culture. HL60 cells are relatively rich in transferrin receptors. FIGURE 1 A and B shows the Scatchard analyses of ^{125}I-labeled transferrin and ^{125}I-labeled L5.1 binding, respectively, to HL60 cells. HL60 cells have a steady-state binding of 3.64×10^5 molecules of transferrin/cell and a K_d of 1.71×10^8. The linear nature of the plot (correlation coefficient, 0.83) suggests a single type or a predominant type of one receptor. The binding of L5.1 to HL60 cells indicates that the cells contain 5.46×10^4 surface binding sites. Because measurement of transferrin binding at 37° C includes ligand bound to the surface plus ligand internalized, we calculated that the ratio of ligand internalized $(LR)_I$ to surface ligand $(LR)_s$ is approximately 7.0.

The transferrin receptor is not expressed homogeneously in all cells throughout the cell cycle. FIGURE 2 shows an analysis using the 50HH cytofluorograph cell sorter and double-labeling of the cells with fluoresceinated antibody and with propidium iodide.

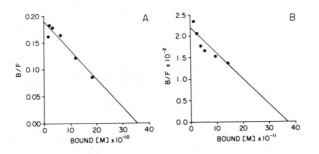

FIGURE 1. Effect of increasing concentrations of ^{125}I-labeled transferrin (**A**) and ^{125}I-labeled L5.1 (**B**) to receptor binding of exponentially growing HL60 cells.

The population of exponentially growing HL60 cells that were positive for L5.1 antibody represents approximately 45% of the total population. However, the G_2 population is almost 65% positive, and the S population is 54% positive. The G_1 population is less than 30% positive. TPA treatment of HL60 cells produces a relatively rapid loss of the receptor: after 12 hours only 3% of the population remains positive for the L5.1 antibody.

The reduction in number of receptor molecules present on the surface of HL60 cells was confirmed by studies in which direct binding of ^{125}I-labeled transferrin and ^{125}I-labeled L5.1 was measured in HL60 cells at different times after TPA treatment (FIG. 3). Loss of the transferrin receptor is already detectable at 3 hours after TPA induction and increases with time.

The disappearance of the transferrin receptor precedes by several hours the changes that can be detected in the cell cycle of HL60 cells. Only after 72 hours is there evidence that the cells without transferrin receptors have altered their growth pattern and have accumulated in the G_1 phase of the cell cycle (FIG. 4). These data confirm previous work done using autoradiography and Feulgen staining analysis of TPA-treated cells.[14]

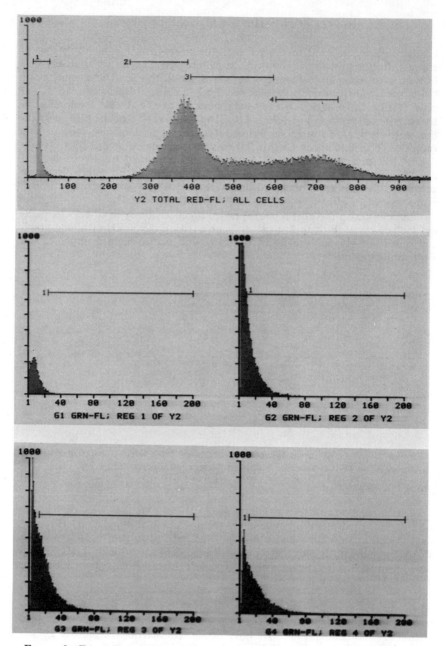

FIGURE 2. Expression of L5.1 on the surface of HL60 cells during the cell cycle. Cells were treated with L5.1 and FITC-conjugated goat anti-mouse F(ab′)₂, fixed with 1% paraformaldehyde, and incubated with propidium iodide. X-axis = intensity of fluorescence; y-axis = number of cells. Y2 (*top*), red fluorescence (propidium iodide staining). Bars indicate cell cycle subpopulations: 1, negative propidium iodide staining population; 2, G_1 phase population; 3, S phase population; 4, G_2 phase population. G1 (*middle left*), green fluorescence of negative population; G2 (*middle right*), green fluorescence of G_1 phase population; G3 (*bottom left*), green fluorescence of S phase population; G4 (*bottom right*), green fluorescence of G_2 phase population. Bar indicates limit within which 99% of control population is fluorescence-negative.

Discussion

The data presented here indicate that TPA-treated human promyelocytic leukemia cells HL60 differentiate into cells that have several markers of monocytes but maintain several myeloid-specific surface markers. The incomplete expression of the differentiation program of TPA-treated HL60 cells could be due (1) to genetic alterations in HL60 cells that do not allow expression of particular markers, (2) to inadequacy of TPA as an inducer of monocytic differentiation, (3) to the fact that monocytes do not normally derive from promyelocytes but from more immature cells, or (4) to the possibility that monocytes and macrophages do not necessarily express the same surface markers even if they are related. It is possible that each of these conditions plays some role in the development of the atypical phenotype observed in TPA-treated HL60 cells. TPA treatment of other cell lines such as ML3 and KG1 leukemic cells results in the expression of slightly different phenotypes when evaluated with the same monoclonal antibodies. It also appears that some markers such as the DR surface antigen that are normally turned off in the promyelocytic stage remain turned off in the differentiated cells. However, if DR is not turned

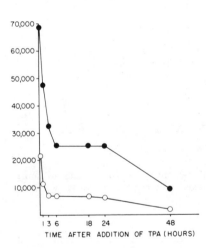

FIGURE 3. ^{125}I-labeled transferrin (●—●) and ^{125}I-labeled L5.1 (○—○) binding to HL60 cells at different times after treatment with 1.7×10^{-8} M TPA. X-axis = time after treatment (hours); y-axis = ^{125}I cpm bound to its cell.

TIME AFTER ADDITION OF TPA (HOURS)

off initially (as in the KG1 line), then DR is expressed in TPA-treated cells. Similarly, if myeloid-specific markers are not expressed in cells (as in some primary cultures of myeloblastic leukemia), then TPA treatment does not induce myeloid-specific markers. An important characteristic of the process of TPA-induced differentiation of myeloid leukemia cells is that the treated cells irreversibly cease to proliferate at a TPA concentration of 1×10^{-8} M.

Studies using the monoclonal antibody L5.1, as well as other antitransferrin receptor antibodies,[27] indicate that TPA treatment of HL60 cells results in a rapid loss of the transferrin receptor from the cell surface. Transferrin is a molecule that is essential for proliferation of these cells in culture.[22] The loss of the transferrin receptor from the surface of TPA-treated HL60 cells is not due to a direct effect of TPA on the receptor. Other leukemic cell lines of different

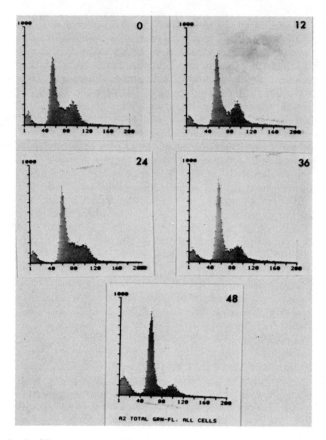

FIGURE 4. Acridine orange staining of HL60 cells at 0, 12, 24, 36, and 48 hours after treatment with TPA ($1.7 \times 10^{-8} M$). X-axis = fluorescence intensity; y-axis = number of cells.

lineage, such as the null cell line Nalm 1, express the transferrin receptor, but TPA has no effect on the receptor or on proliferative activity.[28] Future investigations of the events that lead to the loss of the transferrin receptor in sensitive cells may also yield useful information on the mechanism of action of TPA on myeloblastic leukemia cells. The loss of proliferative activity and the development of cytotoxic activity against tumor cells in TPA-treated HL60 cells suggest the potential use of phorbol diesters in treating acute myeloblastic leukemias. However, the activity of these agents as tumor-promoters, their high toxicity *in vivo* when injected intravenously, and their metabolic instability precludes any meaningful *in vivo* experiment. Because TPA can induce differentiation even after brief treatment of the cells,[1] and because TPA has no effect on the multipotent stem cells of the mouse (CFUs),[23] it is possible to design an experimental model in which treatment of leukemic bone marrow is done *in vitro*. The bone marrow, depleted of myeloid leukemic and normal myeloid cells, but not of CFUs, by TPA treatment *in vitro,* can be returned to lethally irradiated recipients. We are presently investigating this approach using an experimentally transplantable murine myeloid leukemia.

SUMMARY

Treatment with 12-*O*-tetradecanoyl-phorbol-13-acetate (TPA) of acute myeloblastic leukemia cells halts proliferation and induces expression of monocyte/macrophage markers. Surface characteristics of leukemic HL60 cells, as defined using a panel of monoclonal antibodies, were found to be similar to those of normal human promyelocytes. TPA treatment, however, induced a phenotype that, unlike normal monocytes, contained several myeloid-specific markers and lacked several monocyte-specific markers. TPA treatment of HL60 cells causes the rapid disappearance of the transferrin receptor from the cell surface. Because transferrin is essential for HL60 cell proliferation in culture, the disappearance of this receptor is followed by an irreversible accumulation of the cells in the G_1 phase of the cell cycle. The TPA-induced arrest of cell proliferation suggests the potential of this agent in experimentally treating myeloblastic leukemias.

ACKNOWLEDGMENTS

We thank Connie Moody for typing and Marina Hoffman for editing the manuscript. We thank Drs. Zenon Steplewski and Hilary Koprowski for the gift of monoclonal antibodies WGHS-291 and WCDK-6.

REFERENCES

1. ROVERA, G., D. SANTOLI & C. DAMSKY. 1979. Proc. Natl. Acad. Sci. USA **76:** 2779–2783.
2. ROVERA, G., T. O'BRIEN & L. DIAMOND. 1979. Science **204:** 868–870.
3. LOTEM, J. & L. SACHS. 1979. Proc. Natl. Acad. Sci. USA **76:** 5158–5162.
4. PEGORARO, L., J. ABRAHAM, R. A. COOPER, A. LEVIS, B. LANGE, P. MEO & G. ROVERA. 1980. Blood **55:** 859–862.
5. KOEFFLER, H. P., M. BAR-ELO & M. TEVITO. 1980. J. Clin. Invest. **66:** 1101–1108.
6. FIBACH, E. & E. A. RACHMIKIVITZ. 1981. Br. J. Haematol. **47:** 203–210.
7. COLLINS, S. J., R. C. GALLO & R. E. GALLAGHER. 1977. Nature **270:** 347–349.
8. VORBRODT, A., P. MEO & G. ROVERA. 1979. J. Cell Biol. **83:** 303–307.
9. NEWBURGER, P. E., R. D. BAKER, S. L. HANSEN, R. A. DUNCAN & J. S. GREENBERGER. 1981. Cancer Res. **41:** 1861–1865.
10. PERUSSIA, B., D. LEBMAN, B. LANGE, J. FAUST, G. TRINCHIERI & G. ROVERA. 1982. *In* Differentiation and Cancer. A. Pontieri & R. Revoltella, Eds. Raven Press. New York, NY.
11. WEINBERG, J. B. 1981. Science **213:** 655–657.
12. LIEBERMAN, D., D. HOFFMAN, B. LIEBERMAN & L. SACHS. 1981. Int. J. Cancer **28:** 285–291.
13. HUBERMAN, E. & M. F. CALLAHAN. 1979. Proc. Natl. Acad. Sci. USA **76:** 1293–1297.
14. ROVERA G., N. OLASHAW & P. MEO. 1980. Nature **284:** 69–70.

15. PERUSSIA, B., G. TRINCHIERI, D. LEBMAN, J. JANKIEWICZ, B. LANGE & G. ROVERA. 1982. Blood **59**: 382–392.
16. LEBMAN, D., M. TRUCCO, L. BOTTERO, B. LANGE, S. PESSANO & G. ROVERA. 1982. Blood **59**: 671–678.
17. PERUSSIA, B., D. LEBMAN, S. H. IP, G. ROVERA & G. TRINCHIERI. 1981. Blood **58**: 836–843.
18. UGOLINI, V., G. NUMEZ, R. G. SMITH, P. STASTNY & J. D. CAPRA. 1980. Proc. Natl. Acad. Sci. USA **77**: 6764–6768.
19. BREARD, J., E. L. REINHERZ, P. C. KUNG, G. GOLDSTEIN & S. F. SCHLOSSMAN. 1980. J. Immunol. **124**: 1943–1947.
20. HUNTER, W. M. & F. C. GREENWOOD. 1962. Nature **194**: 495–496.
21. SCATCHARD, G. 1949. Ann. N.Y. Acad. Sci. **51**: 660–672.
22. BREITMAN, T. R., S. J. COLLINS & B. R. KEENE. 1980. Exp. Cell Res. **126**: 494–498.
23. PERUSSIA, B., D. LEBMAN, G. PEGORARO, B. LANGE, C. DAMSKY, D. ADEN, J. VARTIKAR, G. TRINCHIERI & G. ROVERA. 1982. *In* Maturation Factors and Cancer. M. A. S. Moore, Ed.: 273–292. Raven Press, New York, NY.
24. ABRAHAM, S., E. VONDERHEID, S. ZIETZ, F. M. KENDALL & C. NICOLINI. 1980. Cell Biophysics **2**: 352–371.
25. STEPLEWSKI, Z. & H. KOPROWSKI. Unpublished material.
26. FERRERO, D., H. E. BROXMEYER, G. L. PAGLIARDI, B. LANGE, S. PESSANO & G. ROVERA. Submitted for publication.
27. LEBMAN, D., *et al.* Unpublished material.
28. LEBMAN, D., *et al.* Unpublished material.
29. MAGNANI, J. L., M. BROCKHAUS, D. SMITH, V. GINSBURG, M. BLASZCZYK, K. MITCHELL, Z. STEPLEWSKI & H. KOPROWSKI. 1981. Science **212**: 55–56.
30. PESSANO, S. *et al.* Unpublished material.
31. PESSANO, S. *et al.* Submitted for publication.
32. GRISSMAN, H. A. & J. A. STEINKAMP. 1973. J. Cell Biol. **59**: 67A.

REGULATION OF THE LEVELS OF CELLULAR TRANSCRIPTS BY SV40 LARGE T ANTIGEN *

R. Robinson, T. Schutzbank, M. Oren, and A. J. Levine

Department of Microbiology
School of Medicine
State University of New York at Stony Brook
Stony Brook, New York 11794

INTRODUCTION

The SV40 large tumor antigen (T antigen) has been shown to have a number of functions during productive infection of monkey cells or in a variety of transformed cells.[1] During lytic infection the large T antigen is required to initiate each round of viral DNA replication [2] and acts by binding to several specific sites on the viral chromosome at or near the origin of DNA replication.[3, 4] In addition, the large T antigen stimulates the levels of cellular deoxyprimidine kinases [5] and cellular DNA synthesis.[6, 7] The large T antigen regulates the rate of its own synthesis [8] by "modulating down" the levels of early gene transcription.[9] The normally high levels of late viral gene transcription do not occur in the absence of a functional large T antigen and so this protein is at least indirectly required to initiate or "modulate up" late viral gene expression.[10, 11] Perhaps employing one or more of these mechanisms, the SV40 large T antigen is required for the initiation and maintenance of the transformed phenotype in cell culture.[12-16]

Transformed cells differ from their normal counterparts in a large number of ways.[1] Any explanation of how the SV40 large T antigen acts in transformed cells must address these differences. Because of this, experiments were designed to determine whether the SV40 large T antigen could regulate cellular gene expression. The results of the experiments presented here demonstrate that the SV40 large T antigen can modulate, in a positive fashion, the levels of some cellular transcripts.

ISOLATION OF cDNA CLONES COMPLEMENTARY TO mRNA FROM SV40 TRANSFORMED CELLS

In order to obtain a cDNA cloned library of an SV40 transformed cell line, the cytoplasmic, poly (A) selected mRNA fraction from SV3T3-T2 cells was isolated.[17] The 17S RNA fraction was used for the synthesis of double-stranded cDNA according to the procedures of Villa-Komaroff et al.[18] This involved the use of poly (dC) and poly (dG) tailing reactions and insertion into the Pst I site of pBR322. The association of the cDNA inserts with pBR322 and their transformation into E. coli HB101 were carried out as described previously.[19] In this

* This research was supported by Grant CA 28146–02 from the National Institutes of Health. R. R. and T. S. were postdoctoral fellows supported by Grant 09176–05 from the National Cancer Institute.

221

way a plasmid library was established of cDNA clones derived from a 17S fraction of mRNA from SV3T3-T2 cells. To search for cellular transcripts that were present at higher levels in SV40 transformed 3T3 cells than in 3T3 cells, the bacterial colonies were plated and replicas were transferred to nitrocellulose filters.[20] Cytoplasmic mRNA from 3T3 cells and SV3T3 cells was obtained,[17] sheared by mild alkali treatment, and labeled with polynucleotide kinase and [γ-^{32}P] ATP.[21] These labeled mRNAs were then employed as a probe in hybridization to filters of the lysed bacterial colonies containing the cDNA plasmids.[22] Following hybridization and autoradiography, a number of colonies demonstrated positive hybridization with the ^{32}P-SV3T3 mRNA probe, but little or no hybridization with the ^{32}P-mRNA from 3T3 cells. After selection of these positive colonies and large-scale preparation of their plasmid DNAs, the purified pBR322 cDNAs were employed to repeat this experiment, using the dot-blot hybridization procedure.[23] FIGURE 1 presents the autoradiogram of dot-blot hybridizations using ^{32}P-mRNA from 3T3 or SV3T3-T2 cells for ten cDNA clones identified in this study. With the cDNA clones numbered A17, 104, 397, 403, 218, B50, 105 and 348, the ^{32}P-mRNA from SV3T3-T2 cells was in much greater abundance than the 3T3 cell mRNA. With clones 192 and 85, the mRNA levels complementary to these cDNA inserts were similar in 3T3 and SV3T3 cells. In all cases the ^{32}P-mRNA from 3T3 or SV3T3 cells failed to hybridize to pBR322 sequences without any cDNA inserts.

To provide a more quantitative measure of the steady-state levels of mRNA in 3T3 and SV3T3-T2 cells, the dot-blot hybridization filters from an experiment similar to that shown in FIGURE 1 were cut out and counted by liquid scintillation spectroscopy. TABLE 1 presents the results of this experiment. Seven of the cDNA clones (A17, 104, 397, 403, 218, B50 and 105) detected RNA complementary to the cDNA insert sequences in SV3T3-T2 cells, but not in 3T3 cells, while three cDNA clones (192, 348 and 85) detected less RNA in 3T3 cells than in SV3T3-T2 cells. Because this procedure detects only moderately abundant RNA classes, the failure to detect hybridization of 3T3 RNA to these cDNA inserts does not imply the total absence of these RNA species in these cells. While the results in FIGURE 1 and TABLE 1 do reflect the relative abundance levels of these RNAs in SV3T3 and 3T3 cells, other factors such as the cDNA insert sizes may affect the efficiency of hybridization observed here. Even with these qualifications the results indicate that the levels of some RNA species in SV3T3 cells are greater than 100-fold more abundant than the levels

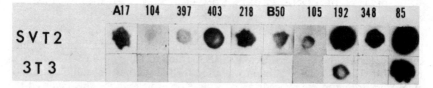

FIGURE 1. Autoradiogram of dot-blot hybridization of cytoplasmic RNA to cDNA clones. Cytoplasmic RNA was extracted from 3T3 cells and SV3T3-T2 cells [17] and labeled with [γ-^{32}P]-ATP and polynucleotide kinase.[21] Equal amounts of RNA from 3T3 and SV3T3 cells (1.66 μg/ml, 2–6 $\times$ 10[7] cpm per μg) were hybridized to the DNA inserts from 10 cloned cDNAs. pBR322 DNA with no insert failed to hybridize any detectable RNA from these preparations. An autoradiogram of the dot blot hybridizations is presented.

TABLE 1

SV40 T-ANTIGEN-REGULATED RNA SPECIES

| | | | Hybridized | | | | | |
| | | | tsA58 | | tsA7 | | | |
Clone No.	SV3T3 (cpm)	3T3 (cpm)	32° C (cpm)	39° C (cpm)	33° C (cpm)	39° C (cpm)	Tumor (cpm)	Liver (cpm)
A17	340	0	350	0	675	0	453	0
104	241	0	717	0	381	0	224	0
397	870	0	1,083	0	1,234	0	—	–
403	776	0	819	0	675	103	192	0
218	1,172	0	1,358	0	1,381	211	302	0
B50	5,103	0	643	0	523	298	926	5
105	511	0	599	62	1,780	241	147	0
192	14,280	707	6,162	849	2,358	1,842	1,846	394
348	6,469	412	2,387	611	533	40	460	17
85	7,412	1,520	35,695	6,862	2,272	1,805	2,275	311

of these RNAs in 3T3 cells. Hybridization between the ten cDNA clones listed in TABLE 1 demonstrated that all ten contained different cDNA insert sequences.

THE LEVELS OF SOME CELLULAR RNA SPECIES ARE REGULATED BY SV40 LARGE T ANTIGEN

In attempting to demonstrate that the levels of cellular mRNA species can be regulated by SV40 large T antigen, we must note two problems with the comparison between 3T3 and SV3T3 cells as presented in FIGURE 1. First, while the SV3T3-T2 cell line employed here was derived from the 3T3 cell line via viral transformation,[24] these two cell lines were obtained 14 years ago. In the interim they have been subcloned many times and thus there has been ample opportunity for many of their properties to diverge. Consequently, the 3T3 and SV3T3 cell lines employed here cannot be considered isogenic, with the only difference between them being the transformed state. Second, the SV3T3 cell line contains SV40-encoded transcripts that are not present in the 3T3 cell line. It is possible that one or more of the cDNA clones under study contain viral encoded cDNA inserts. To address these problems the dot blot hybridization experiments were carried out with ^{32}P-labeled RNA derived from cell lines transformed with SV40tsA mutants (defective in the large T antigen gene). The SV40tsA58 Cb cell line[25] and the SV40tsA7 Balb 3T3 cell line[26] are transformed when grown at 32° C or 33° C, but have a normal phenotype at 39° C. The mRNAs from both of these cell lines grown at 32° or 33° C and at 39° C were extracted, labeled with [γ-^{32}P]-ATP by treatment with polynucleotide kinase and hybridized to the cDNA inserts of the ten clones under study (TABLE 1). On the basis of the results of this experiment, the ten cloned inserts could be divided into three groups. Clones A17, 104 and 397 hybridized with mRNAs from the three (SV3T3, SV40tsA58, SV40tsA7 at 32° or 33° C) transformed cell lines, but did not detect RNA in the nontransformed cell lines (3T3, tsA58 and tsA7 at 39° C). Clones 403, 218 and B50 hybridized with

RNA from SV3T3 and SV40tsA58 at 32° C, but not 3T3 or SV40tsA58 at 39° C. However, with these clones a much smaller differential in RNA levels was found between the SV40tsA7 transformed cells at 33° C and normal cells at 39° C. Clones 105, 192, 348 and 85, while hybridizing with 4- to 20-fold higher concentrations of RNA in SV3T3 versus 3T3 cells, showed little or no temperature regulation of these RNA species in the SV40tsA58 or SV40tsA7 cell lines. This experiment eliminates the possibility that these cDNA inserts are SV40 nucleotide sequences, because the viral mRNA is synthesized in larger amounts at the nonpermissive temperature than at the permissive temperature in SV40tsA transformed cell lines.[9, 10] Second, the use of the SV40tsA transformed cell lines assures that a single cloned cell line (at two temperatures) supplies RNA for this analysis. The multitude of differences between two different cell lines (3T3 versus SV40 3T3) are therefore eliminated by this experimental protocol. For clones A17, 104 and 397, then, it is clear that the SV40 large T antigen can regulate the levels of cellular RNAs complementary to their cDNA insert sequences. To determine whether SV40-induced tumor tissue also expresses these RNA species, RNA preparations from tumors in mice, as well as from normal liver tissue of the same mouse, were labeled and hybridized to the cDNA clones. The results, presented in TABLE 1, demonstrate that the cDNA clones with inserts complementary to RNA species regulated by the SV40 large T antigen (A17, 104, 403, 218, B50, 105 and 348) detect RNAs present in the tumor tissue and not in the normal mouse liver tissue. These results extend the regulation of cellular RNA species by SV40 to the *in vivo* situation (that is, tumors in animals).

CHARACTERIZATION OF THE SV40 LARGE T-ANTIGEN-REGULATED RNA SPECIES

The cDNA clones listed in TABLE 1 were next employed as probes for hybridization to cytoplasmic RNA species from 3T3, SV3T3, SV40tsA58, and SV40tsA7 (at 32° C or 39° C) utilizing the northern gel electrophoresis analysis.[22] In all cases the northern hybridization results were consistent with and confirmed the differential levels of RNA detected in the dot-blot experiments (TABLE 1; FIG. 1). Several cloned inserts detected a single stable RNA species in transformed cells (A17, 403, B50, 105), while other cDNA clones hybridized with two to five different-sized RNA species in these cells (TABLE 2). The relative abundance of these multiple RNA species detected by a single cloned insert varied and the size of the most abundant species is underlined in TABLE 2. On the basis of results of this northern gel analysis several additional features became apparent. When total cytoplasmic RNA from any of the cell lines studied in TABLE 1 was hybridized using dot blots to clone 85 cDNA, little or no regulation by SV40 T antigen was apparent (TABLE 1; FIG. 1). However, when the steady-state levels of cytoplasmic RNA from SV40tsA7 cells at 33° C and 39° C were studied by northern gel analysis, five distinct RNA species were detected with clone 85 cDNA probe (TABLE 2). The relative abundance of each of these five RNA species was determined by densitometer tracings of the autoradiogram from the Northern gel analysis and these results are presented in TABLE 3. The most abundant RNA (1.2 Kb) is regulated poorly by T antigen, while the less abundant RNAs (1.6, 2.0, 2.2 and 2.4 Kb) are regulated to a greater extent by temperature shifts with this cell line. These results suggest that the SV40 T antigen may differentially regulate these five

TABLE 2

CHARACTERIZATION OF THE T-ANTIGEN-REGULATED RNA SPECIES

Clone No.	Number and Size of RNA Species
A17	1; 1.4 Kb
104	4; 2.2, 2.0, <u>1.7</u> <u>1.3</u> Kb
397	3; <u>1.7</u>, <u>1.2</u>, <u>1.0</u>, Kb
403	1; 1.2 Kb
218	2; 1.5, <u>1.2</u> Kb
B50	1; 1.1 Kb
105	1; 1.7 Kb
192	2; 1.7, <u>1.2</u> Kb
348	2; 1.7, <u>1.2</u> Kb
85	5; 2.4, 2.2, 2.0, 1.6, <u>1.2</u> Kb

related (by nucleotide sequence) RNA species. It remains possible, however, that the larger RNA moieties are precursors of the small RNAs and that temperature (not functional T-antigen levels) can affect the rate of RNA processing in clone 85 RNA.

DISCUSSION

This study examines some of the cellular RNA species detected in SV40 transformed cells and tumors. Ten cDNA clones were selected from a library of 420 clones derived from mRNAs found in SV3T3-T2 cells in culture. Three of these cDNA inserts (A17, 104, 397) detect RNA in SV3T3 but not in 3T3 cells, in SV40tsA58 and SV40tsA7 transformed cells at 32–33° C (transformed) but not at 39° C (nontransformed), and in SV40-induced tumor tissue but not in mouse liver tissue (TABLE 1; FIG. 1). These data indicate a greater than 100–200-fold difference in the concentration of these RNA species in the transformed cells compared with that of the nontransformed cells. The labeling of RNA with $[\gamma\text{-}^{32}P]$-ATP and polynucleotide kinase *in vitro* measures (via filter hybridization) the steady-state levels of RNA species (TABLE 1) as does

TABLE 3

RELATIVE ABUNDANCES OF CLONE 85 RNAs REGULATED BY T ANTIGEN

Clone No.	Transcript	Cell Line	
		tsA7	
		39° C	33° C
85	2.4 Kb	0	4
	2.2 Kb	0	5
	2.0 Kb	6	23
	1.6 Kb	4	21
	1.2 Kb	146	212

the northern blot hybridization experiments. The evidence that the SV40 large T antigen regulates the steady-state levels of these RNA species rests upon the temperature-sensitive SV40tsA mutant studies (TABLE 1). It remains possible that some cellular functions, in addition to the SV40 large T antigen, could behave in a temperature-sensitive fashion in any one of these cell lines. To overcome this problem, two independently derived cell lines (SV40tsA7 and SV40tsA58) [25, 26] containing two different A-gene or T-antigen alleles were employed. These cell lines also have different developmental and genetic (129 or BALB) backgrounds as well.[25, 26] The presence of high levels of RNA complementary to the A17, 104 and 397 cloned cDNA inserts in tumor tissue and not liver tissue extends these results *in vivo* and supports the conclusions of these experiments. Finally, SV40 infection of 3T3 cells in culture results in a stimulation of these RNA species complementary to the cloned cDNAs (unpublished observations) and this is independent of temperature shifts. It therefore appears likely that the SV40 large T antigen can regulate the levels of some cellular RNA species. In this context it is interesting to note that SV40 large T antigen stimulates ribosomal RNA synthesis as well.[27, 28]

On the basis of these results, it is not possible to determine whether SV40 T antigen stimulates gene transcription or enhances RNA stability, either of which would increase the steady-state levels of the RNA species detected in this study. Whatever the mechanism, it is selective in that some cellular RNAs are elevated by T antigen while others are not (TABLE 1; FIG. 1). SV40 large T antigen regulates the transformed phenotype [12–16] and by regulating the expression of cellular genes as well, this could explain the large number of differences between normal and transformed cells.[1]

Some cDNA clones (403, 218, B50) contain inserts complementary to RNA species which are regulated with temperature shifts in SV40tsA58 cells but not in SV40tsA7 cells. These differences could be due to a number of reasons: (1) SV40tsA58 and SV40tsA7 are different alleles of the viral A gene (T antigen); (2) the tsA58 and tsA7 cell lines are independent isolates in different developmental and genetic backgrounds,[25, 26] which could have an effect upon gene regulation; and (3) thermolabile factors other than T antigen could affect certain RNA species differently in these two cell lines. While not completely ruled out, this third alternative seems unlikely on the basis of the considerations discussed earlier.

The multiple RNA special detected by northern gel hybridization with some cloned probes (TABLE 2) could arise from: (1) presursor–product relationships between these RNA species; or (2) different transcripts with common nucleotide sequences in either the coding or noncoding (that is, 3' untranslated region) regions of the mRNA. The precursor-product hypothesis appears less likely because cytoplasmic RNA has been employed in this analysis (although nuclear leakage of RNA is possible), and in some cases (clones 398, 104) more than one of the RNA species are found to have an equal and high abundance at steady-state levels.

The results presented here demonstrate that some cellular RNA species are regulated in a positive fashion by SV40 large T antigen in transformed cells. In the SV40tsA transformed cells these RNAs are regulated in a temperature-sensitive fashion. After infection of 3T3 cells with SV40, the levels of these RNA species increase dramatically in the absence of a temperature shift (unpublished results). In SV40 transformed cells (SV3T3-T2) and tumor tissue these RNA species are 100–200-fold more abundant than in nontransformed 3T3 cells or liver tissue. It will now be important to investigate the function of these cellular genes and to determine the mechanism by which T antigen regulates these cellular genes.

ACKNOWLEDGMENTS

We thank R. Pashley, C. Sullivan, and A. K. Teresky for skillful technical assistance and G. Urban for assistance with the manuscript.

REFERENCES

1. TOOZE, J., Ed. 1980. Molecular Biology of Tumor Viruses, 2nd ed. Part II. DNA Tumor Viruses. Cold Spring Harbor Laboratory, NY.
2. TEGTMEYER, P. 1972. Simian virus 40 deoxyribonucleic acid synthesis: The viral replicon. J. Virol. **10:** 591–598.
3. TJIAN, R. 1978. The binding site on SV40 DNA for a T-antigen related protein. Cell **13:** 165–179.
4. SHORTLE, D. R., R. F. MARGOLSKEE & D. NATHANS. 1979. Mutational analysis of the simian virus 40 replicon: Pseudo-revertants of mutants with a defective replication origin. Proc. Natl. Acad. Sci. USA **76:** 6128–6131.
5. POSTEL, E. H. & A. J. LEVINE. 1976. The requirement of simian virus 40 gene A product for the stimulation of cellular thymidine kinase activity after viral infection. Virology **73:** 206–215.
6. CHOU, J. V. & R. G. MARTIN. 1975. DNA infectivity and the induction of host DNA synthesis with temperature-sensitive mutants of SV40. J. Virol. **15:** 145–160.
7. TJIAN, R., G. FEY & A. GRAESSMAN. 1978. Biological activity of purified simian virus 40 T-Antigen proteins. Proc. Natl. Acad. Sci. USA **75:** 1279–1283.
8. TEGTMEYER, P., M. SCHWARTZ, J. K. COLLINS & K. RUNDELL. 1975. Regulation of tumor antigen synthesis by simian virus 40 gene A. J. Virol. **16:** 168–178.
9. REED, S. I., G. R. STARK & J. C. ALWINE. 1976. Autoregulation of simian virus 40 gene A by T-antigen. Proc. Natl. Acad. Sci. USA **73:** 3083–3087.
10. ALWINE, J. C., S. I. REED & G. R. STARK. 1977. Characterization of the autoregulation of simian virus 40 gene A. J. Virol. **24:** 22–29.
11. KHOURY, G. & E. MAY. 1977. Regulation of early and late simian virus 40 transcription: Overproduction of early RNA in the absence of a functional T-antigen. J. Virol. **77:** 167–176.
12. KIMURA, G. & A. ITAGKI. 1975. Initiation and maintenance of cell transformation by SV40: A viral genetic property. Proc. Natl. Acad. Sci. USA **72:** 673–677.
13. MARTIN, R. G. & J. Y. CHOU. 1975. Simian virus 40 functions required for the establishment and maintenance of malignant transformation. J. Virol. **15:** 599–612.
14. TEGTMEYER, P. 1975. Function of simian virus 40 gene A in transforming infection. J. Virol. **15:** 613–618.
15. BRUGGE, J. S. & J. S. BUTEL. 1975. Role of simian virus 40 gene A function in maintenance of transformation. J. Virol. **15:** 619–636.
16. OSBORN, M. & K. WEBER. 1975. Simian virus 40 gene A function and maintenance of transformation. J. Virol. **15:** 636–644.
17. OREN, M., W. MALTZMAN & A. J. LEVINE. 1981. Post translational regulation of the 54K cellular tumor antigen in normal and transformed cells. Mol. Cell. Biol. **1:** 101–110.

18. VILLA-KOMAROFF, U., A. EFSTRADIADIS, S. BROOME, P. LOMEDICA, R. TIZARD, S. P. NABER, W. L. CHICK & W. GILBERT. 1978. A bacterial clone synthesizing proinsulin. Proc. Natl. Acad. Sci. USA **75:** 3727–3731.

19. DAGERT, M. & S. D. EHRILICH. 1979. Prolonged incubation in calcium chloride improves the competence of *Escherichia coli* cells. Gene **6:** 23–28.

20. THAYER, R. E. 1979. An improved method for detecting foreign DNA in plasmids of *Escherichia coli*. Anal. Biochem. **98:** 60–63.

21. SPRADLING, A. C., M. E. BIGAN, A. P. MAHOWALD, M. SCOTT & E. A. CRAIG. 1980. Two clusters of genes for major chorion proteins in Drosophila melanogaster. Cell **19:** 905–914.

22. THOMAS, P. S. 1980. Hybridization of denatured RNA and small DNA fragments transferred to nitrocellulose. Proc. Natl. Acad. Sci. USA **77:** 5201–5205.

23. KAFATOS, F. C., C. W. JONES & A. EFSTRATIADIS. 1979. Determination of nucleic acid sequence homologies and relative concentrations by a dot hybridization procedure. Nucleic Acids Res. **7:** 1541–1552.

24. AARONSON, S. A. & G. J. TODARO. 1968. Development of 3T3-like lines from Balb/c mouse embryo cultures; Transformation susceptibility to SV40. J. Cell Physiol. **72:** 141–148.

25. MALTZMAN, W., D. I. H. LINZER, D. BROWN, A. K. TERESKY, M. ROSENSTRAUS & A. J. LEVINE. 1979. Permanent teratocarcinoma derived cell lines stabilized by transformation with SV40 and SV40tsA mutant viruses. J. Int. Cytol. Suppl. **10:** 173–189.

26. BROCKMAN, W. W. 1978. Transformation of Balb/c 3T3 cells by tsA mutants of SV40: Temperature sensitivity of the transformed phenotype and retransformation of wild type virus. J. Virol. **25:** 860–868.

27. WHELLY, S., T. IDE & R. BASERGA. 1978. Stimulation of RNA synthesis in isolated nuclei by preparations of SV40 T-antigen. Virology **88:** 82–91.

28. IDE, T., S. WHELLY & R. BASERGA. 1977. Stimulation of RNA synthesis in isolated nuclei by partially purified preparations of SV40 T-antigen. Proc. Natl. Acad. Sci. USA **74:** 3189–3192.

MOLECULAR DISSECTION OF MHC COMPLEX AND OF SV40-INDUCED SURFACE ANTIGEN *

PART I: V. B. Reddy,† M. J. Tevethia,‡ S. S. Tevethia,‡ and
S. M. Weissman §

PART II: P. A. Biro,§ J. Pan,§ H. Das,§ A. K. Sood,§
S. M. Weissman,§ J. Barbosa,‖ M. Kamarck, ‖ and F. Ruddle ‖

*Departments of § Human Genetics and ‖ Biology
Yale University School of Medicine
New Haven, Connecticut 06510*

† *Southern Medical and Pharmaceutical Corporation
Tampa, Florida 33612*

‡ *The Milton S. Hershey Medical Center
The Pennsylvania State University
Hershey, Pennsylvania 17033*

INTRODUCTION

Papovaviruses such as SV40 and polyoma can induce tumors *in vivo* and transform cells to a tumorigenic state *in vitro*.[1] These malignant cells may be rejected by immunologic defense mechanisms in appropriately immunized hosts. The immune reactions appear to be directed against virus-encoded proteins, since immunization with any one of several types of cells infected with SV40 will protect the animals against SV40 tumors, but not against polyoma tumors, and *vice versa*.

The immunizing antigen is probably a variant of the SV40 "T antigen" or "A protein" that, in an incompletely understood fashion, reaches the cell surface. In addition, at least for cell-mediated cytotoxicity, the immune reaction is strictly dependent[2] upon the presence on the cell surface of specific host-encoded proteins derived from genes of the major histocompatibility (MHC) complex.[3] In conventional assays, killer lymphocytes can only destroy the cells bearing a foreign antigen if the cells also share one of the surface antigens encoded in the MHC with the cytotoxic lymphocytes, in addition to displaying the foreign antigen determinants on the surface. The nature of the interactions between foreign antigen and MHC products is unknown, but is a subject of intense current investigation.

We have initiated two lines of investigation to apply techniques of modern molecular genetics to the analysis and modification of the model system of host immunologic rejection of virus-induced tumors. On the one hand, investigators in Dr. Tevethia's laboratory and in Dr. Weissman's have begun joint studies to generate cell lines that express modified segments of SV40 early protein in order to investigate both their physiological roles in the

* This investigation was supported by Grant CA 16038 awarded by the National Cancer Institute (Part I), and by Grant 5-P50 GM 20124 from the National Institute of General Medical Sciences (Part II), National Institutes of Health, Department of Health and Human Services, Bethesda, Maryland.

0077-8923/82/0397-0229 $01.75/0 © 1982, NYAS

cell and particularly their roles as antigens in cell-mediated cytotoxicity reactions and tumor rejection. On the other hand, we have cloned extensive regions of the human MHC complex and are in the process of sequencing genes for the serologically identified products with the intention that these genes could then be modified and/or coupled to other DNA segments encoding known antigens such as the SV40 A protein, and reintroduced in cells so as to alter or enhance the immune response of the host to these cells.

PART I

Construction of SV40 Eukaryotic Cloning Vectors

We have studied the expression of SV40 DNA sequences encoding peptides corresponding to fragments of SV40 T antigen in mouse L cells. To do this, we constructed a series of plasmids carrying the ampicillin gene and replication systems of plasmid pBR322 linked to the *Bam* H1 fragment of herpes virus DNA containing the thymidine kinase gene. These in turn were linked to a fragment of SV40 extending from 0.73 to 0.67 map units on the SV40 genome [4] which contained the origin of replication, the adjacent tandem repeated sequences, and the remaining components of the early viral promoter (pZC 265, FIG. 1). Downstream, in the direction of transcription of the early genes of SV40, and immediately adjacent to the origin fragment, any one of several other segments of SV40 early region were inserted. Finally, beyond the inserted segments, all plasmids contained the region of SV40 early from either .17 or .194 through to .144. This region was inserted so that all transcripts initiating from the SV40 promoter would extend through the SV40 early segments to the polyadenylation signals between approximately 0.17 and 0.12 on the SV40 genome [4] (FIG. 1).

Different plasmids were so constructed as to contain coding regions for the various segments of the SV40 early genes between the early promoter and the early polyadenylation sites, together with the intervening sequence and splice junctions contained in the early SV40 genetic region. Plasmids so constructed contained DNA encoding either: (1) the entire early region (pVBE), or (2) truncated portions of large T and the entire small t antigens (pVB t TK-1 and pVB t I), or (3) the short amino terminal segment of large T antigen which is shared with small t, plus the entire small t antigen (p VB t-2; FIG. 1). These plasmids were used to transform TK- mouse L cells. We had noticed earlier that the SV40 origin sequences placed at either end of the thymidine kinase gene, in either orientation, enhanced transformation of TK- L cells by a factor of 10–30-fold.[5] Initially, some but not all laboratories had trouble in reproducing this effect. Some of the difficulties have now been explained by Professor M. Botchan, who has shown that high expression of the herpes virus thymidine kinase leads to inhibition of DNA replication, presumably because of feedback inhibition of ribonucleotide reductase by phosphorylated thymidine derivatives. The effects of the origin sequences have been more precisely characterized by Chambon,[6] Schaffner,[7] and Khoury[8] and their respective colleagues, who have shown that tandem repeats at the SV40 origin have an enhancing effect on transcription of inserted genes independent of their orientation or proximity to remaining components of the promoter.[6] Each of the plasmids we constructed was efficient in transforming the LMTK- cells to thymidine kinase positivity, and this was used as a selection procedure for cells which incorporated the recombinant plasmid.

Cells transformed with the plasmid containing the SV40 early region (pVB t1) could be assayed for production of T antigen. Of nine clones individually examined, one was negative for T antigen and one showed some T-antigen-

SV40 SEGMENTS

SV40
Map Units (a)

(a) Numbers refer to map units of SV40 relative to unique Eco RI site. Two numbers over the same vertical line imply that fragments with ends at these two coordinates were level.

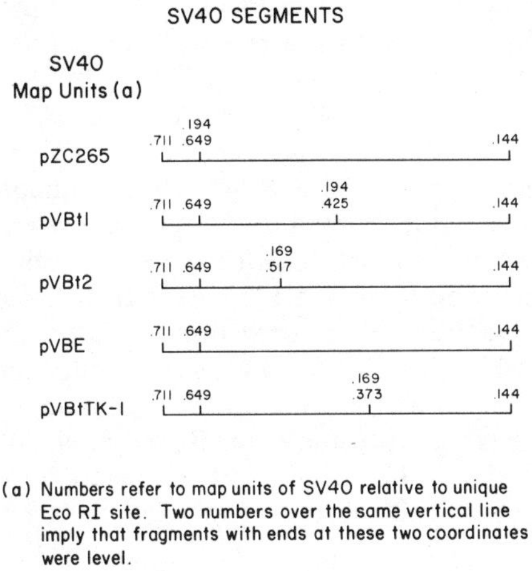

FIGURE 1. SV40 segments incorporated into recombinant pBR 322 herpes TK plasmids. pZC 265 refers to the parental construct containing the SV40 origin of promoter sequences between mapping at .711 and point .649 fused to HindIII site to the SV40 polyadenylation signals contained at map units .194 and .144. pVBt1 contained the first half of the SV40 early region inserted at the .194–.1649 HindIII site. pVBT2 contained a slightly shorter SV40 early region. pVBE contained the entire SV40 early region and pVBTK-1 contained essentially only the segment coding for little t antigen and the amino terminal segment common to little and large T. NOTE: DNA segments are not drawn to scale.

negative cells, while every cell of the remaining seven clones was positive for T antigen. Immunoprecipitation of these cells after labeling with ^{35}S-methionine showed that they synthesized both SV40 large T and small t antigens. Cells transformed by pVB-t-TK-1 (the plasmid lacking the segment of the SV40 early region between .37 and .17 map units) produced only small t antigen, but no detectable amounts of the 40-K truncated large T antigen. This effect could either be due to marked instability of the 40-K peptide or to preferential splicing to produce small t antigen, but has not been further studied. Cells transformed by pVB-t-1, a plasmid containing SV40 early region from the origin through the HindIII site at .425 map units,[4] did not show immunofluorescence, but did produce substantial amounts of a 33-K T-antigen-related peptide as well as small t antigen. Cells transformed by pVB-t-2 containing only the coding regions of small t (and the amino terminal region of large T shared with small t) were found to produce predominantly the short amino terminal segment of large T antigen, as though the predominant form of mRNA splicing was the large T rather than the small t splice. The short amino terminal segment of large T antigen was produced in large amounts and was relatively stable in the cell.[5]

These results show that peptides corresponding to rather arbitrarily chosen short regions from within a large protein may still be relatively stable and accumulate in substantial amounts within cells expressing the truncated gene.

They also caution that the stability of the protein may not be simply related to the amount of the normal coding region retained or to the size of the protein product. In addition, unanticipated effects on the relative efficiency of the formation of alternative splices must be examined and compensated for before one can produce specific products in large amounts from reconstructed genes.

The biological effects of the plasmid encoded in SV40 proteins were examined in two ways. First, plasmids were tested for their ability to immortalize cells or to produce morphologic transformation of mouse 3T3 cells. M. J. and S.S. Tevethia found that the plasmid containing the full-length early region transformed efficiently, but no transformation was detected with any of the plasmids containing truncated T regions.

Secondly, it was found that the plasmid (pVB t TK-1) which produced the 33-K truncated T antigen caused the mouse L cells to become sensitive to T-cell-mediated cell killing by cells immunized against SV40 TSTA (tumor-specific transplantation antigen), as measured by chromium-51 release *in vitro,* whereas the other plasmids containing truncated segments of the early region did not produce this effect. Cells transformed by pVB t TK-1 were then tested for their ability to immunize animals against SV40-induced tumor cells. Two of the plasmids were entirely negative, while the plasmid causing the production of SV40 3T3 truncated T proteins showed rather variable and marginal induction of immunologic protection. In one experiment, for example, the reduction was from more than 90% in animals killed by the control tumor to 60% mortality in animals previously immunized with the cells producing the truncated T peptide.

These results provide strong additional confirmation that the TSTA directly involves SV40 early-region encoded products, and, secondly, they suggest that it may be possible to generate a variety of immunogenic cell lines which are capable of protecting animals against SV40 tumors but do not themselves produce intact transforming protein. Further studies are directed towards enhancing this effect, particularly towards reconstructing the SV40 early gene fragments so as to obtain a larger portion of protein expressed on the cell surface and also to obtain expression of fused products between MHC loci genes and SV40 T antigen segments.

PART II

Analysis of Genes of the Human Major Histocompatibility Complex:
Cloning and Structure of Human MHC Genes

The human MHC complex is a region of DNA covering several recombination units. The exact size of the complex cannot be calibrated, but on the basis of recombination frequency between markers, it may represent several million base pairs and would appear to be larger than the murine MHC. The genes of the human and mouse MHC are individually very similar, but the arrangement of DNA seems to be different in some important respects. For example, both complexes encode the class I antigens present on all cell types, the class II antigens which are correlated with immune response genes, and the class III proteins that include certain components of the major and alternative complement pathways. However, the order of these classes of genes differs in man and mouse.

Our technical approach for cloning the scarce messenger RNAs corresponding to surface antigens encoded in the major histocompatibility complex has been previously described.[9] Essentially, we used available fragmentary amino acid sequence data to design DNA probes partially complementary to the messenger RNA. These DNA probes were annealed to messenger RNA and elongated in the presence of three deoxynucleoside triphosphates and one dideoxynucleoside triphosphates to serve as a chain terminator. In this way a series of products of different lengths was obtained, each corresponding to a different subset of mRNAs. Limited sequence analysis of a few products rapidly served to identify the precise sequence of the segment of the mRNA encoding the known antigen and the appropriate extension products in turn were used as a probe for either cDNA libraries or genomic libraries. By use of this method we have isolated a cDNA clone complementary to most of the messenger RNA sequence of HLA-B7 and also directly isolated a genomic clone encoding the whole of the human DR antigen P34 (heavy chain).

The genomic representation of sequences complementary to the class I heavy-chain HLA-B7 antigen mRNA and those complementary to the class II heavy-chain (HLA-D P34) mRNA was very different. Thus, there were at least 15 *Eco* RI fragments complementary to the class I mRNA in digests of human DNA [10] and in almost every case these fragments have been confirmed to contain either a complete gene or pseudogene. In contrast, there was a single fragment complementary to the P34 mRNA sequences. The analysis of the genes for the class I and class II antigens represents two different sets of problems. In the case of the HLA-D antigen, cloning of the single fragment complementary to the mRNA was readily accomplished and sequence analysis of this fragment has confirmed that it does contain sequences identical to those contained in an isolated cDNA clone [11] and therefore identical to those in HLA-D P34 mRNA.

In contrast, many different clones covering a total of approximately 500,000 kilobases of genomic DNA were obtained when the lambda and cosmid libraries of genomic DNA were screened with the HLA-B7 cDNA probe. We have performed complete sequence analysis of one six-kilobase fragment showing strong complementarity to the B-7 cDNA and partial analysis of four other fragments of similar length.[12]

The completely sequenced DNA proved to encode a pseudogene that showed extensive homology with the entire coding region HLA-B7 cDNA. This homology also extended through most of the 3' untranslated region. Since the nucleotide sequence of the 5' untranslated portion of HLA-B7 cDNA is not known, it is not possible to evaluate the degree of homology in this region. This genomic sequence also showed the characteristic organization that has been identified in both the human and murine class I MHC genes.[13-15] The coding regions were separated by at least eight intervening sequences, the first of which divided the hydrophobic leader segment from the first-domain amino acid residues. Other intervening sequences occurred at amino acid residues 93, 183, and 272, so as to divide the coding regions almost exactly into the three domains suggested from protein chemical studies. The intervening sequence between the DNA encoding the second and third domain of the mature protein has been the largest of the seven in all the human and mouse genes studied. An additional intervening sequence separated the third domain from the coding region for the hydrophilic intramembranous portion of the protein. The short cytoplasmic hydrophilic component was separated into at least two additional domains; but it was impossible to determine whether there could be more than two.

Finally, an intervening sequence divided the coding regions for the cytoplasmic domains from the 3′ untranslated portion of the messenger RNA. This structure is rather unusual; in most cases intervening sequences separate the 5′, not the 3′, untranslated region from coding regions. The same pattern of intervening sequences, including the possible complexities in the cytoplasmic and hydrophilic domains, has also been noted in the other genes we have examined and in two genes from the mouse recently studied by Hood [13, 14] and his colleagues and by Seidman [15] and his colleagues. As also noted by Hood, the most homologous regions between the genes seem to overlap the third coding domain.

Another curious feature of the gene is the long poly(A) track which precedes the putative template for the 5′ untranslated region of the RNA. In most cases, poly(A) tracks noted in human DNA have been linked to the repetitious DNA sequence elements of the *Alu* family. This is not the case in the *Alu* track preceding the pseudogene. The oligo(A)s of the *Alu* families have been implicated in the mechanism of transposition in possible RNA-directed gene conversion.[16] It remains to be seen whether there is any analogy between the possible roles for the oligo(A)s in *Alu* sequences and in their occurrence preceding the MHC gene.

An additional clone was isolated that contained a single *Eco*RI fragment of 11 kilobases. Restriction cutting showed that all the infrequent cutting sites in this second clone corresponded to the sites present in two adjacent *Eco*RI fragments of the first clone whose total length is also 11 kilobases with the exception of the internal *Eco*RI site. Partial sequence analysis showed that the second clone was over 95% homologous to the first pair, both in the coding and in the intervening and flanking regions. Thus, there appear to be relatively long-range repeats in the MHC sequences. Except for the single change at the *Eco*RI site, these clones would have been considered identical. This indicates that considerable caution is needed in interpreting the order of restriction fragments within the MHC by the use of overlapping clones.

In spite of the strong homology to B-7 cDNA and the apparently intact organization of the gene segments, the initial sequences proved to be pseudogenes. This is shown most dramatically by a single base deletion that causes a shift in the reading frame within the first exon of the first domain of what would have been the mature protein in the true gene. Because of the possibility that this might be an artifact that occurred during cloning, the corresponding gene was isolated from the DNA of a second cell line of known HLA type, the JY cell line. Partial sequence analysis of this clone showed that the same base was missing, so as to cause the reading frame to shift. Furthermore, the two pseudogenes isolated from subjects of different ethnic backgrounds showed greater than 99% homology—more than would be expected to be found in the coding regions for different genes for different HLA-B or HLA-A types.

Partial sequence analysis of other genomic clones has revealed several additional pseudogenes that deviate to greater or lesser extent from the HLA-B7 cDNA. However, analysis of one of the genomic clones from a cell line expressing HLA-B7 showed perfect agreement between nucleotide sequences in the genome and the known nucleotide sequences of HLA-B7 cDNA. Thus, by definitive sequence analysis, we have identified the cloned genes for one of the human class I MHC antigens and for the heavy chains of class II MHC antigens.

In a separate series of experiments, TK⁻ L cells were cotransfected with herpes virus TK DNA [17] and individual cosmid, lambda phage, or plasmid clones containing inserts of MHC DNA. These transfected cells were tested by immunofluorescence for ability to bind the monoclonal antibody W6/32 directed against HLA class I antigens (FIG. 2).[18] Two clones were found that induced surface antigens reactive with W6/32. One turned out to be the B7 clone and

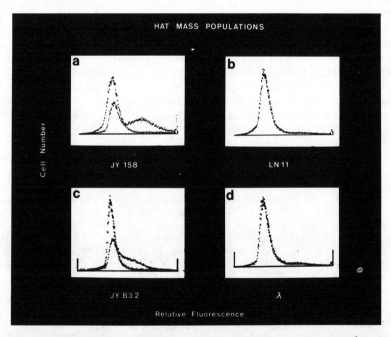

FIGURE 2. HLA-A, B, C expression of LTK⁻ cells which have been transfected with HLA genomic DNA. Cotransfection of 1.5×10^6 cells was performed with μg quantities of Charon 4A vector containing HLA genomic sequences and μg quantities of plasmid (HSV-TK in pBR 322).[19] HAT selection was applied to the transfected cells 60 hours after DMGT, and a large resistant population was recovered 2 weeks later. Indirect immunofluorescence analysis of HLA-A, B, C expression was performed with monoclonal antibody W632 and the fluorescence-activated cell sorter.[20] Each panel compared specific staining with W632 and control staining with myeloma supernatants. HAT mass population generated by cotransfection with (**a**) genomic clone JY158 (HLAB7); (**b**) genomic clone LH11; (**c**) genomic clone B3.2 (HLA-A2); (**d**) lambda DNA. Q. Photomultiplier voltages were converted by logarithmic amplifier for display on the multichannel analyzer.

the other induced an antigen that reacted with anti-A2 antisera. Thus, it appears that the clones for the HLA-A and HLA-B genes have been identified as well as for HLA-D heavy chain. In addition, A. Calman has obtained genomic clones corresponding to the beta-2 microglobulin gene. Current cloning efforts are under way to obtain the genomic clones for the class II light chains.

The precise division of the DNA by introns into segments corresponding to protein domains is of interest in two respects. First, the DNA encoding the cytoplasmic, hydrophilic segment of the HLA antigens is divided into at least two segments, and the sequence suggests that there is a potential for alternate splices in this region. This raises the possibility that alternate forms of mRNA may be produced, resulting in proteins with different cytoplasmic domains, and also suggests that the cytoplasmic segment of the protein may be divided into two short functional regions.

The second point of interest is that the location of intervening sequences makes it technically convenient to isolate subgenomic segments encoding individual domains of these proteins. It may prove relatively convenient to use recombinant DNA techniques to exchange domains between proteins. For example, experiments are under way to create a pseudo-HLA antigen by inserting an additional coding segment corresponding to a portion of SV40 T antigen between the HLA domains. It will be of interest to see whether the HLA-MHC gene framework and coding regions can be used as vehicles to export amino acid sequences corresponding to other proteins to the cell and to enhance their immunologic activity because of their presence on the cell surface and their proximity to domains of MHC proteins.

REFERENCES

1. TOOZE, E., Ed. 1981. Molecular Biology of Tumor Viruses, 2nd ed. Cold Spring Harbor Laboratory. Cold Spring Harbor, NY.
2. ZINKERNAGEL, R. M. & P. C. DOHERTY. 1979. Adv. Immunol. **27:** 51–177.
3. PLOEGH, H. L., H. T. ORR & J. STROMINGER. 1981. Cell **24:** 287–299.
4. REDDY, V. B., B. THIMMAPPAYA, R. DHAR, K. N. SUBRAMANIAN, B. S. ZAIN, P. K. GHOSH, J. PAN, M. L. CELMA & S. M. WEISSMAN. 1978. The Genome of SV40. Science **200:** 494–502.
5. REDDY, V. B., S. S. TEVETHIA, M. J. TEVETHIA & S. M. WEISSMAN. Non-selective expression of SV40 T antigen fragments in mouse cells. Proc. Natl. Acad. Sci. USA. In press.
6. BENOIST, C. & P. CHAMBON. 1981. Nature **290:** 304–310.
7. BANERJI, J., S. RUSCONI & W. SCHAFFNER. 1981. Cell **27:** 299–308.
8. GRUSS, P., R. DHAR & G. KHOURY. 1981. Proc. Natl. Acad. Sci. USA **78:** 943–947.
9. SOOD, A. K., D. PEREIRA & S. M. WEISSMAN. 1981. Isolation of a specific cDNA probe for the human histocompatibility genes by the use of an oligodeoxynucleotide primer. Proc. Natl. Acad. Sci. USA **78:** 616–620.
10. BIRO, P. A., D. PEREIRA, A. K. SOOD, B. DE MARTINVILLE, U. FRANCKE & S. M. WEISSMAN. 1981. The structure of the human major histocompatibility locus. *In* ICN-UCLA Symposium Molecular Biology, Vol. XX: Immunoglobular Idiotypes. E. Janeway, C. A. Setcarc, E. E. and H. Wigzell, Eds.' 315–326. Academic Press. New York, NY.
11. ERLICH, H. *et al.* Manuscript in preparation.

12. WEISSMAN, S. M., P. A. BIRO, A. K. SOOD, D. PEREIRA, V. B. REDDY & J. PAN. 1981. Genes of the human major histocompatibility complex. *In* Medicine in Transition: The Centennial of the University of Illinois College of Medicine. Edward P. Cohen, Ed.: 137–147. University of Illinois Press. Chicago, IL.
13. STEINMETZ, M., K. W. MOORE, J. G. FRELINGER, B. T. SHER, F.-W. SHEN, E. A. BOYSE & L. E. HOOD. 1981. Cell **25:** 683–692.
14. MOORE, K. W., B. T. SHER, H. Y. SUN, K. A. EAKLE & L. E. HOOD. 1982. Science **215:** 679–682.
15. EVANS, G. A., D. H. MARGULIES, D. CAMERINI-OTERO, K. OZATO & J. G. SEIDMAN. Proc. Natl. Acad. Sci. USA. Submitted for publication.
16. JAGADEESWARAN, P., B. G. FORGET & S. M. WEISSMAN. 1981. Cell **26:** 141–142.
17. SCANGOS, G. A., K. M. HUTTNER, D. K. JURICEK & F. RUDDLE. 1981. Mol. Cell. Biol. **1:** 111–120.
18. KAMARCK, M. E., J. A. BARBOSA & F. RUDDLE. Somatic Cell Genet. In press.
19. SCANGOS, *et al.* 1981.
20. KAMARCK, M., J. BARBOSA & F. RUDDLE. Somatic Cell Genetics. In press.

MICROINJECTION OF CLONED SV40 DNA FRAGMENTS IN THE STUDY OF CELL PROLIFERATION

Norbel Galanti,* Kenneth Soprano,† Gerald Jonak,‡ and
Renato Baserga

*Department of Pathology and Fels Research Institute
Temple University Medical School
Philadelphia, Pennsylvania 19140*

INTRODUCTION

During the last decade, the development of the concepts and the techniques of recombinant DNA, DNA sequencing, and the auxiliary methods needed for the identification of particular DNA fragments made possible the investigation of the anatomy of prokaryotic and eukaryotic chromosomes. Likewise, procedures that introduce recombinant DNA into a biologically functional host cell have permitted the study of the function of entire genes or even fragments of genes.

There are many uses for the recombinant DNA technology in the study of cell proliferation. One possibility is to look for genes known to participate in a series of events needed for DNA replication, such as a gene that corrects a temperature-sensitive defect during the prereplicative phase of the cell cycle. A second possibility is to identify specific DNA sequences present in transformed cells and absent in the normal, original cell line. A third possibility is to isolate viral oncogenic genes that induce cellular DNA replication in resting host cells.

With regard to the introduction of an isolated, cloned DNA fragment into a recipient cell, several techniques have been developed in the last 15 years. These include cell fusion, DNA transfection, manual microinjection, and the use of liposomes. However, the manual microinjection technique appears at the present time to be the most suitable.[1, 2]

The Manual Microinjection Technique

As just mentioned, the capacity to introduce informational molecules into a biologically functional mammalian cell makes it possible to study the role of particular genes or gene products on the series of events leading to cell proliferation. The manual microinjection technique offers unique advantages to such studies since expression of the introduced molecule can be followed at definite

* Present address: Departamento de Biología Celular y Genética, Facultad de Medicina, Universidad de Chile, Casilla 6556, Santiago 7, Chile.

† Present address: Department of Microbiology, Temple University Medical School, Philadelphia, Pennsylvania 19140.

‡ Present address: Dupont Experimental Station, Bldg. 328, Room 369, Wilmington, Delaware 19898.

0077–8923/82/0397–0238 $01.75/0 © 1982, NYAS

end points, such as incorporation of ^{3}H-labeled thymidine into cellular DNA (which can be detected by autoradiography under a light microscope) or the appearance of a protein (easily identified by direct or indirect immunofluorescence). It is also possible to follow polypeptide synthesis in only a few cells after manual microinjection of DNA, cRNA or mRNA, by two-dimensional gel electrophoresis.[3, 4]

Indeed, using the manual microinjection technique it is possible to deliver a known, purified molecule or macromolecule directly into the nucleus or the cytoplasm of a particular mammalian cell, preserving its integrity and viability. Thus, this technique not only permits the introduction of a single molecular species into the cell, but also provides precise placement of these molecules, whether in an aqueous or in a nonaqueous solvent, within different compartments of an individual cell.[5]

Manual microinjection integrates the techniques of cell culture, micromanipulation, and phase-contrast light microscopy. It is performed under a phase-contrast microscope by guiding a glass micropipet (tip diameter ~0.5 μm). with a micromanipulator into a cell attached to a cover-slip placed in a petri dish. The glass micropipet is connected to a syringe as the source of negative pressure (to charge the micropipet with the solution to be microinjected) or positive pressure (to discharge the solution into the selected cellular compartment). Volumes of about 10 femtoliters of very highly concentrated solutions may be microinjected.

With this technique, minute amounts of material to be microinjected are required and cells can be monitored, examined, detached, cloned, or analyzed immediately or at any time after microinjection.[5] For studies of cell proliferation, resting cells or synchronized cells at specific times in their cell cycle can be easily microinjected and followed in time-course experiments.

SV40 Virus and Cell Proliferation

The DNA of SV40 virus is a covalently closed, double-stranded circle with a molecular weight of 3.4×10^6. Its 5243 nucleotides have been completely sequenced.[6] There are two regions in this molecule. One extends from the origin of replication (nucleotide 5235, 0.66 map units [m.u.]) counterclockwise to nucleotide 2693 (0.17 m.u.) (early gene). The other region is found between the origin of replication clockwise to nucleotide 2591 (0.16 m.u.) (late gene).

When SV40 virus infects permissive cells, expression of its genes occurs in two phases.[7] During the first phase, two mRNAs are synthesized through different processing of a common precursor transcribed from the early gene. One of the mRNAs codes for a protein of 90,000 daltons (large T). The other mRNA codes for a protein of 17,000 daltons (small t). Shortly after the appearance of these proteins, cell DNA synthesis is induced. If integration of viral DNA into the cellular genome occurs, the host cells become transformed.

Large T antigen is a multifunctional protein which induces cellular DNA synthesis, regulates transcription of its own mRNA, stimulates viral DNA replication, and produces reactivation of nucleolar genes in the host cell. Several domains can be identified in this protein, which can be recognized with specific antibodies (U, TSTA and T) or by growing human adenovirus in monkey cells (helper function).[6, 7, 23]

Early work by Graessmann and his associates[8-10] have shown that the entire protein was required for viral replication, while the amino acid sequence coded by a nucleotide fragment of the early gene that extends from nucleotide 346 (0.725 m.u.) counterclockwise to nucleotide 3733 (0.373 m.u.) was sufficient to make T antigen detectable by the specific antiserum. The adenovirus helper function plus the U and TSTA determinants were coded by 538 base pairs extending from nucleotide 3204 (0.272 m.u.) counterclockwise to nucleotide 2666 (0.169 m.u.). The sequences of the SV40 early gene sufficient for stimulation of cellular DNA synthesis "mapped" between nucleotide 346 (0.725 m.u.) counterclockwise to nucleotide 3204 (0.272 m.u.).

In this paper, we present data on the identification of DNA sequences in the early gene of SV40 virus that are responsible for cell DNA replication and for cell growth in size. These data were obtained by using the recombinant DNA technique to isolate and clone definite, specific fragments of the viral gene, and manual microinjection to introduce the recombinant clones, or fragments, into recipient cells.

MATERIALS AND METHODS

Culture of Cells and Preparation of Viral and Plasmid DNA

ts13 cells, a G_1-specific temperature-sensitive (ts) mutant originally derived from BHK,[11] were grown on glass slides at the permissive temperature of 34° C, as previously described.[12] Before microinjection, ts13 cells were made quiescent by allowing them to grow for 7 days in Dulbecco's modified essential medium supplemented with 1% calf serum. After microinjection, cells were incubated for 24 hours in the same medium at 34° C. All media were prewarmed to the temperature of incubation before use.

NIH-3T3 cells were made quiescent by culturing them in 1% calf serum for 2 days at 37° C. After microinjection, cells were incubated at the same temperature without changing the medium.

TC-7 monkey cells were grown in 5% fetal calf serum at 37° C. They were microinjected while growing exponentially.

Human > mouse hybrid cells (#55–54)[13] were cultured in Dulbecco's medium supplemented with 10% fetal bovine serum. This cell line contains all the human chromosomes and 18 different mouse chromosomes, including those where the mouse rRNA genes are located (#12, 15 and 18).[14]

For the preparation of viral SV40 DNA, CV-1 cells grown in Dulbecco's medium with 10% fetal calf serum were infected with SV40 DNA at m.o.i of 0.02. After 6 days, viral DNA was extracted from infected cells by the Hirt procedure.[15]

Plasmid DNA (pBR322) was obtained from host *E. coli* HB 101 using the technique of Bolivar *et al.*[16]

Cloning of SV40 DNA Fragments

Selected SV40 DNA fragments were obtained with restriction endonucleases and recombined with appropriate pBR322 fragments, as previously described.[17] Specifically, the following recombinant clones were constructed:

(1) a clone, pSV2G, containing the EcoRl-BamHl fragment extending from nucleotide 1782 (1.00 m.u.) to nucleotide 2533 (0.144 m.u.); (2) a clone, pSVPstI, containing the EcoRl-PstI fragment extending from nucleotide 1782 (1.00 m.u.) to nucleotide 3204 (0.272 m.u.); (3) a clone, pSVPvu, containing the PvuII fragment from nucleotide 270 (0.71 m.u.) to nucleotide 3506 (0.33 m.u.); (4) a clone, pSVHpaI, containing the PvuII/HpaIB fragment from nucleotide 270 (0.71 m.u.) to nucleotide 3733 (0.373 m.u.); (5) a clone, pVR200, containing the SV40 sequences from nucleotide 270 (0.71 m.u.) to nucleotide 4002 (0.425 m.u.) and from nucleotide 2799 (0.194 m.u.) to nucleotide 2533 (0.144 m.u.), and (6) several deletion mutants of SV40 cloned in pBR322.§ The structure of all recombinant plasmids was confirmed by restriction analysis.

Microinjection of DNA

DNA fragments recovered from agarose gels by electrodialysis or cloned recombinant DNA fragments were delivered directly into nuclei of cells using the glass capillary manual microinjection technique as described by Graessmann and coworkers.[10] Other technical conditions were as previously described.[17, 21]

Detection of T Antigen and Cell DNA Synthesis

SV40 T antigen was detected by indirect immunofluorescence using the technique of Graessmann *et al.*[18] Cells were continuously labeled with ³H-thymidine (0.7 μCi/ml) during the entire incubation period. Autoradiographs were made and analyzed as described by Baserga and Malamud.[19] Nonmicro-injected cells outside the place of microinjection served as control.

Reactivation of rRNA genes in Human > Mouse Hybrid Cells

This was carried out in exactly the same manner as described by Soprano *et al.*[20]

RESULTS AND DISCUSSION

In a previous paper we have demonstrated that the incorporation of ³H-thymidine detected by autoradiography after microinjection of SV40 DNA is due to replication of cellular DNA.[21] Moreover, ³H-thymidine incorporation is inhibited by the simultaneous microinjection of antibodies against T antigen, suggesting that this effect of the microinjected SV40 DNA is mediated through the large T antigen.

By manual microinjection of SV40 DNA fragments generated from the early gene by restriction endonucleases, or of similar fragments cloned in pBR322 plasmid, or of deletion mutants in the SV40 DNA early gene, we have

§ These deletion mutants were cloned by Dr. J. Pipas and Dr. Daniel Nathans, Department of Microbiology, Johns Hopkins University Medical School, Baltimore, Maryland 21205.

mapped the base sequences necessary and sufficient for the following functions of large T antigen: induction of cellular DNA synthesis, reactivation of silent nucleolar genes, and major T antigen determinant.

For recipient cells we have used quiescent ts13 (hamster) and 3T3 (mouse) cells for the analysis of stimulation of cellular DNA synthesis, a human > mouse hybrid cell (#55–54) for the study of nucleolar reactivation, and TC-7 (monkey) cells to examine the maximal efficiency of expression of the T antigen determinant.

Cellular DNA Replication

d12005 is a mutant of SV40 virus that has a deletion in the region of the early gene coding for the small t (nucleotides 4867–4602, 0.59–0.54 m.u.). This mutant does not produce small t,[22] yet induces cellular DNA replication (TABLE 1). Therefore small t is not required for this function. This fact is further confirmed when a recombinant plasmid of SV40 DNA (pSV3D), also carrying a deletion in the region coding for small t (between nucleotides 5171 to 4442), was microinjected. This recombinant induces cellular DNA replication in the recipient cell (not shown).[17]

In previous work, Graessmann and coworkers [8, 9] had concluded that the sequences of the early gene downstream from nucleotide 3204 (0.27 m.u.) were not necessary for the induction of cell DNA replication. However, this work was done by microinjection of a restriction fragment eluted from agarose

TABLE 1

INDUCTION OF CELL DNA SYNTHESIS IN CELLS MICROINJECTED WITH DIFFERENT FRAGMENTS OF THE SV40 EARLY GENE

DNA Microinjected	Early Gene Sequences from Nucleotide 5235 (0.66 m.u.) to:		% of Cells in DNA Synthesis	
	Nucleotide	Map Units	ts13	3T3
None	—	—	7.5	8.0
pBR322	—	—	6.5	7.5
pSV2G	2533	0.14	78.0	74.0
HpaII/PstI *	3204	0.27	59.0	Not done
pSVPstI	3204	0.27	63.0	56.0
HpaII/PstI †	3204	0.27	46.0	74.0
pSVPvu	3506	0.33	40.0	43.0
HpaIB	3733	0.37	53.0	Not done
pSVHpaI	3733	0.37	52.0	40.0
pVR200	4002	0.42	30.0	64.0
d12005	Δ4867/4602	0.59/0.54	64.0	Not done

NOTE: DNA was manually microinjected into nuclei of cells. After 24 hours in the presence of ^{3}H-labeled thymidine, cells were fixed, T antigen was detected by indirect immunofluorescence, and cells in DNA synthesis were counted as described in the MATERIALS AND METHODS section.

* From pSV2G.
† From pSVPstI.

Table 2

Ability of Cloned Deletion Mutants of SV40 to Express T Antigen and to
Stimulate Cell DNA Synthesis

| Clone | Deleted SV40 DNA Sequences in: | | % T⁺ Cells | % Cells in DNA Synthesis |
	Nucleotides	Map Units		
None	—	—	0	4
pBR322	—	—	0	5
pSVB3	Intact SV40 DNA		98	96
pSV1136	5067/4262	0.63/0.48	0	5
pSV1046 *	4198/3880	0.46–0.42	0	45
pSV1001 †	4006	0.425	60	70
pSV1151 *	3798/3472	0.38/0.32	29	50

Note: Cloned DNA was manually microinjected into ts13 or 3T3 cells. After 24 hours in the presence of ³H-thymidine, cells were processed for T antigen detection and for autoradiography as described in the Materials and Methods section. Clone pSV1001 (†) terminates at nucleotide 4006 (0.425 m.u.).

* In phase deletions.

gels. These preparations can sometimes be contaminated with minute amounts of undigested material, or with other fragments, or their biological activity can occasionally be restrained. Therefore, we repeated the aforementioned experiments using both purified and cloned fragments missing the nucleotide sequence 3′ of nucleotide 3204 (0.27 m.u.). All of these fragments or recombinant plasmids were able to induce cellular DNA replication (Table 1). These results thus confirm data from Graessmann *et al.*[8, 9]

On the other hand, microinjection of the PvuIIA or the HpaIB fragments as well as the pSVPvu, pSVHpaI or pVR200 clones led to stimulation of cell DNA synthesis (Table 1). We therefore conclude that the nucleotide sequence 3′ of nucleotide 4002 (0.42 m.u.) is not necessary for the induction of cell DNA replication in ts13 and 3T3 cells. Since the SV40 deletion mutant d12005 (Δ from nucleotide 4867 to 4602) is fully active (Table 1), as is pSV3D (Δ from nucleotide 5171 to 4442),[17] the base sequences of the early gene needed for cell DNA replication seem to be located between nucleotide 4442 counterclockwise to nucleotide 4002 plus a short sequence near the origin of replication.

To map in greater detail the sequences critical for stimulation of cell DNA synthesis, we also microinjected into recipient cells, cloned mutants of SV40 DNA carrying deletions in different regions of the early gene. Results of this experiment are shown in Table 2. These data together with those from Table 1 show that the minimal sequence needed for cell DNA stimulation codes between nucleotides 4350 to 4190 (0.49–0.46 m.u.). Moreover, clone pSV1046 carrying a deletion between nucleotides 4190 to 3880 (0.46–0.42 m.u.) does not code for the major T antigen determinant, while still inducing cell DNA replication. Thus, the sequence coding for the T antigen major determinant is proximate but separate from the sequence coding for stimulation of cellular DNA synthesis.

Reactivation of rRNA Genes

We have previously demonstrated that the SV40 early gene is capable of reactivating silent mouse rRNA genes in human > mouse hybrid cells #55–54.[23, 24] These hybrid cells contain both human and mouse rRNA genes, but express only human rRNA, even under optimal growth conditions.[14, 25] As we have shown in a recent publication, with the use of nondefective adeno-SV40 hybrid viruses and the manual microinjection of some restriction fragments we were able to determine that the sequences from nucleotide 5235 (0.661 m.u.) downstream to nucleotide 3823 (0.39 m.u.) and from nucleotide 3204 (0.27 m.u.) down to nucleotide 2533 (0.144 m.u.) are not necessary for the reactivation of silent rRNA genes.[20] Data shown in TABLE 3 are the results of microinjection of several restriction fragments or recombinant DNA with different SV40 DNA fragments into nuclei of human > mouse hybrid cells. From these data we conclude that the sequence encoding the information for the reactivation of silent rRNA genes is located between nucleotides 3823 (0.39 m.u.) and 3506 (0.33 m.u.).

When cloned deletion mutants of SV40 DNA early gene are microinjected into #55–54 human > mouse hybrid cells, it was found that clone pSV1001, which terminates prior to nucleotide 3828 (0.39 m.u.) and clone pSV1151, with a deletion between nucleotides 3828 to 3506 (0.39–0.33 m.u.), failed to reactivate silent mouse rRNA genes (TABLE 4). These results confirm that the sequence critical for nucleolar activation is located between nucleotide 3828 (0.39 m.u.) and nucleotide 3506 (0.33 m.u.).

Different Domains for Cell DNA Replication, Nucleolar Activation, and the Major T Antigen Determinant

Taken together, the results presented in TABLES 1, 2, 3 and 4 clearly show that the information for cell DNA replication, reactivation of rRNA genes,

TABLE 3

REACTIVATION OF SILENT rRNA GENES IN CELLS MICROINJECTED WITH DIFFERENT FRAGMENTS OF THE SV40 EARLY GENE

DNA Microinjected	Early Gene Sequences from Nucleotide 5235 (0.66 m.u.) to:		Reactivation of Silent rRNA Genes
	Nucleotide	Map Units	
None	—	—	No
pBR322	—	—	No
pSV2G	2533	0.14	Yes
HpaII/PstI	3204	0.27	Yes
PvuIIA	3506	0.33	Yes (weak)
HpaIB	3733	0.37	No
pVR200	4002	0.42	No
d12005	Δ4867/4602	0.59/0.54	Yes
Ad2+ND5(ins.)	3823/2355	0.39/0.11	Yes

NOTE: DNA was manually microinjected into nuclei of human > mouse hybrid cells. After 16 hours, rRNA was extracted and analyzed as described by Soprano et al.[20] Δ = deletion; ins. = insert of SV40 DNA.

TABLE 4

ABILITY OF CLONED DELETION MUTANTS OF SV40 TO REACTIVATE rRNA GENES

Clone	Deleted SV40 Sequences in:		Reactivation of rRNA Genes
	Nucleotides	Map Units	
None	—	—	No
pBR322	—	—	No
pSVB3	Intact SV40 DNA		Yes
pSV1001, ends	4006	0.425	No
pSV1046 *	4190/3880	0.46/0.42	Yes
pSV1151 *	3798/3472	0.38/0.32	No
pSV1061	3048/2906	0.24/0.21	Yes

NOTE: Cloned DNA was manually microinjected into human > mouse hybrid cells. After 16 hours rRNA was extracted and analyzed as described by Soprano *et al.*[20] pSV1001 terminates at nucleotide 4006 (0.424 m.u.).

* In phase deletions.

and the major T antigen determinant are encoded in separate domains of the early gene of SV40 virus.

Particularly clear are the results obtained with recombinants pSV1046 and pSV1001. The first clone presents a deletion between nucleotides 4198 to 3880 (0.46–0.42 m.u.). This recombinant induces cell DNA replication upon microinjection, but the cells remain T-antigen-negative. Clone pSV1001, which terminates at nucleotide 4006 (0.425 m.u.), induces both cell DNA synthesis and the appearance of the immunologically detectable T antigen (TABLE 2).

On the other hand, clones pSV1046 and pSV1151 stimulate cell DNA replication. Clone pSV1046, with a deletion in phase between nucleotides 4190 to 3880 (0.46–0.42 m.u.), reactivates the silent mouse rRNA genes in human > mouse hybrid cells. Clone pSV1151, with a deletion in phase between nucleotides 3798 to 3472, fails to reactivate rRNA genes (TABLE 4).

These examples confirm the existence of different domains for these three functions in the early gene of the SV40 virus.

DNA Synthesis and Growth in Size

Our results show that the information for cell DNA replication and for reactivation of rRNA genes are encoded in separate domains on the early gene.

Since an increase in cell size is regularly accompanied by an increase in the cellular amount of ribosomal RNA, rRNA genes should be a target for growth-in-size signals. Therefore, large T antigen contains in its amino acid sequence a domain responsible for cell growth in size, and another separate but proximate region coding for cellular DNA replication.

From our results it is not clear whether T antigen acts independently on rRNA genes and on the gene(s) responsible for the initiation of cell DNA replication. If so, it should trigger two parallel pathways leading to rRNA or DNA synthesis, respectively. It may also be possible that nucleolar reactivation is an event previous to, and necessary for, cell DNA synthesis. However, experimental data suggest that rRNA synthesis and cellular DNA replication are separate events. In fact, control of cell size and control of cell DNA synthesis can be dissociated. In the developing rat liver, the RNA/DNA ratio increases from 1.18 on day 16 of fetal development to 3.45 two weeks after birth.[26] In some temperature-sensitive mutants (ts) of mammalian cells that are arrested in G_1, at the restrictive temperature, cell size increases while the cells are arrested in G_1.[27] In quiescent tsAF8 cells, infection by adenovirus 2 causes cell DNA synthesis without a concomitant increase in cell size.[28] On the contrary, platelet-derived growth factor (PDGF) induces stimulation of cellular rRNA synthesis, but not of cell DNA replication.[29]

Thus, growth in cell size can be dissociated from cell DNA replication, at least in the aforementioned examples as well as in others not discussed here. Considering these data and our results, we suggest that cell growth in size and cell DNA synthesis are under separate genetic control, although both pathways should be connected in one or more points during a normal cell cycle.

Another conclusion we obtain from the present results is that the sequence downstream from nucleotide 3506 (0.33 m.u.) is not necessary for either the stimulation of cell DNA replication or for nucleolar reactivation. Considering that the polyA signal in the SV40 early gene is located at nucleotide 2693 (0.18 m.u.), we conclude that the signal for polyA addition is not necessary for these two functions.

It seems of interest to establish correlations between the functions of T antigen we have mapped and the tertiary structure of the early SV40 gene. Interestingly enough, major hairpin loops were identified in the SV40 DNA at or near the origin of DNA replication, immediately before the translation initiation codon for large and small T antigens as well as at nucleotide 2666 (very near the polyA signal) and at nucleotide 3146 (proximate to the PstI site at nucleotide 3204).[30] If such unusual sequences have a biological role, we suggest that the one located around nucleotide 2666 may be related to polyadenylation of large T, while the second one (at nucleotide 3146) may be the signal that separates in the mature protein the helper function plus TSTA and U determinants from the nucleolar activation and cellular DNA synthesis functions.

Another observation is that some of these domains in the early gene seem to be related to other features of the DNA molecule. Thus, it is accepted that in the host cell SV40 DNA exists in its superhelical configuration (DNA I).[6] This DNA form contains an increased free energy and tends to denature locally, behaving in these regions as single-stranded.[6] Surprisingly, the location of one of these regions maps approximately in the same boundaries in which we have found the sequence that codes for cell DNA replication.[6] We cannot explain whether there exists a true relationship between the single-stranded behavior of this fragment and its ability to code for a domain in the large T responsible for the induction of cellular DNA synthesis.

In conclusion, several domains exist in the SV40 early gene coding for different functions of the large T antigen. Thus, sequences coding for nucleolar activation, cellular DNA replication, and the major T antigen determinant are proximate but separate in the early gene. Moreover, polyadenylation seems not to be a necessary event for the full expression of these functions.

Finally, a correlation between the tertiary structure of the early SV40 gene and the functions encoded in its sequence emerges as a reasonable possibility.

SUMMARY

DNA recombinant technology and the manual microinjection technique were used to study the base sequences in the SV40 early gene coding for cell DNA replication and nucleolar activation.

Sequences critical for rRNA gene activation are located between nucleotides 3826 to 3506 (0.39–0.33 m.u.). Base sequences from nucleotide 4350 to 4190 (0.49–0.46 m.u.) are required for cellular DNA replication. Major T antigen determinant is coded by a sequence extending from nucleotide 4190 to 3880 (0.46–0.42 m.u.).

Considering that an increase in cell size is regularly accompanied by an increase in the cellular amount of rRNA, nucleolar genes should be a target for growth-in-size signals. Therefore, the SV40 early gene presents a domain responsible for cell growth in size, and another separate but proximate region coding for cellular DNA replication.

REFERENCES

1. BASERGA, R. 1980. *In* Introduction of Macromolecules Into Viable Mammalian Cells. R. Baserga, C. Croce, and G. Rovera, Eds. The Wistar Symposium Series, Vol. 1: 79–83. Alan R. Liss, Inc. New York, NY.
2. FRALEY, R. & D. PAPAHADJOPOULOS. 1981. TIBS **6:** 77–80.
3. CELIS, J., K. KALTOFT & R. BRAVO. 1980. *In* Introduction of Macromolecules Into Viable Mammalian Cells[1]: 99–123.
4. CELIS, J. & R. BRAVO. 1981. TIBS **6:** 197–201.
5. DIACUMAKOS, E. 1980. *In* Introduction of Macromolecules Into Viable Mammalian Cells[1]: 85–98.
6. LEBOWITZ, P. & S. WEISSMAN. 1979. Curr. Top. Microbiol. Immunol. **87:** 44–172.
7. ACHESON, N. H. 1980. *In* DNA Tumor Viruses. J. Tooze, Ed. Cold Spring Harbor Labs.: 125–204. Cold Spring Harbor, NY.
8. MULLER, C., A. GRAESSMANN & M. GRAESSMANN. 1980. *In* Introduction of Macromolecules Into Viable Mammalian Cells[1]: 135–144.
9. GRAESSMANN, A., M. GRAESSMANN & C. MULLER. 1979. Curr. Top. Microbiol. Immunol. **87:** 1–21.
10. GRAESSMAN, A., M. GRAESSMANN & C. MULLER. 1980. *In* Methods in Enzymology. L. Grossman and K. Moldase, Eds. **65:** 816–825.
11. MEISS, H. & C. BASILICO. 1972. Nature New Biol. **239:** 66–68.
12. FLOROS, J., T. ASHIHARA & R. BASERGA. 1978. Cell Biol. Intern. Rep. **2:** 259–269.
13. CROCE, C. 1976. Proc. Natl. Acad. Sci. USA **73:** 3248–3252.
14. CROCE, C., A. TALAVERA & C. BASILICO. 1977. Proc. Natl. Acad. Sci. USA **74:** 694–697.
15. HIRT, B. 1967. J. Mol. Biol. **26:** 365–369.
16. BOLIVAR, R., R. RODRIQUEZ, P. GREENE, M. BETLACH, H. HEYNECKER & H. BOYER. 1977. Gene **2:** 95–113.
17. GALANTI, N., G. JONAK, K. SOPRANO, J. FLOROS, L. KACZMAREK, S. WEISSMANN, V. B. REDDY, S. TILGHMAN & R. BASERGA. 1981. J. Biol. Chem. **256:** 6469–6474.
18. GRAESSMANN, A., M. GRAESSMANN, R. BOBRIK, E. HOFFMAN, F. LAUPPE & C. MULLER. 1976. Febs Lett. **61:** 81–84.
19. BASERGA, R. & D. MALAMUD. 1969. Autoradiography. Technique and Application. Harper and Row. New York, NY.

20. SOPRANO, K., G. JONAK, N. GALANTI & R. BASERGA. 1981. Virology **109:** 127–136.
21. FLOROS, J., G. JONAK, N. GALANTI & R. BASERGA. 1981. Exp. Cell Res. **132:** 215–223.
22. SLEIGH, M., W. TOPP, R. HANICH & J. SAMBROOK. 1978. Cell **14:** 79–88.
23. SOPRANO, K., V. DEV, C. CROCE & R. BASERGA. 1979. Proc. Nat. Acad. Sci. USA **76:** 3885–3889.
24. SOPRANO, K., M. ROSSINI, C. CROCE & R. BASERGA. 1980. Virology **102:** 317–326.
25. PERRY, R., D. KELLEY, U. SCHIBLER, K. HUEBNER & C. CROCE. 1979. J. Cell Physiol. **98:** 553–560.
26. LAFARGE, C. & C. FRAYSSINET. 1964. Bull. Soc. Chim. Biol. **46:** 1045–1057.
27. ASHIHARA, T., F. TRAGANOS, R. BASERGA & Z. DARZYNKIEWIEZ. 1978. Cancer Res. **38:** 2514–2518.
28. POCHRON, S., M. ROSSINI, Z. DARZYNKIEWIEZ, F. TRAGANOS & R. BASERGA. 1980. J. Biol. Chem. **255:** 4411–4413.
29. ABELSON, H., H. ANTONIADES & C. SCHER. 1979. Biochim. Biophys. Acta **561:** 269–275.
30. GRIFFIN, B. 1980. *In* DNA Tumor Viruses[7]: 61–123.

X CHROMOSOME CONTROL OF CHROMOSOME SEGREGATION IN MOUSE/HAMSTER HYBRID CELL POPULATIONS

Dimitrina D. Pravtcheva * and Frank H. Ruddle

Department of Biology
Yale University
New Haven, Connecticut 06511

Interspecific somatic cell hybrids gradually lose chromosomes of one of the parents.[1,2] The direction and rate of chromosome segregation varies with different parental combinations.[3,4] All the hybrids of a given parental cross, however, segregate the chromosomes of one parent (the only exception known to us was reported by Jami *et al.*[5]) Attempts to manipulate and reverse the direction of chromosome segregation have been mostly unsuccessful.[6-9]

The mechanisms of chromosome segregation are at present unknown. Late replication of the chromosomes of one parent,[10] differential attachment to the mitotic spindle,[11] and eukaryotic restriction/modification enzymes [12] have been proposed as factors determining chromosome segregation, but so far there is no experimental evidence to support the proposed mechanisms.[11,13,14] In human/rodent hybrids chromosome segregation is associated with suppression of the rRNA and histone synthesis of the parent whose chromosomes are eliminated.[15-18] In rodent/rodent hybrids, rRNA of both parents is found in the hybrid.[19-21]

In some recent hybridizations involving X-containing microcell hybrids of the Chinese hamster line E36, we observed a previously unknown property of mouse X chromosomes to reverse segregation in mouse/Chinese hamster somatic cell hybrids. Interestingly, the ability of the mouse X chromosome to regulate segregation appears to be controlled in a specific way which involves recognition of differences in the active X-encoded genes among cell types, which by our present criteria would be considered identical.

MATERIALS AND METHODS

Cell Lines

Meth Aa and Meth As are cell lines established from the ascites and solid forms of the Meth A tumor. Meth A is a BALB/c sarcoma induced by MCA.[22] CMS4 is a cell line established from another MCA-induced BALB/c sarcoma.[23] CMS4T6 is a HPRT⁻ clone of CMS4 (resistant to 30 μg/ml 6-thioguanine) isolated by us. THO is a HPRT⁻- and ouabain-resistant clone of BALB/3T3, clone A31.[24] E36 is a HPRT⁻- and ouabain-resistant Chinese hamster line established from lung cells.[25]

* Recipient of the Oliver E. Spencer Fellowship for Cancer Immunology from the Cancer Research Institute, New York, New York.

249

0077–8923/82/0397–0249 $01.75/0 © 1982, NYAS

Microcell Hybrids

Hybrids mAE were produced by fusion of Meth-Aa-derived microcells with E36. mAE 19 contains only mouse chromosomes X and 1 on E36 background. mAE 29 has only mouse chromosomes 14 and X. Hybrid ms5 was isolated after fusing Meth-As-derived microcells with E36; it contains only the mouse X chromosome. A more detailed account of the production and analysis of mAE and ms hybrids has been presented elsewhere.[26] Hybrid 3mCE1 was produced by hybridization of microcells from CMS4 with E36; it contains only the X^{CMS4} chromosome.[27]

Cell Hybridization

The parental cells were plated in a common T25 flask and 6–24 hours later hybridization was carried out with β-propiolactone-inactivated Sendai virus. 24 hours later the cells were plated out at densities calculated to give less than ten colonies (parental and/or hybrid) per flask. Nonselective or HAT medium[28] was used depending on the parental combination. After 7–10 days, individual colonies were examined and those whose cells differed morphologically from the parental cells were picked by cloning rings.

Chromosome Analysis

Chromosome slides from the hybrid lines were analyzed after G-banding by a modification of the method of Wang and Federoff.[28] 10–50 metaphases were analyzed on the slide for chromosome segregation and banding patterns of their X chromosomes. In addition, at least 10 cells were karyotyped from the ms5 × CMS4T6, mAE 29 × CMS4T6, and 3mCE1 × CMS4T6 hybrids.

Isozyme Analysis

The hybrids were analyzed for the presence of the mouse and Chinese hamster forms of the following enzymes: peptidase 3 (EC 3.4.13), peptidase 1 (EC 3.4.13), nucleoside phosphorylase (EC 2.4.2.1), phosphoglucomutase 2 (EC 2.7.5.1), peptidase 2 (EC 3.4.13), mannose phosphate isomerase (EC 5.3.1.8), adenine phosphoribosyltransferase (EC 2.4.2.7), uridine phosphorylase (EC 2.4.2.3), glyoxalase 1 (EC 4.4.1.5), galactokinase (EC 2.7.1.6), malic enzyme (EC 1.1.1.39), 6-phosphogluconate dehydrogenase (EC 1.1.1.43), glucosophosphate isomerase (EC 5.3.1.9), glutathione reductase (EC 1.6.4.2), triosophosphate isomerase (EC 5.3.1.1), esterase 10, adenosine kinase (EC 2.7.1.20), acid phosphate 1 (EC 3.1.3.2), α-galactosidase (EC 3.2.1.22), lactate dehydrogenase A (EC 1.1.1.27), and enolase (EC 2.4.1.11). The techniques for the enzyme assays have been described.[30]

RESULTS

The general strategy employed to define the effect of X$^{Meth\ A}$ and X^{CMS4} on segregation was (1) to produce simple two-parent mouse/Chinese hamster hybrids (for example, THO × E36, CMS4 × E36), (2) to produce hybrids of the same mouse lines (THO, CMS4, or CMS4T6) with the microcell hybrids of E36, which contain the X chromosome from either Meth Aa, Meth As, or CMS4 (that is, mAE 19, mAE 29, ms5, 3mCE1), and (3) to compare the direction of segregation between corresponding members of the two groups of hybrids.

Five independent hybrid clones were produced between the Chinese hamster line E36 and the mouse line THO. The E36 cells are predominantly near diploid (chromosome number 21–22). 55% of the THO cells have chromosome numbers between 40–50, the rest of the cells representing a continuous range from subtriploid to pentaploid cells. Since the two lines have identical markers (6-thioguanine and ouabain resistance), hybrids were isolated on the basis of morphology after the cells were plated at low density. The clones were analyzed for the presence of Chinese hamster and mouse enzyme markers 1 to 3 months after isolation. All of the clones showed loss of mouse isozymes (and thus mouse chromosomes).

THO cells were then hybridized with mAE 19 ($=$E36 $+$ X$^{Meth\ Aa}$ $+$ 1$^{Meth\ Aa}$). The HPRT$^-$ THO cells have no normal X chromosome and this makes possible the identification of the cytologically normal foreign X (X$^{Meth\ Aa}$) chromosome. Seven independent clones were isolated on HAT medium, which kills the HPRT$^-$ THO cells, but allows the growth of mAE 19 or mAE 19 $\times$ THO hybrids. The latter are easily distinguishable from mAE 19 by both colony and cell morphology. G-banded chromosome slides were analyzed for the presence of the foreign X$^{Meth\ Aa}$ chromosome in the hybrid and to determine the direction of chromosome segregation. All of the hybrids had, in addition to the rearranged X chromosome of THO, a normal X$^{Meth\ Aa}$ chromosome introduced by mAE 19. Because 1$^{Meth\ Aa}$ was indistinguishable from chromosome #1 in the THO cells, we could not monitor its presence in the hybrids. All of the clones showed loss of Chinese hamster chromosomes, with many cells having less than haploid numbers of the latter. Two of the clones were analyzed for segregation of enzyme markers and showed loss of Chinese hamster isozymes. Thus, the addition of X$^{Meth\ Aa}$ (and 1$^{Meth\ Aa}$) to an E36 $\times$ THO hybrid caused a reversion of the direction of chromosome loss (from segregating mouse to segregating Chinese hamster chromosomes).

To determine which of the two mouse chromosomes present in mAE 19 (X$^{Meth\ Aa}$, 1$^{Meth\ Aa}$) was responsible for the reversion of chromosome segregation, we produced hybrids between mAE 29 and THO. mAE 29 has an X$^{Meth\ Aa}$ chromosome (in common with mAE 19), but the second chromosome present in this hybrid is No. 14. Thus, if reversion of segregation does again occur, it would have to be attributed to X$^{Meth\ Aa}$. Using a selection identical to that described above, we isolated seven independent THO $\times$ mAE 29 hybrid clones. By chromosome analysis, all of them showed segregation of Chinese hamster chromosomes. For two of them the direction of segregation was confirmed by isozyme analysis. With the exception of clone 1, in which 30% of the cells had a normal X chromosome, no intact X$^{Meth\ Aa}$ chromosome was seen in any of the other chromosomally analyzed five clones. Since a normal X is present in about 70% of the mAE 29 cells (the rest of the population representing mostly segregants existing because of metabolic cooperation), the absence of a normal X in most of the mAE 29 $\times$ THO hybrids is most probably a result of its rearrangement after hybridization. Despite the absence of an intact X$^{Meth\ Aa}$ in the mAE 29 $\times$ THO hybrids, we can conclude that the reversion is caused by $X^{Meth \; Aa}$, since this is the only common chromosome which mAE 19 and mAE 29 add to the E36 and THO chromosome sets.

To determine whether the X chromosome of the related Meth As line has also the ability to reverse chromosome segregation, we produced five hybrids between ms5 ($=$E36 $+$ $X^{Meth \; As}$) and THO. All of the hybrids had the normal Meth-As-derived X chromosome. The chromosome and isozyme analysis showed that four of the clones segregated Chinese hamster chromosomes (that is, have segregation opposite to that of E36 $\times$ THO hybrids), while one of them segregated mouse chromosomes (that is, had chromosome segregation identical to that of E36 $\times$ THO hybrids).

To determine if the ability to reverse segregation is limited to the X chromosomes of Meth A, we produced hybrids between 3mCE1 ($=$E36 $+$ X^{CMS4}) and THO. Seven independent clones were analyzed by G-banding. All of them had the X^{CMS4} chromosome and all of them showed loss of Chinese hamster chromosomes. Three of the clones were also found to segregate Chinese hamster enzyme markers. Thus, the X^{CMS4} chromosome, like $X^{Meth \; Aa}$ and $X^{Meth \; As}$, caused a reversion in the chromosome segregation of THO $\times$ E36 hybrids.

One way to explain the observed switch in segregation was that the X chromosomes of the two transformed mouse lines Meth A and CMS4 conferred to THO the ability to segregate Chinese hamster chromosomes. This possibility appeared particularly likely because whole-cell hybrids between Meth A and E36 or CMS4 and E36 segregate Chinese hamster chromosomes [26] (see below). To test this possibility, we analyzed the effect of $X^{Meth \; A}$ and X^{CMS4} on hybrids that (unlike E36 $\times$ THO hybrids) spontaneously segregate Chinese hamster chromosomes.

Eight clones of an E36 $\times$ CMS4 cross were isolated on HAT and ouabain selection. All eight clones showed segregation of Chinese hamster enzyme markers. The same direction of chromosome loss was established in a hybrid between E36 and a HPRT$^-$ clone of CMS4—CMS4T6 (isolated without selection on the basis of morphology).

Six independent hybrid clones between ms5 ($=$E36 $+$ $X^{Meth \; As}$) and CMS4T6 were isolated in HAT on the basis of morphology different from that of the surviving ms5 parent. CMS4T6, unlike the CMS4 line from which it is derived, has no normal X chromosome. Thus, we were again able to identify the normal X chromosomes, introduced into CMS4T6 by the microcell hybrids of E36. Six ms5 $\times$ CMS4T6 clones were karyotyped and five of them were analyzed in addition for segregation of enzyme markers. All of the clones contained the normal Meth-As-derived X chromosome. Five of them showed segregation of mouse chromosomes (that is, had segregation opposite to that of E36 $\times$ CMS4 or E36 $\times$ CMS4T6 hybrids) and one showed segregation of Chinese hamster chromosomes (like E36 $\times$ CMS4 hybrids).

One hybrid was produced between mAE 29 ($=$E36 $+$ $X^{Meth \; Aa}$ $+$ $14^{Meth \; Aa}$) and CMS4T6. The karyotype analysis showed that the hybrid contained the $X^{Meth \; Aa}$ chromosome and segregated mouse chromosomes (again opposite to the segregation of E36 $\times$ CMS4T6 hybrids). Segregation of mouse chromosomes was also found by enzyme analysis.

Eight hybrid clones were produced of a 3mCE1 ($=$E36 $+$ X^{CMS4}) $\times$ CMS4T6 cross. All of the hybrids had the CMS4-derived X chromosome and all of them segregated Chinese hamster chromosomes (like E36 $\times$ CMS4 or

E36 × CMS4T6 hybrids). Four of the clones were analyzed for segregation of enzyme markers and all of them showed loss of Chinese hamster isozymes.

DISCUSSION

The results of the experiments described here can be summarized as follows:

1. Hybrids between the Chinese hamster cell line E36 and the mouse 3T3 line THO segregate mouse chromosomes. The addition of a single foreign X chromosome, derived from either of the mouse sarcoma lines Meth Aa, Meth As, or CMS4, reverses the direction of chromosome loss (that is, establishes segregation of Chinese hamster chromosomes).

2. Hybrids between E36 and the mouse sarcoma line CMS4 (or its HPRT⁻ clone CMS4T6) segregate Chinese hamster chromosomes. The addition of a single X chromosome from the sarcoma lines Meth Aa or Meth As reverses the direction of chromosome loss (establishing loss of mouse chromosomes). The addition of an X chromosome from CMS4 has no effect on the direction of chromosome segregation.

The fact that X^{CMS4} is unable to reverse the segregation of E36 × CMS4T6 hybrids rules out the possibility that the X chromosomes acquire their property to reverse segregation during the time they spent in the E36 cells.

Our results suggest that the ability of X to reverse segregation is manifested only if the mouse parent in the hybridization is different from the line from which X originated. $X^{Meth\ Aa}$ and $X^{Meth\ As}$ reverse the segregation of both E36 × THO and E36 × CMS4T6 hybrids—$X^{Meth\ Aa}$ and $X^{Meth\ As}$ are foreign to both the THO and CMS4T6 lines. X^{CMS4} reverses the segregation of E36 × THO hybrids (X^{CMS4} is foreign to THO), but has no effect on the segregation of E36 × CMS4T6 hybrids (it is derived from CMS4). Reversion of segregation occurs without regard to the original direction of segregation, and thus cannot be explained as transfer (through the X chromosome) of the property to segregate in a particular direction.

One can consider two possible reasons for the inability of X^{CMS4} to reverse the segregation of CMS4T6 × E36 hybrids. First, the reversion of segregation of E36 × THO hybrids and of E36 × CMS4T6 hybrids could be caused by two different genetic factors, both of which are active on $X^{Meth\ Aa}$ and $X^{Meth\ As}$, but only one of which (the one affecting THO × E36 hybrids) is active on X^{CMS4}. Second, it is possible that on $X^{Meth\ A}$ and X^{CMS4} there is a single (but nonidentical) factor reversing segregation in both sets of hybrids. Its effect on segregation, however, is not manifested in the X's "native" environment because of suppression or some form of neutralization of the X factor by another product present in that environment.

The fact that reversion of segregation did not occur in one out of five THO × ms5 hybrids and one out of six CMS4T6 × ms5 hybrids could be a result of cytologically undetectable deletions or alterations of some of the $X^{Meth\ As}$ chromosomes in ms5. An alternative explanation would be that some of the ms5 cells contain in addition to $X^{Meth\ As}$ an undetectable chromosome fragment from Meth As, encoding a product which "neutralizes" the effect of X on segregation. At present we cannot distinguish between these two possibilities.

It appears unlikely that the ability to reverse segregation is some property randomly acquired by the X chromosomes during the *in vitro* culture of the sarcoma lines because: (1) the property to reverse segregation of foreign mouse cells is manifested by the X chromosomes of two independently established lines; (2) the ability to switch segregation is common to $X^{Meth\ Aa}$ and $X^{Meth\ As}$, despite the fact that Meth Aa and Meth As were established from the ascites and solid forms of the Meth A tumor about 20 years ago. Thus, the factor responsible for the reversion of segregation was most likely present on the X chromosome of the tumor and retained by the two lines established from it.

Our results suggest the existence of previously unknown differences in the active X-encoded genes even between closely related lines. All lines used in the present study are of BALB/c origin, and thus the ability of the cells to recognize the foreign X chromosome (and to respond to its presence by a switch in segregation) cannot be explained with strain differences of some X-encoded product. Moreover, CMS4 and Meth A are both established from MCA-induced BALB/c sarcomas, and thus the ability of CMS4T6 cells to distinguish their own X (X^{CMS4}) from $X^{Meth\ Aa}$ and $X^{Meth\ As}$ (and reverse its segregation pattern only in the presence of the latter two) indicates that differences in the transformation status and tissue type cannot be the basis for the recognition. Most probably, the differences between the X chromosomes are a manifestation of previously unknown heterogeneity among what now appear identical cell types. More specifically, this heterogeneity appears to be caused by differences in the active members of a group of X-encoded genes revealed in our experimental system by their effect on segregation. The normal function of these genes is at present unknown. The heterogeneity created by them could provide a way for fine regulation of cell growth and differentiation.

REFERENCES

1. RINGERTZ, N. R. & R. E. SAVAGE. 1976. Cell Hybrids. Academic Press. New York, NY.
2. CREAGAN, R. P. & F. H. RUDDLE. 1977. New approaches to human gene mapping by somatic cell genetics. In Molecular Structure of Human Chromosomes. J. Yunis, Ed.: 89–142. Academic Press. New York, NY.
3. WEISS, M. C. & H. GREEN. 1967. Human-mouse hybrid cell lines containing partial complements of human chromosomes and functional human genes. Proc. Natl. Acad. Sci. USA 58: 1104–1111.
4. CROCE, C. M. 1976. Loss of mouse chromosomes in somatic cell hybrids between HT 1080 human fibrosarcoma cells and mouse peritoneal macrophages. Proc. Natl. Acad. Sci. USA 73: 3248–3252.
5. JAMI, J., S. GRANDCHAMP & B. EPHRUSSI. 1971. The karyologic behavior of human x mouse cellular hybrids. C. R. Hebd. Seances Acad. Sci., Ser. D 272: 323–326.
6. PONTECORVO, G. 1971. Induction of directional chromosomal elimination in somatic cell hybrids. Nature (London) 230: 367–369.
7. PONTECORVO, G. 1974. Induced chromosome elimination in hybrid cells. In Somatic Cell Hybridization. R. L. Davidson and F. de la Cruz, Eds.: 65–69. Raven Press. New York, NY.
8. MARSHALL, GRAVES, J. A. 1980. Evidence for an indirect effect of radiation on mammalian chromosomes. Exp. Cell Res. 125: 483–486.
9. COLLINS, J. J., A. T. DESTREE, C. J. MARSHALL & I. A. MACPHERSON. 1975. Selective depletion of chromosomes in a stable mouse-Chinese hamster hybrid cell line using antisera against species-specific antigens. J. Cell. Physiol. 86: 605–620.
10. GREEN, H. 1969. Prospects for the chromosomal location of human genes in human-mouse somatic cell hybrids. Wistar Inst. Symp. Monogr. 9: 51–58.

11. HANDMAKER, S. D. 1973. Hybridization of eukaryotic cells. Ann. Rev. Microbiol. **27:** 189–204.

12. SAGER, R. & R. KITCHIN. 1975. Selective silencing of eukaryotic genes. Science **189:** 426–433.

13. MARIN, G. & P. MANDUCA. 1972. Synchronous replication of the parental chromosomes in Chinese hamster-mouse cell hybrids. Exp. Cell Res. **75:** 290–293.

14. LABELLA, T., G. COLLETTA & G. MARIN. 1976. Asynchronous DNA replication and asymmetrical chromosome loss in Chinese hamster-mouse somatic cell hybrids. Somat. Cell Genet. **2:** 1–10.

15. ELICIERI, G. L. & H. GREEN. 1969. Ribosomal RNA synthesis in human/mouse hybrid cells. J. Mol. Biol. **41:** 253–260.

16. PERRY, R. P., D. E. KELLEY, U. SCHIBLER, K. HUEBNER & C. CROCE. 1979. Selective suppression of the transcription of ribosomal genes in mouse-human hybrid cells. J. Cell. Physiol. **98:** 553–559.

17. AJIRO, K., T. BORUN & C. CROCE. 1978. Species-specific suppression of histone H1 and H2B production in human/mouse hybrids. Proc. Natl. Acad. Sci. USA **75:** 5599–5603.

18. HOHMANN, P., L. K. HOHMANN & T. B. SHOWS. 1980. Expression of H1 histone genes in mouse-human somatic cell hybrids. Somat. Cell Genet. **6:** 653–662.

19. ELICIERI, G. L. 1972. The ribosomal RNA of hamster-mouse hybrid cells. J. Cell Biol. **53:** 177–184.

20. MILLER, O. J., V. G. DEV, D. A. MILLER, R. TANTRAVAHI & G. L. ELICIERI. 1978. Transcription and processing of both mouse and Syrian hamster ribosomal RNA genes in individual somatic hybrid cells. Exp. Cell Res. **115:** 457–460.

21. WEIDE, L. G., V. G. DEV & C. S. RUPERT. 1979. Activity of both mouse and Chinese hamster ribosomal RNA genes in somatic cell hybrids. Exp. Cell Res. **123:** 424–429.

22. OLD, L. J., E. A. BOYSE, D. A. CLARKE & E. GARSWELL. 1962. Antigenic properties of chemically induced tumors. Ann. New York Acad. Sci. **101:** 80–106.

23. DE LEO, A. B., H. SHIKU, T. TAKAHASHI, M. JOHN, & L. J. OLD. 1977. Cell surface antigens of chemically induced sarcomas of the mouse. I. Murine leukemia virus-related and alloantigens on cultured fibroblasts and sarcoma cells. Description of a unique antigen on BALB/c Meth A sarcoma. J. Exp. Med. **146:** 720–734.

24. JHA, K. K. & H. L. OZER. 1976. Expression of transformation in cell hybrids. I. Isolation and application of density-inhibited BALB/3T3 cells deficient in hypoxanthine phosphoriboridtransferase and resistant to ouabain. Somat. Cell Genet. **2:** 215–233.

25. GILLIN, F. D., D. J. ROUFA, A. L. BEAUDET & C. T. CASKEY. 1972. 8-azaguanine resistance in mammalian cells. I. Hypoxanthine-guanine phosphoribosyltransferase. Genetics **72:** 239–252.

26. PRAVTCHEVA, D., A. DE LEO, F. H. RUDDLE & L. J. OLD. 1981. Chromosome assignment of the tumor-specific antigen of a 3-methylcholanthrene-induced mouse sarcoma. J. Exp. Med. **154:** 964–977.

27. PRAVTCHEVA, D. & F. H. RUDDLE. Unpublished material.

28. LITTLEFIELD, J. W. 1964. Selection of hybrids from matings of fibroblasts in vitro and their presumed recombinants. Science **145:** 709–710.

29. WANG, H. C. & S. FEDEROFF. 1971. Banding of human chromosomes treated with trypsin. Nature (London) New Biol. **235:** 52–54.

30. NICHOLS, E. A. & F. H. RUDDLE. 1973. A review of enzyme polymorphism, linkage and electrophoretic conditions for mouse and somatic cell hybrids in starch gels. J. Histochem. Cytochem. **21:** 1066–1088.

INDUCIBLE PROTECTIVE PROTEINS:
A POTENTIALLY NOVEL APPROACH
TO CHEMOTHERAPY *

Robert A. Tobey,† M. Duane Enger,‡ Jeffrey K. Griffith,‡
and C. Edgar Hildebrand ‡

*† Toxicology and ‡ Genetics Groups, Life Sciences Division
Los Alamos National Laboratory
Los Alamos, New Mexico 87545*

INTRODUCTION

Alkylating agents represent an extremely useful class of anticancer drugs which are effective against a wide range of tumors. A major problem associated with their employment, however, is their toxicity for hematopoietic tissue, which results in cumulative myelosuppression.[1, 2] To enhance the usefulness of alkylating agents in a clinical setting, it would be helpful if a technique could be developed that would increase selectively the resistance of normal cells over that of tumor cells in a manner analogous to that achieved in high-dose methotrexate therapy.[3, 4]

A possible approach to achieving this goal involves inducible protective proteins. A number of toxic physical and chemical agents (including alkylating agents) elicit the induction of a series of protein species,[5–10] some of which react with certain agents and render them nontoxic. A few of the induced species (for example, metallothionein) are rich in sulfhydryl groups that might be expected to react with alkylating agents and play a role in their detoxification. If a means could be found to induce the synthesis of alkylating-agent-reactive species safely and prior to exposure to the drug, then those induced species would be capable of increasing cellular resistance to toxicity from alkylating agents.

As part of a long-term program to investigate inducible protective proteins, we have examined the capacity of several trace elements to serve as inducers of a protective response in line CHO Chinese hamster cells and several cadmium-resistant variants against subsequently administered alkylating agents such as iodoacetate and melphalan. Zinc, selenium, copper, and arsenic all were able to increase the resistance of cells (monitored as colony-forming ability) to alkylating-agent toxicity, and there were indications that different agents elicited different domains of responses. Thus, it appears that resistance to alkylating agents can be modulated by manipulation of the level of available trace elements. On the basis of reported differences in inducibility of protective proteins in normal and in tumor cells, a novel approach to alkylating agent chemotherapy is proposed.

MATERIALS AND METHODS

The cells utilized in this report were all derived from line CHO Chinese hamster cells and were selected by exposing the cells to ever-increasing concen-

* This work was sponsored by the United States Department of Energy.

trations of $CdCl_2$ (0.2 to 30 μM), after which cultures exhibiting the control (untreated) growth rate were cloned.[11] The derived variants, which were resistant to 2-, 20-, or 30-μM $CdCl_2$ were designated Cd^{r}2C10, Cd^{r}20F4, and Cd^{r}30F9, respectively, and they were shown to maintain their resistance to cadmium during a 6-month period of maintenance in Cd-free medium.[11] Suspension cultures of cells were grown in F–10 medium supplemented with 15% neonate calf serum, penicillin, and streptomycin.

Stock solutions of $ZnCl_2$, K_2SeO_3 and $CuSO_4$ were prepared in 0.01 N HCl, sterilized by filtration through a 0.22-μ filter, dispensed into polyethylene tubes, and stored at either −20° C ($ZnCl_2$ and K_2SeO_3) or at room temperature ($CuSO_4$); dilutions were prepared in distilled water. Sodium arsenite was weighed out immediately prior to use, dissolved in distilled water, and sterilized by filtration. Solutions of iodoacetate were prepared immediately prior to utilization by dissolving the alkylating agent in serum-free medium, sterilization by filtration, and dilution in sterile serum-free medium. Melphalan (L-PAM, sarcolysin, L-phenylalanine mustard), NSC 8806, was generously provided by Dr. David Abraham, Investigational Drug Branch, National Cancer Institute, Bethesda, MD. Solutions of melphalan were prepared immediately prior to use by dissolving the drug in acidic ethanol (70% ethanol in 0.05 N HCl) prior to dilution in serum-free medium and sterilization by filtration.

Because of the sensitivity of line CHO and its derivatives to serum-free medium, dilutions of alkylating agent were added directly to cells in complete (serum-containing) medium for the exposure studies. The presence of serum did not adversely affect melphalan activity, judging from observed linear decreases in survival over the exposure periods utilized and a minimal experiment-to-experiment variability in survival measurements. In this regard, O'Neill *et al.*[12] have demonstrated that the mutagenicity and cytotoxicity resulting from exposure of CHO cells to a variety of alkylating agents are not affected by the presence of serum. We have noted, however, that the absolute survival rate varies somewhat with the batch of serum employed (unpublished preliminary observations); a single batch of serum was utilized for all of the experiments described in this report.

For survival studies, aliquots of alkylating-agent-exposed cells were removed from suspension, pelleted by centrifugation, resuspended in drug-free medium, counted in a Coulter counter, and diluted and plated into 60-mm tissue culture dishes. Following a 1-week incubation period, the dishes were washed, fixed, and stained with crystal violet prior to determination of colonies (50 or more cells). Plating efficiencies (P.E.) ranged from 80% to 96%, with no significant differences in P.E. observed between trace-element-treated control cultures, except for the one high level of $NaAsO_2$ cited in TABLE 1. It should be emphasized that the utilization of suspension cultures for exposure of cells to trace elements and alkylating agents circumvented the need to trypsinize the cells, thereby eliminating possible trypsin-specific effects on survival, which would greatly complicate interpretation of data.

The technique utilized to monitor metallothionein synthesis rate [13] is a variation on a general analytical approach utilized by Steinberg *et al.*[14] In our procedure, Sephadex G–75 column chromatography of cytoplasmic fractions pulse-labeled with [^{35}S]cysteine was employed to separate the [^{35}S]-labeled metallothionein species from larger, ^{35}S-containing cytoplasmic components and from unincorporated amino acid. The relative rate of metallothionein synthesis was then calculated as 100 times the fraction of ^{35}S cpm in the

TABLE 1

EFFECT OF SELENIUM (K₂SeO₃), COPPER (CuSO₄), OR ARSENIC (NaAsO₂)
USED AS AN INDUCER TO ENHANCE RESISTANCE OF CHO CELLS
TO MELPHALAN-SPECIFIC CYTOTOXICITY

Concentration of Inducer (μM)*	Survival (%)	Relative Enhancement of Survival
K_2SeO_3		
0	0.98	—
10	0.95	0
20	6.0	6.1-fold
30	9.6	9.8-fold
$CuSO_4$		
0	3.7	—
75	8.5	2.3-fold
100	8.1	2.2-fold
150	11.4	3.1-fold
$NaAsO_2$		
0	4.1	—
2	6.1	1.6-fold
5	7.9	1.9-fold
10	3.0	— †

* The cells were pretreated for 9 hr with the appropriate level of inducer, then for an additional 3 hr with 8-μM melphalan prior to plating in normal (melphalan-free) medium for colony formation.

† The plating efficiency of the arsenite-pretreated cells prior to addition of melphalan was lower than that of the control culture, indicating that this level of arsenic is, by itself, toxic.

metallothionein peak relative to the counts in nonmetallothionein proteins that eluted prior to metallothionein.

To study uptake and intracellular distribution of labeled iodoacetic acid, cultures of CHO or Cd^{r}20F4 cells, grown in suspension culture in the presence or absence of 100-μM ZnCl$_2$ for 9 hr, were exposed to 100-μM ³H-iodoacetic acid (100–300 mCi/mmol, New England Nuclear Corp., Boston, MA) for 3 hr. Cells were harvested by centrifugation and washed twice with Hank's balanced salt solution. Aliquots of cells and supernatant solutions were removed at each step for analysis of ³H-iodoacetate levels. Washed cell pellets were resuspended at 1.7×10^7 cells/ml in 0.01-M Tris·Cl (pH 7.4), 0.01-M KCl, 0.0015-M MgCl$_2$, and 0.02-M 2-mercaptoethanol, after which the cells were lysed by addition of 1/10 volume of 10% NP–40, and cytoplasmic and nuclear fractions were obtained as detailed elsewhere.[13] Fifty-μl aliquots of cytoplasmic and nuclear fractions, removed for monitoring of ³H-iodoacetate levels, were first digested with 0.5 ml Protosol® (New England Nuclear Corp.) at 37° C for 12–16 hr, then counted in 10 ml of Econofluor® (New England Nuclear Corp.).

To measure binding of ³H-iodoacetic acid to cytoplasmic components, aliquots of cytoplasmic fractions were prepared for polyacrylamide gel electrophoresis as described previously.[15] In some experiments, unlabeled cytoplasmic extracts were mixed with labeled ³H-iodoacetic acid (100 μM) and then prepared for analysis by sodium dodecyl sulfate polyacrylamide gel electrophoresis. Samples were analyzed as described elsewhere.[15]

RESULTS

Our initial attempts to devise a means for increasing the resistance of cells to alkylating agents centered on the expectation that metallothionein might play a role in the detoxification of these agents.[16, 17] Metallothionein (MT) species represent a class of low molecular weight, cysteine-rich proteins that appear to play a role in the regulation of zinc and copper metabolism [18, 19]; they are also involved in detoxification of harmful trace elements such as cadmium and mercury.[20, 21] Given the thiol-rich nature of MT,[22] the expected reactivity of alkylating agents with the sulfhydryl moieties of metallothionein, and the observation that metallothionein synthesis is induced in hepatic tissue of rats treated with alkylating agents,[6] we decided to explore the possibility that synthesis of that protein species could serve as a detoxification mechanism for alkylating agents.

The availability of a series of cultured cell variants of line CHO which differed greatly in their ability to induce synthesis of metallothionein after treatment with $ZnCl_2$[16, 17] provided a means to test directly the correlation between metallothionein inducibility and resistance to alkylating-agent toxicity. The approach utilized was to compare the cytotoxicity resulting from exposure to an alkylating agent in both induced and noninduced cultures of each cell type.

FIGURE 1 presents data on the inducibility of metallothionein by zinc in each

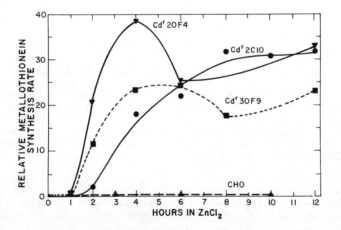

FIGURE 1. Metallothionein-induction kinetics in CHO cells and in a series of CHO-derived, cadmium-resistant variant cells after exposure to zinc. $ZnCl_2$ (100 μM) was added to each culture at t = 0 and maintained throughout the course of the experiment. Experimental details are provided in the MATERIALS AND METHODS section and in Reference 13; ▲ = CHO, ● = 2C10, ▼ = 20F4, and ■ = 30F9. If a maximal binding of 7 g atoms of Cd^{++} per MT molecule is assumed,[22] MT is accumulated at a rate of 1.3×10^6 molecules per cell per hour in the maximally induced (by Cd^{++} or Zn^{++}) 2C10 cell.

of the cells. All three cadmium-resistant variants responded to treatment with $ZnCl_2$ by elaborating synthesis of metallothionein, while zinc was without apparent effect on MT synthesis in the parental CHO cell. If MT actually plays a major role in reducing alkylating-agent cytotoxicity, then the zinc-pretreated 2C10, 20F4 and 30F9 cells, which already possess high levels of metallothionein when the alkylating agent is first added, should exhibit enhanced resistance relative to their noninduced counterparts. In similar fashion, CHO cells should not benefit from pretreatment with zinc, since $ZnCl_2$ failed to induce MT synthesis in that cell. Any variation from that pattern (for example, lack of enhancement of survival in zinc-pretreated cadmium-resistant cells or increased survival of zinc-treated CHO cells) is an indication that MT does not play a major role in the detoxification of alkylating agents.

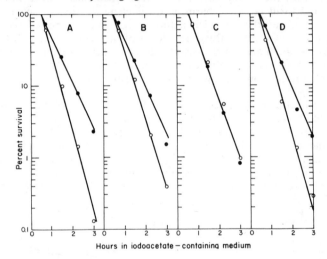

FIGURE 2. Survival of CHO and the Cd^r variant cells exposed to iodoacetate ± a 9-hr pretreatment with zinc chloride. For each cell, a large culture was split into two smaller cultures, and zinc chloride (100 μM) was added to one of those. Nine hours later, both the zinc-pretreated culture (●) and the nontreated control culture (○) received sodium iodoacetate (100 μM), and aliquots were removed from each culture at intervals thereafter for plating in regular F–10 medium to determine survivors via colony formation. The cells examined were (A) Cd^r30F9, (B) Cd^r20F4, (C) Cd^r2C10, and (D) CHO.

FIGURE 2 presents the results obtained when each of the four cell variants was exposed to the alkylating agent, iodoacetate (100 μM) ± a 9-hour pretreatment period with 100-μM $ZnCl_2$. After 3 hours in the presence of iodoacetate, two of the zinc pretreated cadmium-resistant cells, 30F9 (FIG. 2A) and 20F4 (FIG. 2B), exhibited a nearly 10-fold increase in survival. Note, however, that even though zinc pretreatment greatly enhanced the rate of synthesis of MT in 2C10 cells (FIG. 1), there was no evidence that the induced metallothionein reduced the toxicity of iodoacetate in this cell (FIG. 2C), a finding that is incompatible with the notion of a simple correlation between MT inducibility and resistance to toxicity. Even stronger evidence that the protective response does not depend upon MT-inducibility is provided in FIG. 2D, in which zinc

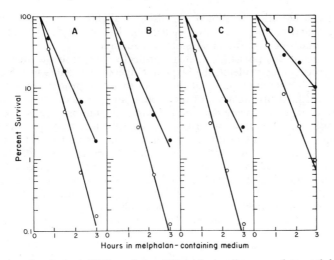

Hours in melphalan-containing medium

FIGURE 3. Survival of CHO and the Cd^r variant cells exposed to melphalan ± a 9-hr pretreatment with zinc chloride. Experimental details and symbols as in FIGURE 2, except that melphalan (8 μM) was substituted for the iodoacetate.

pretreatment greatly enhanced the survival of CHO cells under conditions in which the amount of MT was essentially zero in both induced and uninduced cultures.

Experiments illustrated in FIGURE 3 with a more clinically relevant alkylating agent, melphalan, revealed a generally similar phenomenon, with all four cultures that were pretreated with ZnCl$_2$ exhibiting a nearly 10-fold enhancement in survival relative to the noninduced controls. Taken together, the data in FIGURES 1 to 3 indicate the existence of a zinc-inducible protective response that is not dependent on metallothionein synthesis.

A further indication that resistance and MT synthesis are not related in simple fashion is provided by the data in FIGURE 4, in which a comparison was made between proteins that bind ^{3}H-iodoacetate in induced and noninduced cultures of CHO and 20F9 cells. Analysis of ^{3}H-iodoacetic-acid-binding components from metallothionein-deficient CHO cells or metallothionein induction-proficient 30F9 cells exposed to labeled iodoacetic acid in culture or in extracts (Zn pretreatment) indicates that metallothionein is not a major ^{3}H-binding component. Furthermore, since ^{3}H-iodoacetic acid is not observed to be associated with such a low molecular weight component in CHO cells, the protection against ^{3}H-iodoacetic-acid-mediated cytotoxicity can not be ascribed to the presence of MT. Independent experiments demonstrated that the levels of metallothionein synthesis in the cultures exposed to ^{3}H-iodoacetate in FIGURE 4 were as expected from the data presented in FIGURE 1.

The induction of the protective responses presented in FIGURES 2 and 3 was obtained with 100-μM ZnCl$_2$, a level far removed from normal physiological conditions. The effect of varying the level of zinc utilized as an inducer on the survival of melphalan-treated CHO cells is shown in TABLE 2. While the 100-μM level of zinc yielded the greatest enhancement of survival, there was still a significant increase in resistance obtained in cells that had received only 20-μM

ZnCl$_2$; a concentration of 20-μM zinc is only slightly above the level of Zn normally found in human serum,[23] indicating that the protective response can be elicited under nearly normal physiological conditions.

To eliminate the possibility that the protective response was due to a zinc-induced process that rendered the alkylating agent unavailable to the cells (for example, by facilitating binding of the agent to serum proteins outside the cell or by extracellular precipitation of the agent), an experiment was performed to assess the effect of removing the zinc from the medium prior to addition to the alkylating agent. A culture of CHO cells was split into three parallel cultures, and 100-μM ZnCl$_2$ was added to two of these. Nine hours later, the cells in one of the zinc-treated cultures were resuspended in normal medium, after which melphalan was added to all three cultures. The results presented in FIGURE 5 reveal that removal of the inducer prior to addition of melphalan had little or no effect on the enhanced resistance. This observation indicates that the increased resistance of zinc-pretreated cells is not the result of a zinc-induced, extracellular inactivation of the alkylating agent. The results instead suggest the existence of

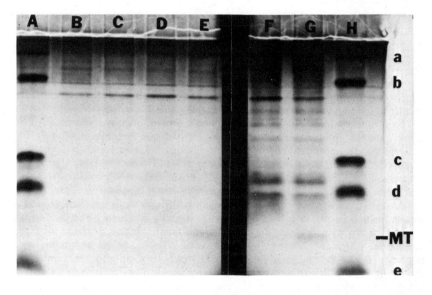

FIGURE 4. SDS-polyacrylamide gel electrophoretic analysis of cytoplasmic components from ^{3}H-iodoacetic-acid-treated cultured cells or cytoplasmic fractions. Lanes A and H represent molecular weight standards, with (a) representing phosphorylase b (92,500 MW), (b) ovalbumin (46,000 MW), (c) lactoglobulin a (18,367 MW), (d) cytochrome c (12,300 MW), and (e) insulin (5800 MW). MT denotes the mobility of metallothionein determined from other gels. Lanes B and C represent cytoplasmic fractions from CHO cells untreated (B) or pretreated with 100-μM ZnCl$_2$ (C) for 9 hr prior to a 3-hr exposure to ^{3}H-iodoacetic acid. Lanes D and E represent cytoplasmic fractions from Cd^{r}30F9 cells untreated (D) or zinc-pretreated (E) for 9 hr prior to exposure for 3 hr to ^{3}H-iodoacetic acid. Lanes F and G represent the cytoplasmic fractions obtained from unlabeled Cd^{r}30F9 cells either untreated (F) or pretreated for 9 hr with ZnCl$_2$ (G) prior to being mixed with ^{3}H-iodoacetic acid prior to analysis by SDS-PAGE.

TABLE 2

EFFECT OF CONCENTRATION OF ZnCL₂ USED AS AN INDUCER TO
ENHANCE RESISTANCE OF CHO CELLS TO
MELPHALAN-SPECIFIC CYTOTOXICITY

Concentration of ZnCl₂ (μM) *	Survival (%)	Relative Enhancement of Survival
0	0.58	—
20	2.6	4.5-fold
40	2.4	4.1-fold
60	1.6	2.8-fold
80	5.1	8.8-fold
100 †	9.5	16.4-fold

* The cells were pretreated for 9 hr with the appropriate level of ZnCl₂, then for an additional 3 hr with 8-μM melphalan prior to plating in normal (melphalan-free) medium for colony formation.

† While a level of 100-μM ZnCl₂ could be tolerated by CHO cells for at least 48 hr with no decrease in survival, slight increases in zinc level to concentrations of 125 μM or 150 μM resulted in decreases in survival (9-hr exposure period) of 33% and 75%, respectively.

an induced product whose functional activity is not immediately lost when the inducer is removed from the culture medium.

While the preceding experiment ruled out the possibility of a zinc-induced decrease in availability of alkylating agent, another possible explanation for the

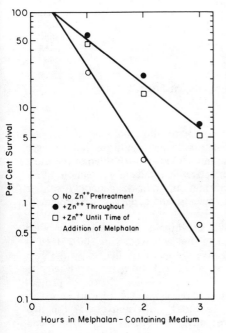

FIGURE 5. Effect of melphalan on survival of induced CHO cells exposed in medium from which the ZnCl₂ inducer had been removed. ZnCl₂ (100 μM) was added to two of three parallel cultures of CHO cells. Nine hours later, the cells in one of the zinc-treated cultures were resuspended in regular F-10 medium, after which melphalan (8 μM) was added to all three cultures. Aliquots were withdrawn from culture at intervals and plated in drug-free medium to determine survivors via colony formation. (○) = the non-Zn-induced control culture; (●) = the induced culture in which the ZnCl₂ was maintained throughout the entire course of the experiment; (□) = the induced culture that was returned to inducer-free medium prior to addition of the melphalan.

results is that the transport of agent into the cell is reduced in the presence of high levels of zinc, with the result that the intracellular level of alkylating agent is lower in induced than in noninduced cells. Measurement of ^{3}H-iodoacetic acid incorporation into induced or uninduced CHO or 20F4 cells (TABLE 3) indicated that pretreatment with zinc enhanced the incorporation of ^{3}H-iodoacetic acid into CHO cells, but not into 20F4 cells. While further studies will be required to delineate the factors responsible for the different patterns of iodoacetic acid uptake into the two cells, it is clear that the protection mediated by zinc cannot be ascribed to a simple reduction in uptake or binding of ^{3}H-iodoacetic acid by zinc-pretreated cells.

Thus far, major attention has been focused on the effects of zinc as an inducer of a protective response against alkylating-agent toxicity, but what about other trace elements suspected of inducing synthesis of batteries of proteins? To investigate the possibility that other trace elements could serve as inducers, cultures of CHO cells were exposed to different levels of selenium (potassium selenite, K_2SeO_3), copper (cupric sulfate, $CuSO_4$), or arsenic (sodium arsenite, $NaAsO_2$) for 9 hr prior to addition of 8-μM melphalan; nonmetal-treated parallel cultures served as controls. At the end of a 3-hr period of exposure to

TABLE 3

EFFECT OF ZINC PRETREATMENT ON UPTAKE OF ^{3}H-IODOACETIC ACID
INTO CHO AND Cd^r 20F4 CELLS *

Cell	Treatment with 100-μM ZnCl$_2$ for 9 hr	^{3}H cpm/10^6 cells		
		Cytoplasm	Nucleus	Total
CHO	−	6875	2733	9608
CHO	+	10269	3399	13668
Cd^{r}20F4	−	5620	3047	8667
Cd^{r}20F4	+	5047	2897	7944

* See MATERIALS AND METHODS section for experimental details.

melphalan, cells were plated in normal medium to allow colonies to develop from the surviving cells. The results presented in TABLE 1 indicate that all three trace elements induce a protective response in CHO cells, with selenite the most effective element and arsenic the least effective in inducing protection. Preliminary experiments, which require confirmation, indicate generally similar quantitative protective responses induced by selenite and copper, but no enhancement induced by arsenite in 20F4 cells.

The degree of enhancement in survival attributable to pretreatment with 30-μM selenite is approximately equivalent to that achieved with 100-μM zinc, raising the possibility that the same protective response is elicited by the two elements. If so, simultaneous treatment of a cell with both zinc and selenite prior to exposure to melphalan should result in an equivalent degree of protection to that achieved with either agent administered singly (that is, no improvement in survival of cells receiving both elements). Alternatively, if the two metals are inducing different domains of response, the level of survival in a cell treated with both metals should increase to a level that is equal to (or, perhaps, greater than) the sum of the survivals afforded by each agent administered singly.

FIGURE 6 presents results obtained when cultures of CHO cells induced with selenite alone, zinc alone, or selenite plus zinc were treated with 8-μM melphalan; an uninduced culture that received only melphalan served as control. The cells that were induced with both metals exhibited an enhanced survival relative to cells treated with either singly administered agent. The survival of the doubly induced cells for the 2-hr and 3-hr samples was approximately equivalent to the sum of survivals achieved in the singly induced cells, suggesting that selenite and zinc induce different protective mechanisms whose effects are additive.

DISCUSSION

These results indicate the existence of a novel, trace-element-inducible response that protects cells against alkylating-agent cytotoxicity. The protective mechanism does not appear to involve decreased extracellular availability of the alkylating agent (FIG. 5), reduced transport of the drug into cells (TABLE 3), or the induction of metallothionein (FIGS. 1–4). In regard to the latter point, Cagen and Klaassen [24] have arrived at a similar conclusion from studies that examined the binding of radiolabeled iodoacetate to metallothionein isolated from hepatic homogenates of rats that had been pretreated with zinc to boost the level of MT. Their findings suggest that while the sulfhydryl groups on MT *can* act as binding sites for alkylating agents, the preferential affinity of alkylating agents for another thiol-rich species, glutathione, indicates that MT does not

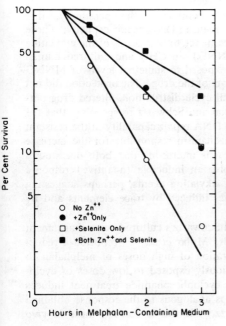

FIGURE 6. Effect of utilization of multiple inducers (Zn and Se) on survival of CHO cells treated with melphalan. Four parallel cultures of CHO cells were set up, and ZnCl₂ (100 μM) was added to one, K₂SeO₃ (30 μM) was added to a second, both ZnCl₂ and K₂SeO₃ were added to a third, and a fourth culture received no inducer. Nine hours later, melphalan (8 μM) was added to each culture, and aliquots were removed from each culture at intervals for plating in regular F-10 medium to determine survivors via colony formation. (◯) = the uninduced control; (●) = the culture induced with zinc only; (☐) = the culture induced with selenite; (■) = the culture induced with both zinc and selenite.

represent a major mechanism for detoxification of alkylating agents. Thus, their *in vivo* results, which monitored binding affinity, are in excellent agreement with our *in vitro* findings, which employed cytotoxicity as the endpoint, indicating that comparable mechanisms are operative in the two systems. Stated differently, the comparability of results suggests that our cultured cells can serve as a useful model system to provide information of relevance to more complex systems, such as intact animals. Given the comparability of results generated in the two analytical systems, our observation (TABLE 2) that the protective response may be elicited at a level of zinc that is only slightly in excess of the normal level of zinc in human serum [23] suggests that if a similar phenomenon can be induced in humans, the level of inducer required should fall within a physiologically reasonable range.

While we have not yet identified the mechanism responsible for the protective response, several speculative possibilities may be proposed for consideration. Zinc could cause an increase in glutathione, a species known to interact readily with alkylating agents. While we have not determined the levels of glutathione in induced and noninduced cultured cells, there was no evidence for a significant enhancement of glutathione levels in kidney and liver tissue from rats exposed to a high level of zinc in the studies of Klaassen and his associates.[24, 25]

Other candidates as trace-element-inducible products include nonmetallo-thionein proteins that might be capable of binding and inactivating alkylating agents or species that enhance alkylating-agent catabolism. In regard to the first possibility, while there is no direct evidence that bears on this notion, stressful conditions that cause the induction of metallothionein also induce the synthesis of a series of proteins whose functions have not yet been established.[7–10] The result of enhanced catabolism of alkylating agents would be to reduce the effective concentration of the active forms of the drugs, thereby preventing them from attacking sensitive intracellular targets.

The studies of Samson and Schwartz [26] point to another possibility: that the trace elements are inducing an enhancement in DNA repair capacity. Those investigators demonstrated an enhanced resistance to high levels of the alkylating agent, *N*-methyl,*N'*-nitrosoguanidine (MNNG), in CHO and cultured human skin fibroblasts that had been previously exposed to sublethal levels of MNNG prior to challenge with a normally toxic level of the drug. The protection did not appear to be attributable to changes in cell cycle distribution, altered drug permeability, or detoxification, leading Samson and Schwartz to speculate that the low levels of MNNG induced an adaptive DNA repair capability in the resistant cells. While the precise nature of the mechanism responsible for the increase in resistance might be open to question, it is interesting that both our studies and those of Samson and Schwartz involve an inducible (adaptive) response which greatly increases the resistance to alkylating agents, perhaps suggesting a similar or identical domain of responses induced by trace elements and by low levels of alkylating agents.

A phenomenon similar to Samson and Schwartz's cultured cell enhancement studies may be occurring in intact animals. Millar *et al.*[27, 28] reported a reduction in toxicity associated with administration of high doses of melphalan to sheep and mice if the animals were previously exposed to low doses of cyclophosphamide. It appears likely that the cyclophosphamide treatment induces an adaptive response in the animals that is analogous to the response obtained in cultured cells by Samson and Schwartz.[26] If this is correct, these *in vivo* studies provide yet another indication that the inducible protective responses are not an artifact arising only in cultured cells.

The studies described in this report suggest that inducible protective responses against alkylating-agent toxicity may indeed occur in humans and intact animals as well as in cultured cells, but if such a system is to be exploited successfully in cancer chemotherapy, there is also a requirement for obtaining a differential response between normal and tumor cells. For optimal effectiveness, a dramatic quantitative difference in response of the two types of cells would be required. Since the precise mechanism underlying the trace-element-induced response is unknown, we can not yet specify the behavior of normal and tumor cells in a clinical setting; however, several observations from other laboratories suggest that clinically exploitable differences may exist that justify continuing studies of the underlying mechanism.

If the protective response is triggered only when an intracellular "threshold" concentration of inducer is exceeded, then differences in the endogenous level of inducer in normal and tumor cells might be extremely important. For example, if the intracellular level of zinc were significantly lower in tumor cells than in their normal cell counterparts, it might be possible to utilize a level of zinc that would preferentially induce only the normal cells to respond.

Regarding this possibility, a number of studies [29–35] have demonstrated reductions in the intracellular levels of zinc in tumor tissue (for example, an approximately 45% reduction in the level of zinc is observed in tumors arising in mice fed diethylnitrosamine [35]). Further increasing the disparity in level of intracellular zinc between normal and tumor tissue is a tendency for the zinc lost from tumor tissue to migrate to normal (that is, nontumor-involved) tissue [36–38]; the net result is an elevation in the zinc level of normal tissue of cancer patients to values in excess of those found in normal tissue from tumor-free individuals. Accordingly, it may be possible to provide a level of zinc to a patient that will specifically "trigger" a protective response in normal but not tumor tissue. Note, however, that a few reports (reviewed by Pories *et al.*[39]) have appeared in which the intracellular level of zinc in neoplastic tissue was equivalent to or slightly greater than that of normal tissue, which indicates that triggering of protective responses may not be feasible in all types of tumors.

That it is possible to utilize a trace element to induce a protective response in normal human cells under conditions in which the response of human tumor cells is quantitatively greatly reduced has been demonstrated by Phillips.[40] Phillips showed that incubation of freshly collected normal human lymphocytes with zinc transferrin (a zinc-binding serum glycopeptide [41]) resulted in induction of levels of metallothionein that were 3.6 to 21 times greater than the levels of MT induced in lymphocytes from leukemic patients. While the protective protein (that is, synthesis of metallothionein) elicited in Phillips' study is clearly not responsible for the zinc-mediated reduction in alkylating-agent toxicity described in this report, Phillips' findings strongly suggest that conditions can be found in which a given level of trace element stimulates synthesis of an inducible protective protein to a much greater extent in normal cells than in tumor cells. If the trace element-inducible substance responsible for protecting cells against alkylating-agent toxicity behaves in similar fashion, pretreatment of a patient with an appropriate level of trace element prior to initiation of alkylating-agent therapy may result in a selective sparing of normal tissue. Note that administration of zinc to animals results in elevated levels of inducible proteins such as metallothionein in the tissue of the treated animals,[24, 25, 42, 43] suggesting the feasibility of inducing protective proteins in humans.

It is obvious that much additional work will be required before the clinical relevance of this type of approach can be determined. If feasible, there are several advantages to utilization of a technique such as this one. In the first place, essential trace elements (such as zinc, selenium, and copper) can be employed at subtoxic levels to elicit the protective response. The observation that the effects of selenite and zinc may be additive (FIG. 6) suggests the possibility of employing combinations of trace elements; utilization of low levels of a number of inducers as opposed to use of a high level of a single inducer should be technically easier to accomplish and less toxic. A second advantage is the rapidity with which such an approach could be applied to the clinic in the event that promising preclinical results were obtained; that is, the trace element technique could be utilized with a variety of existing alkylating agents that have already been approved for human therapy. Finally, if there is an identifiable biochemical species whose synthesis correlates with the protective response (for example, increased enzymatic activity or elevated level of binding protein) and whose induction can be quantitated precisely, it may be possible to monitor the induction capacity in a prospective patient by measuring the level of protective substance induced in cultured lymphocytes derived from a 5- to 10-ml aliquot of blood; this approach would allow identification of patients with a favorable prognosis for this type of therapy.

It should be emphasized that we recognize that tumor cell heterogeneity may be a limiting factor in this type of therapeutic approach. For example, even though all of the leukemic patients examined in the studies of Phillips exhibited a reduced capacity for induction of metallothionein when provided with zinc transferrin relative to that of normal controls,[40] the difference in inducibility between the highest and lowest responder in the leukemic series was nearly seven-fold. Furthermore, examples of tumor lines in which inducible proteins such as metallothionein are readily expressed and subject to hormonal modulation have been reported,[44] which suggests that not all types of tumors will respond favorably in a clinical setting to the trace-element stimulation approach to chemotherapy with alkylating agents.

We are also not advocating a return to single-agent therapy. Instead, we are suggesting that the effectiveness of alkylating agents in standard combination therapy regimens might be enhanced by utilization of the approach outlined in this report, provided, of course, that the efficacy of this approach is first established in preclinical studies.

The specific suggestions outlined in this report represent only one possibility for utilization of inducible biochemical processes. As our knowledge of the range of responses and associated mechanisms of protection increases, a variety of novel approaches to detoxification of hazardous physical and chemical agents may be possible that should allow us: (1) to monitor and minimize the harmful effects of such agents after accidental exposure; and (2) to develop techniques for precisely controlling the behavior of selected toxic substances utilized in the treatment of disease.

SUMMARY

A number of toxic chemical and physical agents elicit the induction of a series of protein species, some of which react with the agents and render them nontoxic. A few of the induced species (such as metallothionein) are rich in thiol groups that might be expected to react with alkylating agents and render them nontoxic. If a safe means could be found for selectively enhancing the synthesis of alkylating-agent-reactive species in normal but not tumor cells, such a procedure would have ramifications in the area of cancer chemotherapy. In this report, we have utilized a variety of trace elements (Zn, Se, Cu, As) as inducers of synthesis of protective species in line CHO Chinese hamster cells and in a number of derived variants to determine whether this type of approach can be utilized to increase resistance to alkylating-agent toxicity. Our results indicate that Zn, Se and Cu elicit a protective response (increased survival, monitored by colony-forming ability) against the toxic effects of iodoacetate or melphalan, and, at least in the case of zinc, at levels that are physiologically reasonable. Arsenite appears to be a marginally effective inducer in the CHO cell and an ineffective inducer in the Cd^{r}20F4 variant cell. The increased survival is not attributable to metallothionein inducibility, decreased availability of the alkylating agent in the medium, or decreased uptake of the drug into the trace-element-pretreated cells. The protective responses induced by zinc or selenite alone are additive in cells receiving both trace elements prior to exposure to alkylating agent, which suggests that different domains of response are elicited by the two metals. In view of reported differences in inducibility of protective proteins between normal and tumor cells, a possibility is raised for a novel approach to alkylating-agent chemotherapy that is somewhat analogous to the protocol utilized in high-dose methotrexate therapy.

ACKNOWLEDGMENTS

We gratefully acknowledge the excellent technical assistance of Joseph G. Valdez, John L. Hanners and A. Christine Munk.

REFERENCES

1. HOOGSTRATEN, K. B., P. R. SCHECHE, J. CUTTNER, T. COOPER, R. A. KYLE, R. A. OBERFIELD, S. R. TOWNSEND, J. B. HARLEY, D. M. HAYES, G. COSTA & J. F. HOLLAND. 1976. Melphalan in multiple myeloma. Blood 30: 74–83.
2. FURNER, R. L. & R. K. BROWN. 1980. L-Phenylalanine mustard (L-PAM): The first 25 years. Cancer Treat. Rep. 64: 559–574.
3. MEAD, J., J. VENDITTI, A. SCHRECKER, A. GOLDIN & J. KERETSZTESY. 1963. The effect of reduced derivatives of folic acid on toxicity and antileukemic effect of methotrexate in mice. Biochem. Pharmacol. 12: 371–383.
4. DJERASSI, I., C. J. ROMINGER, J. S. KIM, J. TURCHI, U. SUVANSRI & D. HUGHES. 1972. Phase I study of high doses of methotrexate with citrovorum factor in patients with lung cancer. Cancer 30: 22–30.
5. OH, S. H., J. T. DEAGEN, P. D. WHANGER & P. H. WESWIG. 1978. Biological function of metallothionein. V. Its induction in rats by various stresses. Am. J. Physiol. 243: 282–285.
6. KOTSONIS, F. N. & C. D. KLAASSEN. 1979. Increase in hepatic metallothionein in rats treated with alkylating agents. Toxicol. Appl. Pharmacol. 51: 19–27.
7. LEVINSON, W., H. OPPERMANN & J. JACKSON. 1980. Transition series metals and sulfhydryl reagents induce the synthesis of four proteins in eukaryotic cells. Biochim. Biophys. Acta 606: 170–180.
8. JOHNSTON, D., H. OPPERMANN, J. JACKSON & W. LEVINSON. 1980. Induction of four proteins in chick embryo cells by sodium arsenite. J. Biol. Chem. 255: 6975–6978.

9. GRIFFITH, J. K., M. D. ENGER, C. E. HILDEBRAND & R. A. WALTERS. 1981. The differential induction by cadmium of a low complexity RNA class in cadmium resistant and cadmium sensitive cells. Biochemistry 20: 4755–4761.

10. HILDEBRAND, C. E., J. K. GRIFFITH, R. A. TOBEY, R. A. WALTERS & M. D. ENGER. 1981. Molecular mechanisms of Cd detoxification of Cd-resistant cultured cells: Role of metallothionein and other inducible factors. In The Biological Role of Metallothionein. E. C. Foulkes, Ed.: 279–303. Elsevier. The Netherlands.

11. HILDEBRAND, C. E., R. A. TOBEY, E. W. CAMPBELL & M. D. ENGER. 1979. A cadmium-resistant variant of the Chinese hamster (CHO) cell with increased metallothionein induction capacity. Exp. Cell Res. 124: 237–246.

12. O'NEILL, J. P., R. L. SCHENLEY & A. W. HSIE. 1979. Cytotoxicity and mutagenicity of alkylating agents in cultured mammalian cells (CHO/HGPRT system): Mutagen treatment in the presence or absence of serum. Mutation Res. 63: 381–385.

13. HILDEBRAND, C. E. & M. D. ENGER. 1980. Regulation of Cd^{2+}/Zn^{2+} stimulated metallothionein synthesis during induction, deinduction and superinduction. Biochemistry 19: 5850–5857.

14. STEINBERG, R. A., B. B. LEVINSON & G. M. TOMKINS. 1975. "Superinduction" of tyrosine aminotransferase by actinomycin D: A re-evaluation. Cell 5: 29–35.

15. ENGER, M. D., L. B. RALL & C. E. HILDEBRAND. 1979. Thionein gene expression in Cd^{++}-resistant variants of the CHO cell: Correlation of thionein synthesis rates with translatable mRNA levels during induction, deinduction and superinduction. Nucleic Acids Res. 7: 271–288.

16. TOBEY, R. A., M. D. ENGER, J. K. GRIFFITH & C. E. HILDEBRAND. 1982. Zinc-induced resistance to alkylating agents: Lack of correlation between cell survival and metallothionein content. Toxicol. Appl. Pharmacol. 64: 72–78.

17. TOBEY, R. A., M. D., ENGER, J. K. GRIFFITH & C. E. HILDEBRAND. 1982. Zinc-induced resistance to alkylating-agent specific toxicity: A potentially novel approach to cancer chemotherapy. Cancer Res. 42: 2980–2984.

18. CHEN, R., D. EAKIN & P. WHANGER. 1974. Biological function of metallothionein. II. Its role in zinc metabolism in the rat. Nutr. Rep. Int. 10: 195–200.

19. EVANS, G. 1971. Function and nomenclature for two mammalian copper proteins. Nutr. Rev. 29: 195–197.

20. NORDBERG, M., B. TROJANOWSKA & G. NORDBERG. 1974. Studies on metal-binding proteins of low molecular weight from renal tissue of rabbits exposed to cadmium or mercury. Environ. Physiol. Biochem. 4: 149–158.

21. PIETROWSKI, J., B. TROJANOWSKA, J. WISNIEOSKA-KYNPL & W. BOLANOWSTRA. 1974. Mercury binding in the liver and kidney of rats repeatedly exposed to mercuric chloride: Induction of metallothionein by mercury and cadmium. Toxicol. Appl. Pharmacol. 27: 11–19.

22. KAJI, J. & B. VALLEE. 1961. Metallothionein: A cadmium- and zinc-containing protein from equine renal cortex. II. Physiochemical properties. J. Biol. Chem. 236: 2435–2442.

23. STIKA, K. M. & G. H. MORRISON. 1981. Analytical methods for the mineral content of human tissues. Fed. Proc. 40: 2115–2119.

24. CAGEN, S. Z. & C. D. KLAASSEN. 1980. Binding of glutathione-depleting agents to metallothionein. Toxicol. Appl Pharmacol. 54: 229–237.

25. WONG, K. L. & C. D. KLAASSEN. 1981. Relationship between liver and kidney levels of glutathione and metallothionein in rats. Toxicology 19: 39–47.

26. SAMSON, L. & J. L. SCHWARTZ. 1980. Evidence for an adaptive DNA repair pathway in CHO and human skin fibroblast cell lines. Nature 287: 861–863.

27. MILLAR, J. L., T. A. PHELPS, R. L. CARTER & T. J. MCELWAIN. 1978. Cyclophosphamide pretreatment reduces the toxic effect of high dose melphalan on intestinal epithelium in sheep. Eur. J. Cancer 14: 1283–1285.

28. MILLAR, J. L., B. N. HUDSPITH, T. J. MCELWAIN & T. A. PHELPS. 1978. The effect of high dose melphalan on bone marrow and intestinal epithelium in mice pretreated with cyclophosphamide. Br. J. Cancer **38**: 137–142.

29. OLSON, K. B., G. HEGGEN, C. F. EDWARDS & L. WHITTINGTON. 1954. Trace element content of cancerous and non-cancerous human liver tissue. Science **119**: 772–773.

30. OLSON, E. B., G. HEGGEN & C. F. EDWARDS. 1958. Analysis of 5 trace elements in the liver of patients dying of cancer and noncancerous disease. Cancer **11**: 554–561.

31. ARNOLD, M. & D. SASSE. 1961. Quantitative and histochemical analysis of Cu, Zn and Fe in spontaneous and induced primary tumors of rats. Cancer Res. **21**: 761–766.

32. FREDRICKS, R. E., K. R. TANAKA & W. N. VALENTINE. 1964. Variations of human blood cell zinc in disease. J. Clin. Invest. **43**: 304–315.

33. WRIGHT, E. G. & T. L. DORMANDY. 1972. Liver zinc in carcinoma. Nature **237**: 166.

34. KEW, M. C. & R. C. MALLETT. 1974. Hepatic zinc concentrations in primary cancer of the liver. Br. J. Cancer **29**: 80–83.

35. BROWN, D. A., K. W. CHATEL, A. Y. CHAN & B. KNIGHT. 1980. Cytosolic levels and distribution of cadmium, copper and zinc in pretumorous livers from diethylnitrosamine-exposed mice and in non-cancerous kidneys from cancer patients. Chem.-Biol. Interactions **32**: 13–27.

36. MORGAN, J. M. 1970. Cadmium and zinc abnormalities in bronchogenic carcinoma. Cancer **25**: 1394–1398.

37. MORGAN, J. M. 1971. Tissue cadmium and zinc content in emphysema and bronchogenic carcinoma. J. Chron. Dis. **24**: 107–110.

38. BROWN, D. A. 1977. Increase of Cd and the Cd:Zn ratio in the high molecular weight protein pool from apparently normal liver of tumor-bearing flounders (*Parophyrs vetulus*). Marine Biol. **44**: 203–212.

39. PORIES, W. J., A. M. VAN RIJ, E. G. MANSOUR & A. FLYNN. 1979. Trace element profiles in cancer patients. Biol. Trace Element Res. **1**: 229–241.

40. PHILLIPS, J. L. 1979. Zinc-induced synthesis of low molecular weight zinc-binding protein by human lymphocytes. Biol. Trace Element Res. **1**: 359–371.

41. BOYETT, J. D. & J. F. SULLIVAN. 1970. Distribution of protein-bound zinc in normal and cirrhotic serum. Metab. Clin. Res. **19**: 148–157.

42. OLAFSON, R. W. 1981. Differential pulse polarographic determination of murine metallothionein induction kinetics. J. Biol. Chem. **256**: 1263–1268.

43. GARVEY, J. S. & C. C. CHANG. 1981. Detection of circulating metallothionein in rats injected with zinc or cadmium. Science **214**: 805–807.

44. GILES, P. J. & R. J. COUSINS. 1982. Hormonal regulation of zinc metabolism in a human prostatic carcinoma cell line (PC-3). Cancer Res. **42**: 2–7.

INSERTION OF NEW GENETIC INFORMATION INTO BONE MARROW CELLS OF MICE: COMPARISON OF TWO SELECTABLE GENES *

Karen E. Mercola, Menashe Bar-Eli, Howard D. Stang, Dennis J. Slamon, and Martin J. Cline

Division of Hematology-Oncology
Department of Medicine
UCLA School of Medicine
Los Angeles, California 90024

Gene transfer in bone marrow cells of living mice has been accomplished using two different selectable systems: (1) transformation by high molecular weight mouse DNA containing gene sequences coding for a mutant drug-resistant enzyme; (2) transformation by purified herpesvirus thymidine kinase (HSVtk) gene sequences. In the first instance the transforming DNA was obtained from a methotrexate (MTX)-resistant cell line containing reiterated gene sequences coding for a mutant dihydrofolate reductase (DHFR).[1-3] This mutant enzyme had a reduced affinity for the folic acid antagonist, MTX.[3] Mouse marrow was transformed *in vitro* with the calcium phosphate technique [4, 5] and injected into irradiated genetically compatible animals. During the period of cellular proliferation required to restore hematopoiesis, MTX was administered to apply selective pressure favoring those few stem cells that had incorporated and expressed new drug resistance genes. The progeny of transformed cells were identified by a karyotype marker, drug resistance,[1, 2] and, in later experiments, by the presence of the electrophoretically distinct mutant DHFR.[3]

In a parallel series of experiments herpesvirus thymidine kinase in a variety of molecular forms was used as the transforming reagent, also utilizing the calcium phosphate technique.[2, 6] Some of the animals receiving transformed bone marrow were treated with MTX; others were left untreated. Insertion and expression of viral gene sequences were analyzed by karyotype analysis, by molecular hybridization techniques, and by assay for the distinctive viral tk enzyme in mammalian cells.[2, 6]

More than 200 mice were examined utilizing these gene insertion and analytical techniques. It is possible, therefore, to compare these two selectable systems in regard to the efficiency and stability of gene insertion and expression.

METHODS

Mouse bone marrow cells (strain CBA) were transformed *in vitro* by the calcium phosphate DNA-mediated gene transfer technique [4, 5] as previously described.[1, 6] DNA from MTX-resistant 3T6R1 mouse cells [3, 7] or cloned herpesvirus tk gene [8] served as the transforming reagents. MTX was administered according to a previously described schedule.[1]

* This work was supported in part by Grants HL27079, CA15619, AM18058, and CA27682 from the National Institutes of Health.

Tk Vectors

A variety of forms of the herpesvirus tk gene were used, including (FIG. 1) a 3.5-Kb tk fragment inserted in the Bam site of plasmid pBR322 (a gift of Dr. L. Enquist); a mixture of excised 3.5-Kb tk Bam fragments and plasmid; concatemers of ligated tk Bam fragments free of plasmid sequences; three recombinant molecules made with HSVtk and a human beta-globin clone Hβ1 (a gift from T. Maniatis). Chimeras 1 and 2 were made with the 4.4-Kb Pst fragment of the beta-globin gene inserted in either of two orientations into the Pst site of pBR322 and the Bam fragment of HSVtk inserted into one of the Bam sites. In chimera 1, tk and Hβ1 were read in the same direction; in chimera 2, tk and Hβ1 were on opposite strands of DNA. A third recombinant molecule, 3, was made by first cutting with Sal and then ligating together HSVtk in pBR322 and Hβ1 in pBR322 in a ratio of tk:Hβ1 of 1 to 1.5.

Tk Analysis

Spleen DNA was extracted for HSVtk analysis, cut with EcoR1, Pst or Bam H1 (Bethesda Research Laboratories), subjected to agarose gel electrophoresis, transferred to nitrocellulose filter strips, and hybridized with ^{32}P-labeled 3.5-Kb HSVtk Bam H1 fragment as described by Southern.[9] Alternatively, the DNA

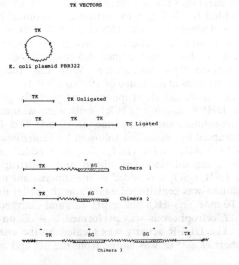

FIGURE 1. Forms of herpes virus thymidine kinase gene (TK) used in DNA-mediated transformation of mouse bone marrow cells: a 3.5-Kb TK fragment inserted in the Bam site of *E. coli* plasmid pBR 322; excised 3.5-Kb TK Bam fragment; TK Bam fragments ligated by DNA ligase. Chimeras 1 and 2 were made with the 4.4-Kb Pst fragment of human beta globin gene inserted in either of two orientations into the Pst site of pBR 322 and the Bam fragment of TK inserted into one of the Bam sites. Chimera 3 was made by first cutting with Sal and then ligating TK in pBR 322 and human beta globin in pBR 322 in a ratio of 1 to 1.5 TK:beta globin.

was spotted on filters and analyzed by the hybridization technique of Brandsma and Miller.[10] *In vitro* labeling of the tk probe was performed as described by Summers *et al.*[11] to yield a specific activity of 0.5 to 1 $\times$ 10[8] cpm/μg.

Herpes simplex virus tk gene expression was assayed in sonicated spleen fragments in either of two ways. The viral tk is really a pyrimidine kinase, whereas the mammalian enzyme has thymidine as its only defined substrate. In earlier experiments pyrimidine kinase activity was assayed using high specific activity ^{125}I deoxycytidine as a substrate in the presence of Mg and ATP according to the method of Summer and Summer.[12] Deoxycitidine (Sigma, St. Louis, MO) was labeled with carrier-free [125]I (New England Nuclear, Boston, MA) and purified by ion exchange chromatography. In later experiments viral and mammalian enzymes were separated by electrophoresis on polyacrylamide gel.[13]

DHFR

DHFR enzymes were purified by the method of Hanggi and Littlefield [14] as modified by Gupta *et al.*[15] Titration of dihydrofolate reductase with MTX using enzymes purified from MTX-sensitive 3T6 and MTX-resistant 3T6R1 cells was performed as described previously.[3] DHFR activity was assayed at room temperature by a fluorometric method measuring the oxidation of NADPH $\rightarrow$ NADP[+]. The standard assay contained 0.7 ml of 0.15 M Tris–HCl buffer pH 7.5, 50 μl KCl 2.25 M, 50 μl NADPH 1.0 mM, 50 μl 2-mercaptoethanol 0.3 M, and 50 μl dihydrofolic acid 2.0 mM. For assay of inhibition of DHFR activity by MTX, purified enzymes (100 μl) were incubated for 15 min, then 0.5 ml of 0.6 N HCl was added for 3–5 min to destroy any residual NADPH. Samples of 100 μl were mixed vigorously with 150 μl 10 N NaOH in 10 $\times$ 75-mm glass tubes, left for at least 60 min to allow the strongly fluorescent alkaline reaction products of NADP[+] to form, and diluted 6.5-fold with distilled water before reading on an Aminco fluorocolorimeter. With this assay NADP[+] can be measured at concentrations in the range of 10[-5] to 10[-11] M.

Native polyacrylamide gel electrophoresis of partially purified cell extracts was analyzed for DHFR activity. 3T6R1 cells were washed three times with cold buffered saline solution and resuspended in 10 mM Tris–HCl buffer pH 7.5. The cells were disrupted by sonication followed by centrifugation at 20,000 $\times$ g for 30 min at 4° C. After solid $(NH_4)_2SO_4$ was added to the S–100 to a saturation of 40%, the solution was stirred and centrifuged for 15 min at 2,000 $\times$ g. Solid $(NH_4)_2SO_4$ was added to the supernatant to a final saturation of 88%. The solution was centrifuged again and the pellet dissolved in a minimum volume of 10 mM Tris–HCl buffer pH 7.5, and dialyzed overnight against the same buffer. Electrophoresis was performed at 4° C on 7.5% polyacrylamide at pH 8.5. The DHFR activity was located by the enzyme activity stain described by Hiebert *et al.*[16] or was eluted from the gel and assayed.

RESULTS

HSVtk Transforming Vector

In initial studies, the distribution of the T6T6 chromosome marker in recipients of transformed bone marrow was used to identify animals requiring further analysis of gene insertion and expression. When an equal mixture of

T6T6 and Ca bone marrow cells is used to reconstitute hematopoiesis in irradiated CBA/Ca mice, less than half of the dividing marrow cells have the T6 chromosome marker (mean $\pm$ 2SD = 38 $\pm$ 10%) because of the contribution of residual hematopoiesis in recipient mice.[1-3] Since T6T6 marrow cells were transformed with HSVtk in most experiments, predominance of this karyotype pattern was used as initial indirect evidence of transformed gene function. Predominance was defined as a marrow karyotype with $\geq$60% of the cells being T6T6.

TABLE 1 shows data on 93 primary recipients of an equal mixture of HSVtk-transformed T6T6 marrow and mock-transformed Ca marrow, analyzed between 30 and 250 days of marrow inoculation. Thirty-three percent of the animals demonstrated marrow T6T6 predominance at some time during this interval. This percentage varied from 12% to 57%, depending upon the tk vector.

MTX treatment of animals was unnecessary for acquisition of transformed karyotype predominance with any of the vectors except perhaps ligated HSVtk. With this reagent T6T6 predominance was observed in four of nine untreated mice and in four of five MTX-treated mice. With the other vectors, no advantage was associated with MTX administration.

Most animals were sacrificed at preset time intervals for analyses; a few were subjected to repeated karyotype analysis to assess stability of the transformed phenotype. Stable transformation was defined as persistence of $\geq$60% T6T6 for at least 2 months. With ligated HSVtk two of six chronically observed animals demonstrated stable predominance; with the HSVtk Bam fragment as transforming vector, three of four animals demonstrated such stability. When all vectors were examined in 44 recipient animals demonstrating karyotype predominance at some point, stability in the pattern was observed in only 6 (13%), indicating that transformation with tk in plasmid or in chimeric form was rarely stable.

Correlation between Transformed Phenotype and Tk Gene Sequences

DNA was extracted from spleens of 56 animals with high T6 marrow karyotypes and analyzed for the presence of viral gene sequences by blot hybridization analysis.[10] Using either pBR322 and/or tk Bam fragment as

TABLE 1

CORRELATION BETWEEN T6T6 KARYOTYPE PREDOMINANCE IN MARROWS OF
RECIPIENT ANIMALS AND HSVTK VECTOR USED IN TRANSFORMATION

Tk Vector	Animals Receiving Transformed Marrow	Animals with T6T6 Predominance
tk in plasmid	6	2
tk Bam fragment	14	4
tk ligated	14	8
Chimera #1	29	10
Chimera #2	14	4
Sal-cut and ligated	16	2

probe, positive "dot blots" were obtained in 26 of these samples. DNA from twelve control animals was negative in this assay.

Viral Gene Expression

An assay for viral pyrimidine kinase was carried out on spleens from selected animals with a high T6 karyotype and on comparably treated low karyotype controls.[2] Five animals with karyotypes ranging from 70% to 95% T6 had 3.8- to 15-fold background activity of conversion of deoxycytidine to the phosphorylated derivative. Spleens from control mice had less than 2.3 times background activity. One of the spleens demonstrating viral pyrimidine kinase was also analyzed by blot hybridization and found to have viral gene sequences.

3T6R1 DHFR Is a Mutant Enzyme

We performed another series of experiments in which high molecular weight DNA from a MTX-resistant mouse cell line was used as the transforming reagent. A series of drug-resistant cell lines was examined and one was chosen because of its high level of resistance to MTX and suggestive evidence that it had a mutant drug-resistant dihydrofolate reductase. This cell line, designated 3T6R1, was originally described by Kellems et al.[7]

DHFR activity from MTX-resistant 3T6R1 were compared for MTX resistance, heat stability, and electrophoretic mobility. As shown in TABLE 2, the 3T6R1 enzyme was considerably more resistant to the inhibitory effects of the folate antagonist. We have previously reported that the 3T6R1 DHFR also has altered heat stability and electrophoretic mobility relative to the wild-type enzyme.[2, 3, 17] These characteristics suggest that DHFR from 3T6R1 cells is a mutant enzyme.

Transformation of Mouse Bone Marrow with 3T6R1 DNA

Marrow cells from chromosomally marked CBA/T6T6 mice were exposed to 3T6R1 DNA and cells from CBA/Ca mice were exposed to salmon sperm DNA under transforming conditions. After mixing at a ratio of 1:1 the cells

TABLE 2

TITRATION OF DHFR WITH MTX USING PARTIALLY PURIFIED ENZYMES
FROM MTX-SENSITIVE WILD-TYPE AND MTX-RESISTANT 3T6R1 CELLS

Cell Line	Percentage of Residual DHFR Activity $\pm$ SD at MTX Concentration of:				
	0	10^{-8}	10^{-7}	10^{-6}	10^{-5}
3T6WT	100	50.1 ± 1.4 *	0	0	0
3T6R1	100	93.6 ± 3.3	93.5 ± 1.7	84.2 ± 2.4	73.6 ± 1.5

* The residual activity in the presence of the drug is expressed as a percentage of the activity in the absence of the drug.

TABLE 3

PREDOMINANCE OF T6T6 KARYOTYPE IN MICE RECEIVING T6T6 MARROW
TRANSFORMED WITH 3T6R1 DNA *

Duration of MTX Therapy (days)	No. of Mice with T6T6 Predominance	No. of Mice Treated with MTX
30–40	5	9
40–50	7	13
> 50	14	20

* Predominance defined as $\geq$ 60% T6T6.

were injected intravenously into irradiated CBA/Ca mice. In a successful transformation the T6T6 cell type receiving the MTX-resistant DNA showed a growth advantage and came to predominate in recipient animals treated with MTX. TABLE 3 illustrates the type of results obtained in which T6T6 cells transformed with MTX-resistant DNA become the predominant marrow cells after 30 days. Control experiments have demonstrated that such results are not due to an inherent proliferative advantage of either T6T6 or Ca hematopoietic cells.[1-3] Furthermore, the transformed karyotype was only observed in MTX-treated recipients and not in untreated control mice. Once established, the transformed phenotype was generally stable.

DHFR in Transformed Mice

To assess whether MTX-resistant DHFR genes were expressed in hematopoietic or other cells of mice receiving transformed bone marrow, spleens and livers were removed from six recipients of transformed marrow and assayed for DHFR. Five of the recipients had been treated with MTX for 50 to 68 days, and one recipient was never treated by drug.

We have previously shown that three of five treated animals had DHFR activity that was resistant to 10^{-4} M MTX detectable in splenic homogenates.[3, 17] These animals had marrows demonstrating T6T6 karyotypes of 67, 73, and 90%. Electrophoretic analysis showed that spleens of these mice had components of rapidly and slowly migrating DHFR that corresponded to those of 3T6R1 cells and normal mouse cells. Liver cells had only the wild-type mouse DHFR.

Two other treated animals from the same experiments and demonstrating karyotype predominance had no detectable resistant enzyme. The recipient of transformed bone marrow who had never been treated with MTX had no T6T6 karyotype predominance in marrow cells and no detectable resistant enzyme in the spleen. Twelve irradiated MTX-treated control animals had no detectable MTX-resistant DHFR.

Health of Animals and Autopsy Results

Animals receiving tk vectors and 3T6R1 DNA after lethal irradiation were observed for periods of up to 16 months. No animal surviving the initial 3-week period of pancytopenia during reconstitution of hematopoiesis showed any untoward effects other than transient diarrhea and weight loss, which occurred in a few animals receiving MTX. Examination of autopsy specimens of liver, lungs, kidney and heart from randomly chosen experimental animals was normal. Cytospin preparations of marrow and peripheral blood gave no morphologic evidence of leukemia.

DISCUSSION

HSVtk

Adult mice receiving syngeneic bone marrow containing some stem cells transformed with HSVtk gene sequences were followed up to 250 days following DNA-mediated transformation. When a variety of tk vectors were used, 33% of animals demonstrated at least transient predominance of the karyotype of the transformed marrow population; however, with all tk vectors, karyotype predominance was stable for more than 2 months in only 13% of animals. Ligated tk appeared to be the most effiicent transforming vector, and 8 of 14 mice demonstrated T6T6 karyotype predominance.

Methotrexate administration, intended to provide a selective pressure favoring proliferation of transformed hematopoietic stem cells, did not influence transformed phenotype predominance, except possibly with ligated tk as the transforming vector. Both gene insertion and expression were observed in some animals never exposed to MTX.

The mechanism of transformation with viral tk in the absence of drug selection is not known. It may be that in mouse bone marrow the salvage pathway for de novo DNA synthesis is preferentially operational even without drug pressure, and that the more effective viral thymidine kinase enzyme provides transformed cells with a proliferative advantage.

DHFR

Our observations that the DHFR of MTX-resistant 3T6R1 differs in several properties from the enzyme of the wild-type cell line suggests that the 3T6R1 cells contain a structurally altered DHFR.[3, 17] The major features distinguishing the 3T6R1 enzyme are resistance to inhibition by MTX, relative heat stability, and altered pattern of electrophoretic mobility. The MTX titration inhibition curves suggest that the 3T6R1-DHFR has an altered affinity of the enzyme. Similar observations have been made by Haber et al.[18]

A high proportion of MTX-treated mice receiving bone marrow cells exposed to 3T6R1 DNA demonstrate evidence of successful transformation, including predominance of the karyotype of the transformed marrow population and resistance to MTX of hematopoietic tissues. On the other hand, we have been unsuccessful in obtaining evidence for successful transformation of bone marrow when we have used DNA from other MTX-resistant cell lines. These cell lines are thought to contain reiterated copies of wild-type mouse DHFR (MTX[R] L1210 cells) or reiterated copies of a mutant hamster DHFR. The mutant hamster DHFR is, however, far less resistant to MTX than the reductase from 3T6R1 cells.[2] These observations suggest that the successful introduction of new functional DHFR genes into marrow stem cells is most likely the result of the insertion of one or a few copies of a mutant gene producing a highly MTX-resistant dihydrofolate reductase.

Several aspects of the transformation system with mutant DHFR can be contrasted with the results with herpesvirus thymidine kinase. In the DHFR system transforming frequency defined by karyotype predominance was high ($\simeq$70%) and was nearly always stable. Transformation, whether defined by karyotype analysis or analysis for mutant gene product, was only seen in drug-treated animals. The mutant 3T6R1 DHFR gene appeared not to provide hematopoietic cells with a proliferative advantage in the absence of drug selection.

Other Observations

It is noteworthy that two of five mice in the MTX system and 30 of 56 mice in the HSVtk system had karyotype predominance but no detectable gene (tk) or gene product (DHFR). Several explanations of these observations are possible: The karyotype analysis may not accurately reflect transformation; the analysis for HSVtk gene or MTX-resistant gene product may be insufficiently sensitive; the new genes may be unstable in their new environment and expressed only transiently, resulting in stable karyotype predominance but impermanent expression of resistant enzyme.

Intact animals present a highly complex system for analysis of DNA-mediated gene transfer. The tissues available for analysis are limited and, obviously, once the animal is sacrificed no further analyses of gene stability and expression are possible. In the bone marrow either pluripotent stem cells or committed stem cells may be targets of gene insertion. It should be noted that 10 to 100 committed stem cells exist for each pluripotent stem cell in the marrow. Moreover, gene integration and expression may potentially be either transient or stable in either of these target stem cells. Depending upon the target or targets and the degree of stability, analyses for detecting the gene and its direct expression in enzyme or indirect expression in the predominant marrow population are likely to vary with time in any group of experimental animals.

Our observations suggest that it is possible to insert new "selectable" genes into mouse hematopoietic cells and, in some cases, to have these genes expressed selectively in hematopoietic tissues. The superior efficiency and stability of the system utilizing a gene for a mutant drug-resistant dihydrofolate reductase suggest strategies for future studies of genetic transformation of blood-forming stem cells.

Summary

A system for insertion of new genetic information into mouse hematopoietic cells is described. Two selectable genes were examined: herpesvirus thymidine kinase and a mutant mouse dihydrofolate reductase. The DHFR system appears to be superior in terms of the frequency and stability of gene insertion and expression in hematopoietic tissues. About 70% of mice had indirect (karyotypic) evidence of gene insertion; of these, about 60% (three of five) had stable expression of the inserted mutant DHFR. In contrast, only 13% of mice demonstrated stable karyotypic transformation by HSVtk, and of those with stable transformation five of seven showed persistent viral gene sequences in hematopoietic tissues.

ACKNOWLEDGMENTS

We wish to thank Carol Le Fèvre and Debra Morse for excellent technical assistance.

REFERENCES

1. CLINE, M. J., H. STANG, K. E. MERCOLA, L. MORSE, R. RUPRECHT, J. BROWNE & W. SALSER. 1980. Nature **284:** 422–425.
2. SALSER, W., B. D. TONG, H. D. STANG, J. BROWNE, K. MERCOLA, M. BAR-ELI & M. J. CLINE. 1981. *In* Molecular Mechanisms of Hemoglobin Switching. G. Stamatoyannopoulos & S. W. Nienhuis, Eds.: 313–334. Grune & Stratton. New York, NY.
3. BAR-ELI, M., K. E. MERCOLA, H. D. STANG, D. SLAMON, N. MAURITZSON & M. J. CLINE. 1982. J. Cell. Physiol. (Suppl.) In press.
4. BACHETTI, S. & F. I. GRAHAM. 1977. Proc. Natl. Acad. Sci. USA **74:** 1490–1494.
5. WIGLER, M., H. PELLICER, S. SILVERSTEIN & R. AXEL. 1978. Cell **14:** 725–731.
6. MERCOLA, K. E., H. D: STANG, J. BROWNE, W. SALSER & M. J. CLINE. 1980. Science **208:** 1033–1035.
7. KELLEMS, R. E., F. W. ALT & R. T. SCHIMKE. 1976. J. Biol. Chem. **251:** 6987–6993.
8. ENQUIST, L. W., M. J. MADDEN, P. SCHIOP-STANSLY & G. F. VAN DE WOUDE. 1979. Science **203:** 541–544.
9. SOUTHERN, E. M. 1975. J. Molec. Biol. **98:** 503–517.
10. BRANDSMA, J. & G. MILLER. 1980. Proc. Natl. Acad. Sci. USA **77:** 6851–6855.
11. SUMMERS, J., A. O'CONNELL & I. MILLMAN. 1975. Proc. Natl. Acad. Sci. **72:** 4597–4601.
12. SUMMERS, W. C. & W. P. SUMMERS. 1977. J. Virol. **24:** 314–318.
13. CHANG, Y.-C. & W. H. PRUSOFF. 1974. Biochemistry **13:** 1179–1183.
14. HANGGI, U. J. & J. W. LITTLEFIELD. 1974. J. Biol. Chem. **249:** 1390–1397.
15. GUPTA, R. S., W. F. FLINTOFF & L. SIMINOVITCH. 1977. Can. J. Biochem. **55:** 445–452.
16. HIEBERT, M., J. GAULDIE & B. L. HILLCOAT. 1972. Anal. Biochem. **46:** 433–437.
17. BAR-ELI, M., H. D. STANG, K. E. MERCOLA & M. J. CLINE. 1982. Expression of a methotrexate-resistant dihydrofolate reductase gene in transformed hematopoietic cells of mice. Submitted for publication.
18. HABER, D. A., S. M. BEVERLY, M. L. KIELY & R. T. SCHIMKE. 1981. J. Biol. Chem. **256:** 9501–9506.

TUMOR CELL METABOLIC HETEROGENEITY: THE ROLE OF METABOLIC MODIFICATION IN CHEMOTHERAPY

Oliver Alabaster

Department of Medicine
George Washington University
Washington, D.C. 20037

INTRODUCTION

There is clear evidence that sensitivity to cytotoxic drugs is influenced by the growth rate of target cells.[1,2] Tumors with a rapid growth rate and a high growth fraction, such as Burkitt's lymphoma, are more sensitive to chemotherapy than are slow-growing tumors with a low growth fraction, such as multiple myeloma. Similar observations can be made of the bacterial response to antibiotics [3] and the response of plants to light deprivation. These observations suggest that cytotoxic agents mainly act on growth-related biochemical events, and that the rate of these biochemical reactions is significant.

Examination of the biochemical sequence of known events during the cell cycle (FIG. 1) reveals negligible growth-related metabolic activity during early G_1 and obviously none in dormant G_0 cells. These observations would therefore suggest that G_1 cells would be those most likely to survive cycle-dependent chemotherapy.

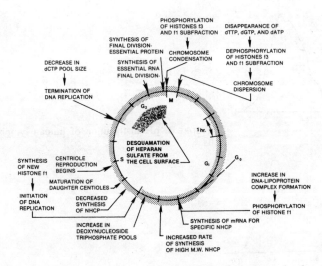

FIGURE 1. Temporal sequence of some biochemical events in the cell cycle.

281

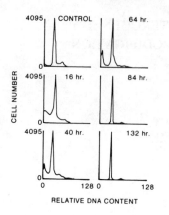

FIGURE 2. Sequential DNA content distributions in Burkitt's lymphoma after COMP induction.

EXPERIMENTAL DATA

Flow cytometric cell cycle analysis of a patient with Burkitt's lymphoma treated with COMP chemotherapy is shown in FIGURE 2. These DNA content distributions were derived from tumor cells harvested from a pleural effusion before and after chemotherapy. Despite a cytoreduction of greater than 99%, nearly all surviving cells had a G_0/G_1 DNA content. Similar observations also have been made in two patients with lymphoma treated with cyclophosphamide alone.[4]

Using the pH-dependent fluorochrome, dicyanohydroquinone,[5] flow cytometric analysis of the intracellular pH distribution of two human lymphoma cell lines was obtained, which are shown in FIGURE 3.

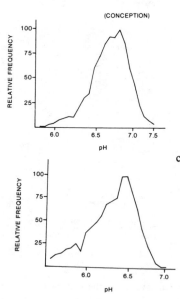

FIGURE 3. pH distribution of human lymphoma cells.

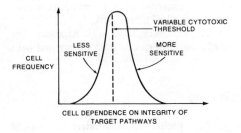

FIGURE 4. Distribution of cell sensitivity to drug action.

DISCUSSION

Since potentially sensitive cells that survive chemotherapy appear to have less growth-related metabolic activity, it would seem reasonable to propose that some cells survive because critical metabolic pathways on which drug cytotoxicity depends are relatively quiescent. This metabolic heterogeneity is supported by the new observation that the intracellular pH of tumor cells is not uniform. Metabolic heterogeneity, whether related to cell cycle distribution, growth rate, nutrient supply, oxygenation or intracellular pH, can be expressed for any active intracellular cytotoxic agent as a relative distribution of cell dependence on the integrity of target metabolic pathways (FIG. 4). It is postulated that this dependence is directly related to the relative rates of these critical biochemical reactions. These concepts can be integrated, and are schematically presented in FIGURE 5.

From this hypothesis it follows that agents that increase the level of activity of the target metabolic pathways for a cytotoxic drug would increase cell-dependence upon them, and thereby would increase cell vulnerability to drug action. However, since the biochemical sequence of events that leads to cell death is not adequately understood, and since we do not know all the biochemical sequelae of drug–cell interaction, it is not yet possible to define approaches to metabolic modification with much certainty. Nevertheless, studies in which insulin was used to alter the metabolism of human breast cancer cells (MCF–7) *in vitro* during treatment with methotrexate resulted in accelerated

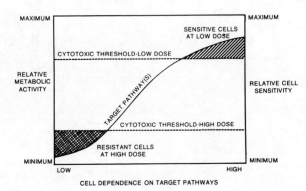

FIGURE 5.

free methotrexate uptake [6] and a 10,000-fold increase in cell sensitivity within the optimal dose range without increasing the level of bound drug.[7]

Despite this early encouragement, it will, however, always be necessary for metabolic modifiers to act more specifically on tumor cells than on normal cells to enhance the therapeutic index.

REFERENCES

1. VALERIOTE, F. & L. VAN PUTTEN. 1975. Proliferation-dependent cytotoxicity of anticancer agents: A review. Cancer Res. **35:** 2619–2630.
2. SHACKNEY, S. E., G. W. McCORMACK & G. J. CUCHURAL. 1978. Growth rate patterns of solid tumors and their relation to responsiveness to therapy: An analytical review. Ann. Intern. Med. **89:** 107–121.
3. PITTILO, R. F., F. M. SCHABEL & H. E. SKIPPER. 1970. The sensitivity of resting and dividing cells. Cancer Chemother. Rep. **54:** 137–142.
4. ALABASTER, O., I. T. MAGRATH, M. C. HABBERSETT & C. J. HERMAN. 1979. Effects of cyclophosphamide on the mithramycin-DNA fluorescence of human lymphoma cells: A possible result of guanine alkylation. J. Histochem. Cytochem. **27:** 500–504.
5. VALET, G., A. RAFFAEL, L. MORODER, E. WUNSCH & G. RUHENSTROTH-BAUER. 1981. Fast intracellular pH determination in single cells by flow cytometry. Naturwissenschaften **68:** S265.
6. SCHILSKY, R. L., B. D. BAILEY & B. A. CHABNER. 1981. Characteristics of membrane transport of methotrexate by cultured human breast cancer cells. Biomed. Pharmacol. **30:** 157.
7. ALABASTER, O., B. K. VONDERHAAR & S. M. SHAFIE. 1981. Metabolic modification by insulin enhances methotrexate cytotoxicity in MCF-7 human breast cancer cells. Eur. J. Cancer Clin. Oncol. **17**(11): 1223.

STUDIES ON THE MECHANISM OF THE ANTIPROLIFERATIVE EFFECT OF INTERFERON

J. A. Bilello and P. M. Pitha

The Johns Hopkins Oncology Center
Baltimore, Maryland 21205

A number of *in vitro* and *in vivo* studies have indicated that cellular proliferation is inhibited after treatment with interferon (IFN). We have undertaken studies to determine the molecular basis for the direct effect of interferon on cell growth. In order to distinguish effectively alterations in cell proliferation from other IFN-induced changes, we have established a series of Friend erythroleukemia cell clones resistant to growth inhibition by interferon *in vitro*. These mutants were selected by continuous passage in 5000 units/ml of purified mouse fibroblast interferon (8.4×10^7 U/mg protein). Clones isolated from IFN-containing methylcellulose were grown in the absence of interferon and then screened for proliferation in the presence and absence of IFN. The clones were concomitantly tested for the production of retrovirus particles by assay of reverse transcriptase in the culture medium. Results with a representative group of clones are shown in TABLE 1. Three classes of clones were isolated: resistant, sensitive, and a single clone, F4–6 R–301, which proliferates more rapidly in the presence of IFN.

Analysis of reverse-transcriptase-containing particles indicated a 100% correlation between the release of virus particles and whether the clone was growth-inhibited or -stimulated by IFN. Cell lines sensitive to growth inhibition by IFN varied in the extent of inhibition of virus release. In some cases (such as F4–6 R–302) virus release as measured by reverse transcriptase was inhibited to a greater degree than cell growth. Whether differences in sensitivity to the inhibition of virus release relates to the rapidity of the growth response to IFN is under study. We have used RNA tumor virus proteins as probes for interferon-induced alterations in protein synthesis, modification, and secretion.

TABLE 1

Cell Line	Proliferation (cells $\times$ 10^{-6})		Reverse Transcriptase Activity (cpm $\times$ 10^{-3})	
	Control	Interferon	Control	Interferon
F4–6	1.19	0.71	34.1	13.8
F4–6 R–1	1.31	1.34	107.0	96.0
F4–6 R–6	0.84	0.77	60.3	83.4
F4–6 R–201	0.87	1.11	—	—
F4–6 R–2013	0.98	0.68	—	—
F4–6 R–301	0.62	2.20	46.1	107.0
F4–6 R–302	0.90	0.74	55.3	14.3
F4–6 R–306	0.85	0.57	82.7	7.8

Synthesis of the putative transformation protein coded for by spleen-focus-forming virus of the Friend virus complex, gp55,[1] was normal at all doses of IFN tested (50–5000 U/ml). Pulse-chase analysis of ^{35}S-methionine-labeled Friend virus envelope glycoprotein precursor, gPr85^{env}, showed that synthesis and processing to gp70 and p15E were indistinguishable in the presence and absence of interferon. The virion matrix protein p15E is processed to p12E and the R pentadecapeptide. One major difference observed was that p12E, which is usually linked by a disulfide bond to gp70, was no longer associated with gp70 in virions. Fully processed p12E accumulates intracellularly in the presence of IFN. The kinetics of secretion of gp70 were identical in control and treated cells, even under conditions where gp70 was not assembled into virions.

In contrast to what has been previously reported,[2] no interferon-induced inhibition of N-linked glycosylation was observed. Analysis of glycolipid fractions indicated that there was no change in the partition of label in organic and aqueous solvents. Biogel® P–10 chromatography of glucosamine labeled glyco-peptides indicated no overt change in the oligosaccharide moieties after treatment with growth-inhibitory levels of IFN.

Two significant changes in membrane structure/function were observed upon exposure of erythroleukemia cells to growth-inhibitory doses of IFN. Transport of methionine and α-amino-isobutyric acid was rapidly decreased after exposure to 5000 U/ml of IFN. In contrast, transport was not decreased in cell lines resistant to the growth-inhibitory effect of interferon. Analysis of membrane fluidity by DPH labeling and fluorescence polarization analysis indicated that 72 hours of exposure to IFN decreased the fluidity of the membrane (control, $p = 0.236$; IFN, $p = 0.250$). Induction of erythroid differentiation with DMSO resulted in a decrease in fluidity ($p = 0.266$), while blockage of erythroid differentiation with IFN resulted in an extremely rigid membrane with p value in excess of 0.275.

Further studies are in progress which will determine whether the decrease in membrane fluidity is directly responsible for the inhibition of cell growth and retrovirus maturation.

REFERENCES

1. BILELLO, J. A., G. COLLETTA, G. WARNECKE, G. KOCH, D. FRISBY, I. B. PRAGNELL & W. OSTERTAG. 1980. Virology 107: 331.
2. MAHESHWARI, R. K., D. K. BANERJEE, C. J. WAECHTER, K. OLDEN & R. M. FRIEDMAN. 1980. Nature 287: 454.

COTRANSFER OF CLONED ADENOVIRAL GENES INTO PERMISSIVE AND NONPERMISSIVE MAMMALIAN CELLS

L. E. Babiss, H. S. Ginsberg, C. S. H. Young,
and P. B. Fisher

Department of Microbiology
Cancer Center/Institute of Cancer Research
Columbia University
College of Physicians and Surgeons
New York, New York 10032

A major objective of our laboratories is to elucidate the roles that early adenovirus gene products play in both the initiation and maintenance of mammalian cell transformation and viral DNA replication. With this goal in mind, the recombinant plasmid pSV2–gpt [1] was modified to contain selected adenovirus DNA fragments encoding early-region E1a (0–4.5 map units [m.u.]), or E1a and E1b (0–15.5 m.u.), or E2a (59.5–78.5 m.u. or 58.5–70.7 m.u.). These plasmids were used separately to transform one or more cell lines permissive for adenovirus infection (human HeLa, KB, 293), and nonpermissive rat (CREF, 3Y1) and mouse (3T3) cell lines. Transformation frequencies were determined directly by selecting cells expressing the gpt gene function in XAT medium. The results indicated that nonpermissive cell lines were transformed at a higher frequency than the permissive cell lines in the order: CREF > 3Y1 > 3T3 > 293 > HeLa > KB. Coexpression of appropriate adenovirus genes could be monitored by one or more of several criteria: morphologic changes, fluorescent-antibody staining, cytoplasmic mRNA production, and complementation of viral host-range mutants. In general, 20 to 50% of the cells expressing gpt functions also expressed one or both virus-specific regions. Southern blot analysis revealed that those cell lines not expressing all or some of the adenovirus gene functions contained deletions within these sequences. Of particular interest were the KB cell lines transfected with a gpt plasmid, pLB206, bearing both E1a and E1b viral sequences. Of the nine clones studied in detail, two appeared to express both viral gene functions, whereas one expressed E1a alone and two expressed solely E1b, as determined by their ability to complement the host-range mutants d1312 (Δ1.2–3.7) and d1315 (Δ3.7–8.7). These KB cell lines can be used to study the effects of cell-encoded E1a and/or E1b gene products upon viral replication, with the standard KB line forming the appropriate negative control. They also have the technical advantages of being adaptable to spinner culture and of being suitable for large-scale viral production.

REFERENCE

1. MULLIGAN, R. B. & E. P. BERG. 1980. Science **209:** 1422.

287

A GENETICALLY DEFINED ROLE FOR PROTEIN PHOSPHORYLATION IN THE REGULATION OF PROLIFERATION BY INSULIN

Robert Fleischmann, Marilyn Murray, and John Pawelek

Department of Dermatology
Yale University School of Medicine
New Haven, Connecticut 06510

The proliferation of Cloudman S91 melanoma cells is affected by insulin, which acts as a potent, reversible inhibitor of the growth of the wild-type cell line. Three phenotypes of insulin response have been established in Cloudman cells: insulin-inhibited (wild type), insulin-resistant, and insulin-dependent. In addition, "revertants" from the insulin-dependent line have been isolated that display the insulin-resistant phenotype.

In order to study the genetics and biochemistry of insulin action we have utilized these mutant cell lines to develop a system of cell hybridization and genetic complementation in conjunction with studies of protein phosphorylation. Two parental insulin-inhibited lines have been established. The first is ouabain-sensitive and hypoxanthine guanine phosphoribosyl transferase-positive (HGPRT+). The second parental line is ouabain-resistant and HGPRT−. Using these cell lines and the insulin phenotype variants selected from these lines, we have shown that insulin inhibition is dominant over insulin resistance and insulin dependence, and that insulin dependence is domiant over insulin resistance. We have also achieved genetic complementation between insulin-resistant variants, which, when fused together, exhibit the wild-type insulin-inhibited phenotype. Two insulin-resistant variants were unable to complement one another, and the fused product exhibited the variant insulin-resistant phenotype.

We are studying the variant cell lines in hopes of identifying phosphoproteins that mediate responses to insulin. Cells cultured in the presence or absence of insulin are lysed, incubated with ^{32}P-ATP and magnesium, and analyzed by SDS-polyacrylamide gel electrophoresis followed by autoradiography. We found that the phosphorylation of a group of proteins in the 27–32,000 MW range is apparently involved in mediating the proliferative response of these cells to insulin. The proteins are found exclusively in a particulate fraction (30,000 g pellet) of the cells. In addition, an insulin-dependent cell line shows an increased phosphorylation of a 105,000 MW phosphoprotein when grown in the absence of insulin. This protein is also found in a particulate fraction of the cells.

We hope that such studies of variant cell lines and hybrids will allow us to correlate changes in specific phosphoproteins with particular phenotypes thus identifying cause/effect relationships in the insulin response.

CONTRASTING EFFECTS OF EGF/UROGASTRONE AND THE TUMOR PROMOTERS, TPA AND DEOXYCHOLIC ACID, ON PREMALIGNANT HUMAN COLONIC EPITHELIAL CELLS

Eileen Friedman

Memorial Sloan-Kettering Cancer Center
New York, New York 10021

There is increasing evidence that many human neoplasms arise through a series of progressive changes and, by inference, a series of premalignant cells. Premalignant epithelial cells in the human colon form a benign tumor called an adenoma, which can grow to several centimeters in diameter due to the slow evolution of this form of cancer. Adenomas have been staged into three classes by their histologic appearance and malignant potential: the *tubular* (early stage, low potential for containing a carcinoma), the *villous* (late premalignant stage with a high probability of becoming malignant), and the *villotubular* (having mixed histologic properties and intermediate likelihood of containing a foci of carcinoma). The cells cultured from villous (late stage) adenomas had more phenotypic markers in common with malignant cells than did those cells cultured from tubular (early stage) adenomas, while villotubular tumors gave rise to epithelial cultures with intermediate characteristics.

Epithelial cells from all three benign tumor classes respond to phorbol ester tumor promoters. In analogy to the two-step model of mouse skin carcinogenesis, the adenomatous epithelial cells are all initiated, but are at different stages in the progression towards frank carcinoma. Surprisingly, TPA had two effects. It increased the fraction of dividing cells in early-stage derived cultures from 34 to 117%. However, its effect on replication of middle- and late-stage cells could not be assayed because of the dramatic morphologic changes it induced at these stages. Cells became multilayered and formed into ridges; then they formed multicellular clusters by partly detaching from the plate. A protease with many properties of a plasminogen activator was released during multilayering. Inhibition of protease activity also inhibited cell clustering, suggesting that the secreted protease caused the morphologic changes by acting directly on the cells.

There is reason to believe that endogenous promoting agents exist and, furthermore, that phorbol esters are their analogs. Accordingly, we have begun to assay for the effects of putative endogenous promoting agents. Epidermal growth factor has a strong structural homology to human urogastrone, a tropic hormone in the intestine. EGF increased stimulation by 58 to 120% of the replication of late- or intermediate-stage cells. EGF also did not alter the morphology of late-stage cultures. EGF and TPA are known to have different receptors. Therefore, while EGF (urogastrone) may enhance tumor production by stimulating the growth of early-stage cells, it does not mimic TPA's effects on late-stage cultures.

Deoxycholic acid (DOC), a secondary bile acid found in the colon, has been implicated in the etiology of colon cancer by several investigators. Increasing the concentration of bile acids in the intestines of laboratory animals pretreated with a carcinogen in all cases caused an increase in the number of colonic tumors. An increase in bile acid concentration was not by itself tumorigenic. Therefore, in analogy to the two-step model of carcinogenesis in mouse skin, bile acids have been postulated to act as promoting agents *in vivo*. Bile acids, cholesterol derivatives that function in fat, cholesterol, and fat-soluble vitamin absorption may also play this role in man. Epidemiologic studies have suggested a link between high-fat diets and a high incidence of human cancer. In studies from this laboratory, DOC markedly stimulated the proliferation of only one class of human premalignant colonic cells, the early-stage cells, by 55 to 150%. It had no effect on the replication, morphology, or extent of plasminogen activator secretion in intermediate- or late-stage premalignant cell cultures.

The designation of human colonic epithelial cells from benign tumors as early-, intermediate-, or late-stage premalignant is based on clinical and histopathologic criteria. This designation has been strengthened by the cells' differential expression of a second-trimester fetal intestinal antigen. The frequency of expression of this antigen increased during the progression of cells through the adenoma to carcinoma sequence. Antigen-positive cells were found in 18% of early-stage cultures, 43% of intermediate-stage cultures, 70% of late-stage premalignant cultures, and 83% of colonic carcinomas. Thus, the extent of expression in late-stage cultures was closest to the malignant phenotype of all premalignant classes.

LITHIUM ENHANCEMENT OF
MEGAKARYOCYTOPOIESIS *

Christina Gamba-Vitalo, Vincent S. Gallicchio,
Thomas D. Watts, and Michael G. Chen

*Department of Therapeutic Radiology
Yale University School of Medicine
New Haven, Connecticut 06520*

Lithium (Li) has been used successfully for many years to reverse symptoms of manic depression. However, one side effect of this therapy is peripheral granulocytosis and thrombocytosis.[1, 2] For this reason, lithium has been proposed as a possible therapeutic drug in alleviating some symptoms of pancytopenia associated with intensive chemotherapy and radiotherapy.

Previously, we and others have shown that Li modulates murine hematopoiesis at the level of pluripotential (CFU-S) and committed (CFU-GM, BFU-E and CFU-E) stem cells. Mechanisms for this granulocytosis have been through a direct effect of Li on stem cells [3, 4] and an indirect action by the production of colony-stimulating factors.[5]

Now we have investigated the effects of Li on the proliferative potential of marrow megakaryocyte stem cells (CFU-Mk) in the presence of optimal (100 μl) and suboptimal levels (as low as 10 μl) of Meg-CSF, obtained from a WEHI–3 tetraploid cell line.[6] To determine the mechanism of Li action on increasing CFU-Mk levels, heterogenous bone marrow was separated into adherent and nonadherent cell populations. This separation procedure would determine whether the observed increase by Li resulted from a direct effect on stem cells or rather represented an indirect stimulatory effect on a macrophage/fibroblastic-like cell population producing Meg-CSF.

CFU-Mk, identified by positive acetylcholinesterase activity, were cultured using a modification of the Williams technique [6] in the presence of increasing concentrations of ultrapure LiCl (0.1 to 5.0 mEq/L). At optimal levels of CM (100 μl) all concentrations of LiCl augmented CFU-Mk numbers. Significant increases of 83 and 81% in CFU-Mk numbers were observed at 1.0 and 3.0 mEq/L, respectively. Suboptimal levels of CM, as low as 10 μl, in the presence of 1 mEq/L LiCl effected a 200% increase above its control level, suggesting a greater sensitivity of stem cells in the presence of Li to stimulatory factors. Furthermore, Meg-CSF is obligatory for Li-induced megakaryocytopoiesis.

The nonadherent cell population, cultured in the presence of optimal CM and LiCl, showed significantly elevated CFU-Mk levels (85%) above control nonadherent cells cultured without Li. These results suggest a direct effect of Li on megakaryocyte progenitor cells. Data obtained from adherent cell population studies suggest that this population contains a small fraction of megakaryocyte stem cells directly responsive to Li as well as a population of macrophage-like cells, which produce CSF acting on these stem cells.

* This work was supported in part by Grants CA–06519 and CA–09259 from the National Institutes of Health.

In vivo experiments comprised of three daily intraperitoneal injections of 0.042 mg per ml of lithium produced a thrombocytosis from days 4 through 15, post lithium. Maximal stimulation (33% above control levels) was observed in circulating platelet levels 6 days post lithium injection. These data correlate well with the observed *in vitro* increase in CFU-Mk, as well as with the previously reported *in vivo* and *in vitro* [8, 9] increases in the granulocytic line.

We have shown for the first time that lithium enhances megakaryocytopoiesis by increasing the number of CFU-Mk. Thus, lithium could be useful in alleviating the severe leukopenia and thrombocytopenia present after chemotherapy and radiotherapy. Modulation of granulopoiesis and megakaryopoiesis could permit longer, more appropriately timed, intensive treatment of malignant diseases.

REFERENCES

1. LYMAN, G. H., C. C. WILLIAMS & D. PRESTON. 1980. N. Engl. J. Med. **302:** 257.
2. BILLIE, P. E., M. K. JENSEN, J. P. K. JENSEN & J. C. POULSEN. 1975. Acta Med. Scand **198:** 281.
3. LEVITT, L. J. & P. J. QUESENBERRY. 1980. N. Engl. J. Med. **302:** 713.
4. GALLICCHIO, V. S. & M. G. CHEN. 1980. Blood **56:** 1150.
5. RAMSEY, R. & E. F. HAYS. 1979. Exp. Hematol. **7:** 245.
6. WILLIAMS, N. & H. JACKSON. 1978. Blood **52:** 163.
7. KARNOVSKY, M. L. & J. ROOTS. 1964. J. Histochem. Cytochem. **12:** 219.
8. GALLICCHIO, V. S. & M. G. CHEN. 1981. Exp. Hematol. **9:** 804.
9. GALLICCHIO, V. S. & M. G. CHEN. 1982. Cell Tissue Kinet. **15:** 179.

BONE MARROW SUPPRESSION FROM DOXORUBICIN AND *CIS*-DIAMMINEDICHLOROPLATINUM IS SUBSTANTIALLY DEPENDENT UPON BOTH CIRCADIAN AND CIRCANNUAL STAGES OF ADMINISTRATION

William J. M. Hrushesky

Section of Medical Oncology
School of Medicine
University of Minnesota
Minneapolis, Minnesota 55455

A circadian rhythm of high amplitude is an essential endogenous property of the cytokinetics of virtually every tissue studied using adequate sampling frequency. Both the proportion of cells within each of the "cell cycle compartments" and the average span of time that these cells spend in each of the compartments have been well documented to be circadian-stage-dependent by American,[1-9] Norwegian,[10-12] and Russian,[13] investigators. Circadian rhythms in cell proliferation were documented in human bone marrow by Mauer [14] in 1965. More recently, using cytofluorometric methods, Laerum [12] has shown that endogenous *circannual,* as well as circadian, rhythmicity characterizes the entry and exit of murine bone marrow cells to and from each of the "cell cycle compartments."

The lethality of seven anticancer agents has been established to be circadian-stage-dependent in murine systems.[15, 16] The toxicity of two of these agents, doxorubicin (D) and *cis*-diamminedichloroplatinum (C), has been studied in 24 patients suffering from widely metastatic ovarian carcinoma or transitional cell carcinoma of the urinary bladder. Initially, 14 previously untreated, ambulatory, diurnally awake (from about 0700 to 2200) adult patients were treated monthly with D, 60 mg/m^2, followed 12 hours later by C, 60 mg/m^2. Patients were randomly assigned to receive chemotherapy beginning at either 0600 (A) or 1800 (B), and then switched to the opposite schedule with a continuing alternation of schedule throughout 9 months of treatment. A three-way analysis of variance for effects on white blood cells of circadian (A or B) and circannual (spring, summer, fall, winter) treatment and time from last chemotherapy course (days 7, 14, 21, 28) showed (1) dependence of toxicity upon circadian stage ($p < 0.001$) and circannual stage ($p < 0.001$) and (2) a strong circadian–circannual treatment time ($p = 0.007$). When circadian treatment schedule A is compared with B on day 28 after treatment, white blood cell recovery is 18% greater in spring, 43% greater in summer, 23% better in fall, but 26% worse in winter.

An additional 10 patients were randomly assigned to receive each monthly course of chemotherapy on circadian schedule A or schedule B. Because of leukopenia, 4 of 5 patients treated on circadian schedule B had to have a >33% dose reduction and 3 of them had to have treatment delays of >2 weeks. None of those treated on circadian schedule A had to have dose reductions or delays in planned chemotherapy treatments. Assessment by linear regression analysis of individuals' white blood cell decrease and recovery (on days 1, 7, 14, and 28) after treatment revealed cumulative bone marrow toxicity in each of the patients treated on circadian schedule B, despite substantial dose reductions. The recovery of WBC on day 28 exhibited a substantial negative slope over all treatment courses in the group of patients treated monthly on circadian schedule B ($r = 0.6$, $p < 0.002$), but not in the group treated monthly on schedule A ($r = 0.2$, $p = 0.2$).

Both acute and cumulative bone marrow toxicity of this combination as reflected by the decrease and recovery of circulating white blood cells, neutrophils, and platelets are circadian-stage-dependent. There is a circannual modulation of the acute toxicity. These susceptibility rhythms have resulted in dose reductions and treatment delays. Since metabolic, excretory, hormonal, and immunobiologic circadian rhythms are also important rhythmic variables, the extent to which endogenous cytokinetic circadian and circannual rhythms within human bone marrow are responsible for these rhythmic susceptibility patterns remains to be further clarified. Nevertheless, consideration of *in vivo* cytokinetic rhythms may be helpful in planning experimentation and interpreting both preclinical and clinical data. Proper *a priori* consideration of these temporal rhythms, as well as of drug sequence and the interval between drugs, in the design of clinical trials may help to render clinically useful the profound advances that cytokineticists are now documenting in *in vitro* systems.

REFERENCES

1. HALBERG, F., E. HAUS & L. E. SCHEVING. 1978. *In* Biomathematics and Cell Kinetics. A. J. Valleron and P. D. M. Macdonald, Eds.: 175–190. North-Holland. Amsterdam.
2. SCHEVING, L. E. 1981. *In* Eleventh International Congress of Anatomy: Biological Rhythms in Structure and Function: 39–79. Alan R. Liss, Inc. New York, NY.
3. SCHEVING, L. A., Y. C. YEH, T. H. TSAI & L. E. SCHEVING. 1980. Endocrinology **106:** 1498–1503.
4. SCHEVING, L. A., Y. C. YEH, T. H. TSAI & L. E. SCHEVING. 1979. Endocrinology **105:** 1475–1480.
5. BURNS, E. R. 1981. Cancer Res. **41:** 2795–2802.
6. BURNS, E. R. 1981. Cell Tissue Kinet. **14:** 219–224.
7. BURNS, E. R. 1982. Oncology **39:** 250–254.
8. RUBIN, N. H. 1982. Radiation Res. **89:** 65–76.
9. IZQUIERDO, J. N. & S. J. GIBBS. 1974. Cell Tissue Kinet **7:** 99–111.
10. CLAUSEN, O. P. F., E. THORUD, R. BJERKNES & E. ELGJO. 1979. Cell Tissue Kinet. **12:** 319–337.
11. THORUD, E., O. P. F. CLAUSEN, R. BJERKNES & E. AARNAES. 1980. Cell Tissue Kinet. **13:** 625–634.
12. LAERUM, O. D. & N. P. AARDAL. 1981. *In* Eleventh International Congress of Anatomy: Biological Rhythms in Structure and Function. E. V. Acosta, *et al.*, Eds.: 87–97. Alan R. Liss, Inc. New York, NY.
13. MAMONTOV, S. G. 1968. Bull. Exp. Biol. Med. **66:** 1277.
14. MAUER, A. M. 1965. Blood **26:** 1–7.

15. LEVI, F., W. HRUSHESKY, E. HAUS, F. HALBERG, L. E. SCHEVING & B. J. KENNEDY. 1980. *In* Proceedings of NATO Advanced Study Institute on the Principles and Application of Chronobiology to Shifts in Schedules with Emphasis on Man: 481–511. Sijthoff and Noordhoff, Alphen aan der Rijn. The Netherlands.
16. HRUSHESKY, W., F. LEVI, F. HALBERG, E. HAUS, L. SCHEVING, S. SANCHEZ, E. MEDINI, H. BROWN & B. J. KENNEDY. 1980. *In* Proceedings of NATO Advanced Study Institute on the Principles and Application of Chronobiology to Shifts in Schedules with Emphasis on Man: 513–533. Sijthoff and Noordhoff, Alphen aan der Rijn. The Netherlands.

ALTERED REGULATION OF PROLIFERATION IN TRANSFORMED LIVER EPITHELIAL CELLS

James B. McMahon and P. Thomas Iype

Chemical Carcinogenesis Program
NCI Frederick Cancer Research Facility
Frederick, Maryland 21701

Relatively little is known about the role of negative growth factors in the regulation of cell proliferation compared with that of nutrients, ions, and positive growth factors. While the existence of such negative factors has been reported in different tissues, it has not been proven unequivocally that their biologic effects are not due to acute cytotoxicity. We used a quantitative colony assay to differentiate between cytotoxic or cytostatic (reversible) actions of test chemicals on liver cells. Using this assay, we reported [1] the partial purification of a factor from rat liver which, while inhibiting cell division in a variety of untransformed rat liver epithelial cell lines, had either no effect, or a growth-promoting activity, on malignant liver cells transformed *in vitro* or *in vivo*. Moreover, this factor could differentiate between mutant transformed liver epithelial cells and nonmalignant liver epithelial cells even in experimental conditions under which the mutant cells exhibited a nonmalignant phenotype.[2] The role of such regulators of cell proliferation can only be studied in detail if such factors are purified to homogeneity. We have recently purified a hepatic protein which reversibly and preferentially inhibits the proliferation of non-malignant rat liver cells.[3] Although the hepatic proliferation regulator (HPR) can be purified to apparent homogeneity by DEAE-cellulose chromatography, this is a time-consuming procedure since the column must be washed extensively before HPR can effectively be isolated by salt elution. After a preliminary dialysis against dilute acetic acid we found anion exchange HPLC to be a more rapid and effective means of purification. Moreover, the factor isolated by this technique possessed all the physical and biologic properties of HPR isolated by DEAE-cellulose chromatography. We report here the biologic and biochemical characteristics of HPR and the preliminary results of its localization studied with monospecific antibodies. The properties of HPR established so far are listed below:

Molecular mass (daltons)	26,000
Isoelectric point	4.65
A_{260}/A_{280}	1.85
Carbohydrate content	None detected
Heat stability	Stable for 30 min at 70°C
Proteolytic stability	Sensitive to trypsin and pronase
Target cell	Nonmalignant rat liver epithelial cells
Effective concentration	10^{-10} to 10^{-9} M

Antisera, raised against HPR in New Zealand white rabbits were purified with protein A–Sepharose and the resultant IgG fraction was shown to be monospecific by double immunodiffusion and electroimmunodiffusion. In preliminary experiments, HPR was localized in normal rat liver epithelial cell lines by indirect immunofluorescence using the monospecific IgG fraction. In fixed rat tissues, HPR was not detected in lung, intestine, or muscle. In the liver of normal Fischer rats, all the hepatocytes within the hepatic lobule contained HPR. In contrast, the distribution of HPR was not uniform in the liver of older Fischer rats. Hyperplastic nodules showed only weak fluorescence compared with that of the adjacent hepatocytes.

The role played by HPR in the carcinogenic process is being studied. In an *in vitro* transformation system, it was found that the inhibition of cell proliferation exerted by HPR on normal liver cells was altered when such cells were maintained in culture after treatment with the hepatocarcinogen aflatoxin B_1. This fact, together with the observations that the HPR content is decreased in hyperplastic nodules (regarded as a preneoplastic change *in vivo*), suggests that the alteration in the response to HPR may be a key event during the carcinogenic process.

REFERENCES

1. McMahon, J. B. & P. T. Iype. 1980. Cancer Res. **40:** 1249.
2. Iype, P. T. & J. B. McMahon. 1981. Cancer Res. **41:** 3352.
3. McMahon, J. B., J. G. Farrelly & P. T. Iype. 1982. Proc. Natl. Acad. Sci. USA **79:** 456.

AN UNEXPECTED ROLE FOR TYROSINASE IN MELANIN BIOSYNTHESIS AND THE AUTODESTRUCTION OF MELANOMA CELLS

Ann Korner and John Pawelek

Department of Dermatology
Yale University School of Medicine
New Haven, Connecticut 06520

Tyrosinase (EC 1.10.3.1) catalyzes the oxidation of tyrosine to dopa and dopa to dopaquinone and initiates the biosynthesis of melanin. We have recently reported three additional factors that control melanin biosynthesis in mammals and in melanomas. Dopachrome conversion factor catalyzes the conversion of dopachrome to 5,6-dihydroxyindole. Indole conversion factor catalyzes the conversion of 5,6-dihydroxindole to melanochrome in extracts of Cloudman S91 melanoma cells that were synthesizing melanin. Extracts of amelanotic cells contain indole blocking factor and inhibit melanin production from 5,6-dihydroxindole.

We now report that indole conversion factor copurifies with tyrosinase from Cloudman S91 melanomas and that purified tyrosinase converts 5,6-dihydroxindole to melanochrome in a reaction that requires dopa as a cofactor and that is inhibited by L-tyrosine, phenylthiourea and diethyldithiocarbamate, two inhibitors specific for enzymes that contain copper. Conversely, 5,6-dihydroxindole inhibits the oxidation of tyrosine to dopa. The inhibition of the conversion of 5,6-dihydroxindole to melanochrome by L-tyrosine is "noncompetitive." It appears, therefore, that L-tyrosine and 5,6-dihydroxindole interact with tyrosinase at separate sites on the enzyme.

It has been demonstrated that the precursors of melanin are toxic to pigment-producing cells and that melanotropin (MSH) enhances the toxicity of such precursors. Under normal conditions pigment cells are protected from these toxic effects. Overproduction of pigment disrupts the protective mechanism. Our results suggest that the relative concentrations of L-tyrosine and 5,6-dihydroxindole may influence the generation of toxic intermediates in the pigment cell through previously unrecognized control of tyrosinase activity.

RHODAMINE-123 IS SELECTIVELY TOXIC AND PREFERENTIALLY RETAINED IN CARCINOMA CELLS *IN VITRO* *

Theodore J. Lampidis, Samuel D. Bernal,
Ian C. Summerhayes, and Lan Bo Chen

Sidney Farber Cancer Institute
Harvard Medical School
Boston, Massachusetts 02115

INTRODUCTION

Rhodamine-123, a cationic fluorescent dye, has previously been shown to localize specifically in mitochondria of living cells.[1] It has also been found to be nontoxic in a variety of cell types studied and has thus become a useful tool for probing mitochondria *in situ*.[2] Recently, however, we have detected a toxic effect of this compound on the function and viability of cardiac muscle cells in culture. Since we have also found that cardiac muscle cells as well as carcinoma cells accumulate and retain more rhodamine-123 than do cardiac-derived fibroblasts or epithelial cells, we were prompted to investigate the cytotoxic effects of this agent on carcinoma cells.

RESULTS

FIGURE 1 shows the difference in the effect of rhodamine-123 on the growth of three epithelial cell lines and one fibroblastic cell line. At two days of treatment a marked cytotoxic effect is seen in a human pancreatic carcinoma cell line, CCL 1420 (FIG. 1A), whereas the growth of human breast carcinoma cell line, MCF–7 (FIG. 1C), is inhibited. As cells are incubated further, 3 days for CCL 1420 and 7 days for MCF–7, the cell number is reduced to less than 10^3/plate in each of the rhodamine-treated cultures. In marked contrast to these results, CV–1 and CCL 149, nontumorigenic cell lines derived from normal African green monkey kidney (epithelial) and normal rat lung (fibroblast), respectively, show no cytotoxicity when exposed to the same dose of rhodamine-123 (FIGS. 1B and D). With even longer exposure (2 weeks at 10 μg/ml) or at higher doses (50 μg/ml $\times$ 7 days) the viability and cell growth of CV–1 and CCL 149 remain unaffected.

In order to determine whether this selective toxicity is a general phenomenon shared by other tumor-derived epithelial cells, a number of carcinoma lines were studied. Seventeen different cell lines were tested for sensitivity to rhodamine-123 by exposing them continuously to various doses. It was found that all of the tumorigenic epithelial cell lines,[9] derived from a variety of carcinomas, were sensitive ($\geq$50% cell death, 2–7 days) when treated with 10, 25 or 50 μg/ml. The nontumorigenic epithelial cell lines derived from normal tissues tested were unaffected by this treatment and continued to grow

* This work was supported by Grants CA 22427, 24771 and 06943 from the National Cancer Institute and by Grant CD 92B from The American Cancer Society.

normally as untreated cells (7–14 days). Primary cultures of cardiac muscle cells were also sensitive to rhodamine-123.

Mitochondria in cardiac muscle cells and myoblast-fused myotubes show unusually long retention of rhodamine-123. Whereas most normal nonmuscle cells (with exceptions, such as embryonic kidney cells) release rhodamine-123 within 1 to 16 hr after staining, muscle cells retain a significant level of dye fluorescence, even after 6 days. Significantly, numerous carcinoma and trans-

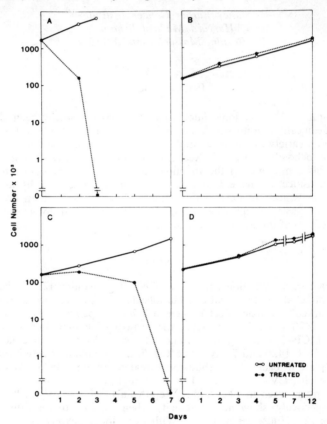

FIGURE 1. Cell counts of carcinoma cell lines, 1420 (**A**) and MCF-7 (**C**), and of untransformed cells, CV-1 (**B**) and CCL 149 (**D**), continuously exposed to rhodamine-123 at 10 μg/ml. Each point represents the average count of triplicate cultures.

formed epithelial cell lines, but not normal epithelial cells or any of the other cell types we have tested, that is, sarcoma, transformed fibroblasts, leukemia, neuroblastoma or glioma, have mitochondria with prolonged rhodamine-123 retention, similar to muscle mitochondria. After screening more than 50-keratin-positive carcinoma or transformed epithelial cell lines, such mitochondria are detected in transitional cell carcinoma and adenocarcinoma lines, in most chemical-carcinogen-transformed epithelial cell lines, and some squamous cell cell carcinoma lines; but not in oat-cell carcinoma (TABLE 1).

TABLE 1

RHODAMINE-123 RETENTION IN HUMAN TUMOR LINES

Tumor Line	Location	Relative Fluorescence after 24 hr in Rhodamine-123-Free Medium
Carcinoma		
MCF–7	Breast, adenocarcinoma	95
T47D	Breast, adenocarcinoma	95
ZR–75–1	Breast, adenocarcinoma	80
BT20	Breast, adenocarcinoma	80
HBL–100	Breast, adenocarcinoma	80
SW480	Colon, adenocarcinoma	80
HeLa	Cervix	70
CaSki	Cervix	90
PaCa–2	Pancreas	90
PC–3	Prostate	90
OD562	Ovary	80
OVCA 433	Ovary	70
SCC–4	Tongue, squamous	60
SCC–9	Tongue, squamous	65
SCC–12	Skin, squamous	60
SCC–13	Skin, squamous	50
SCC–15	Tongue, squamous	40
SCC–25	Tongue, squamous	20
SCC–27	Skin, squamous	50
HUT23	Lung, adenocarcinoma	75
HUT125	Lung, adenocarcinoma	60
A549	Lung, adenocarcinoma	60
U1752	Lung, squamous	60
HUT157	Lung, large cell	0
LX–1	Lung, large cell	0
HUT169C	Lung, oat-cell	0
HUT60	Lung, oat-cell	0
HUT128	Lung, oat-cell	0
HUT231	Lung, oat-cell	0
HUT64	Lung, oat-cell	0
Neuroblastoma		
CHP–100		0
CHP–134		0
CHP–212		0
Leukemia and lymphoma		
HL60		0
U937		0
K562		0
KG1		0
MOLT–4		0
LA2–221		0
CEM		0
LA2–156		0
Osteosarcoma		
N377/H135	Lung metastasis	10

DISCUSSION

The basis for the similarity between cardiac and carcinoma cells in response to rhodamine-123 remains to be investigated. One possibility is that both cell types contain binding sites that allow the dye to accumulate and/or be more readily retained than in normal epithelial cells, which contain fewer such sites. Another possibility relates to the electric potential of the plasma membrane. It is known that cardiac cells have a highly negative resting plasma membrane potential. *In vitro* measurements have placed it at −80 to −90 mV.[3, 4] It has previously been demonstrated that the positive charge of rhodamine-123 is essential for its intracellular accumulation.[5] Thus, a highly negative internal cellular charge may play an important role in the attraction of positively charged rhodamine-123 in cardiac muscle cells as opposed to the potential of other normal cells, which have been estimated to be at significantly lower values.[6] Consequently, it is conceivable that the ability of carcinoma cells to accumulate more positively charged dye than do normal epithelial cells may also be reflective of a higher transmembrane potential in the former as compared to the latter cells. This possibility may also be related to the subsequent sensitivity to rhodamine-123 of carcinoma cells.

Since rhodamine-123 has shown a strong selectivity in killing carcinoma cells *in vitro*, the efficacy of using it as a chemotherapeutic agent *in vivo* is now being tested in animals. In preliminary experiments, mice bearing Ehrlich ascites tumor were injected intraperitoneally with 20 mg/kg of rhodamine-123 on days 1, 3 and 5. This regimen prolonged survival by 220% as compared with that of untreated controls. We are currently investigating the antitumor activity of rhodamine-123 in a variety of animal tumor models.

REFERENCES

1. JOHNSON, L. V., M. L. WALSH & L. B. CHEN. 1980. Proc. Natl. Acad. Sci. USA **77:** 990–994.
2. CHEN, L. B., I. C. SUMMERHAYES, L. V. JOHNSON, M. L. WALSH, S. D. BERNAL & T. J. LAMPIDIS. 1982. Cold Spring Harbor Symp. Quant. Biol. **XLVI:** 141–155.
3. PARKER, J. L. & H. R. ADAMS. 1977. J. Am. Vet. Med. Assoc. **177:** 77.
4. SPERELAKIS, N. 1981. *In* Cardiac Toxicity, Vol. I. T. Balazs, Eds.: 39–108. CRC Press. Boca Raton, Florida.
5. JOHNSON, L. V., M. L. WALSH, B. J. BOCKUS & L. B. CHEN. 1981. J. Cell Biol. **88:** 526–535.
6. FREEDMAN, J. C. & P. C. LARIS. 1981. Int. Rev. Cytol. **12:** 177–246.

EMERGENCE OF 6-THIOGUANINE-RESISTANT LYMPHOCYTES IN PEDIATRIC CANCER PATIENTS *

Beverly J. Lange and J. Eric Prantner

Division of Oncology
Children's Hospital of Philadelphia
Philadelphia, Pennsylvania 19104

This paper describes a prospective study and a simultaneous longitudinal study of the frequency of 6-thioguanine (6-TG)-resistant peripheral blood lymphocytes in children with cancer and in control subjects. The purpose of the work was to measure the effects of cancer therapy on the nonmalignant cells of pediatric cancer patients by assaying the induction of resistance to 6-TG in lymphocytes of patients not receiving 6-TG. Patients were children or adolescents with Hodgkin's disease, Ewing's sarcoma, or rhabdomyosarcoma. Thioguanine resistance was measured autoradiographically by the ability of phytohemagglutinin-stimulated lymphocytes to incorporate tritiated thymidine in the presence or absence of 2×10^{-4} M or 2×10^{-5} M 6-TG.[1] The frequency of 6-TG-resistant cells was calculated according to the following formula:

$$vf = \frac{LI\ (PHA + 6\text{-}TG)}{LI\ (PHA)}$$

where vf is the variant frequency, LI is the labeling index, and PHA is phytohemagglutinin.

The longitudinal study showed that 5 of 29 untreated cancer patients had higher variant frequencies of 6-TG-resistant lymphocytes than any of 116 controls. Patients receiving chemotherapy or radiation therapy showed statistically significantly higher numbers of 6-TG-resistant lymphocytes than did controls, and in some patients abnormally higher frequencies of 6-TG-resistant cells persisted after therapy was discontinued. Among 22 patients studied prospectively before and during therapy, the frequency of 6-TG-resistant lymphocytes was significantly higher during therapy.

To determine whether 6-TG-resistant cells are capable of reproduction, lymphocytes from healthy young adults and from adolescent patients with cancer were examined for their ability to incorporate [^{3}H]thymidine in short-term culture in the presence of phytohemagglutinin and 6-TG. The numbers of labeled nuclei after 72 hours in culture were compared with numbers of labeled nuclei after 30 hours in culture. The numbers of labeled nuclei in the presence of 6-TG increased 6- to 50-fold between 30 and 72 hours. The increases could be accounted for by 4 to 6 cycles of cell division. The data suggest that 6-TG-resistant peripheral blood lymphocytes are capable of reproduction in short-term culture. However, attempts to establish 6-TG-resistant lymphoblastoid cell lines have not been successful.

* This work was supported by Grant RO1 CA26907–04 from the National Cancer Institute, and by JCFC 564 from the American Cancer Society.

303

In previous work, Strauss and Albertini [1] proposed that the emergence of 6-thioguanine-resistant peripheral blood lymphocytes in cancer patients is a potentially useful measure of somatic cell mutation *in vivo* in man. Our data, like those of Albertini, show that some cancer patients have a higher frequency of 6-TG-resistant variant lymphocytes than do healthy controls. Cancer therapy appears to augment this variation, either by selection or mutation, and thus cancer therapy appears to generate further genotypic or phenotypic damage.

REFERENCE

1. STRAUSS, G. H. & R. J. ALBERTINI. 1979. Enumeration of 6-thioguanine peripheral blood lymphocytes in man as a potential test for somatic cell mutations arising in vivo. Mutat. Res. **61**: 353–379.

THE MECHANISM OF CENTROSOMAL SEPARATION INDUCED BY EPIDERMAL GROWTH FACTOR

R. N. Mascardo and P. Sherline

Department of Medicine
University of Connecticut Health Center
Farmington, Connecticut 06032

Epidermal growth factor (EGF), a mitogenic peptide that was originally isolated from mouse submaxillary glands, induces proliferation in a wide variety of cells. As with other peptide hormones, EGF action is initiated by the binding of EGF to high-affinity receptors on the plasma membrane, and is followed, 12 to 15 hours later, by DNA synthesis and subsequently cell replication. However, the intermediate events between the EGF–receptor binding and EGF-induced mitosis are still unclear. Using a rabbit antiserum specific to a high molecular weight microtubule-associated protein (MAP_1) which stains centrosomes in numerous cell lines, we observed, by immunofluorescence microscopy, that perinuclear centrosomal splitting occurs in HeLa cells within 20 minutes after the addition of EGF (100 ng/ml). Centrosomal separation, which was quantitated by scoring cells with centrosomes $>5°$ apart in a double-blind manner, was observed in an increasing number of HeLa cells with longer EGF incubation (unsynchronized cells: 0 min ('), 6%; 20', 19%; 45', 28%; 90', 35%; 180', 35%; 240', 34%; synchronized by serum deprivation and with 2 mM hydroxyurea $\times$ 48 hr: 0', 2%; 20', 12%; 45', 28%; 90', 36%; 180', 48%; 240', 62%). Centrosomal splitting was also observed at lower concentrations of EGF (0.05–50 ng/ml).

To clarify the mechanism by which EGF induces rapid centrosomal separation, we preincubated HeLa cells for 45–60 min in medium containing drugs that are known to affect energy availability, the structure of microtubules and microfilaments, protein synthesis, prostaglandin synthesis, or calcium–calmodulin interaction. Sodium fluoride ($10^{-2}M$) and sodium azide ($5 \times 10^{-4} M$) blocked the EGF effect completely. Colchicine ($10^{-6}M$) induced centrosomal separation alone, and accentuated the effect of EGF. Taxol ($10^{-6}M$), which stabilizes microtubules, and cytochalasin D ($10^{-5}M$), which disrupts microfilaments, blocked the EGF effect completely. A23187 ($10^{-5}M$), a calcium ionophore, induced centrosomal separation alone, but did not enhance EGF-induced centrosomal splitting. Trifluoperazine (TFP, $10^{-5}M$) and chlorpromazine (50 μM), calmodulin inhibitors, blocked the effect of EGF and A23187 on centrosomal splitting. Neither cycloheximide ($10^{-5}M$) nor indomethacin ($10^{-4}M$) blocked the EGF effect.

Using immunofluorescence autoradiography,[1] we found that taxol, TFP, and cytochalasin D blocked the EGF-induced increase in nuclear ^{3}H-thymidine uptake 18 hours after the addition of EGF (labeling index: control, 14%; EGF, 33%; TFP + EGF, 15%; taxol + EGF, 16%; cytochalasin D + EGF, 13%).

In summary, EGF induces rapid centrosomal separation in HeLa cells; this action is energy-dependent, requires calcium and calmodulin, and intact microfilaments, and is enhanced by microtubule disassembly. The exact relationship of this particular EGF effect to the subsequent events in the cell cycle leading to cell replication remains to be elucidated. However, the observation that drugs that stimulate rapid centrosomal migration (for example, EGF and colchicine) also induce DNA synthesis, and drugs that block centrosomal separation (for example, taxol, TFP and cytochalasin D) also suppress DNA synthesis suggests that the early cytostructural change (that is, centrosomal separation) could be a key event in triggering DNA synthesis.

REFERENCE

1. LOCKWOOD, A. H.   1980.   Exp. Cell Res. **128:** 383.

INSULIN ENDOCYTOSIS IS HIGHLY CORRELATED WITH INSULIN REQUIREMENT FOR GROWTH *

Robert F. Murphy, Scott Powers, Charles R. Cantor,
and Robert Pollack

*Departments of Chemistry, Biological Sciences, and
Human Genetics and Development
Columbia University
New York, New York 10027*

In the past few years many of the steps involved in receptor-mediated endocytosis have been clarified using video intensification microscopy to follow the binding, clustering, internalization and subsequent processing of fluorescently labeled hormones.[1] Flow cytometry is a recently developed technique which, like video intensification microscopy, measures the properties of individual cells, and can accurately quantitate these properties for large numbers of cells. We have recently used flow cytometry to measure the binding and internalization by Swiss 3T3 cells of a fluorescein isothiocyanate (FITC) derivative of insulin.[2] We now describe the changes in insulin internalization that accompany the loss of growth control after transformation by SV40.

We have measured insulin internalization by four cell lines, derived from mouse embryo fibroblasts, which differ in their requirement for insulin. 3T3 is contact-inhibited, requires anchorage to a solid substrate for growth, and requires insulin for growth in serum-free medium. SV101 is derived from 3T3 by SV40 transformation, is not contact-inhibited and does not require either anchorage or insulin. Aγ4 is derived from SV101 by negative selection for reversion to a normal serum requirement, but is still similar to SV101 in that it grows well without anchorage. The fourth cell line, 3T6, is not transformed by SV40, but has a diminished insulin requirement while retaining the anchorage requirement. As a measure of the insulin requirement of these cell lines, we define relative growth rate to be the ratio of the growth rate in serum-free medium without insulin to the growth rate with insulin.

Cell monolayers were incubated with 1 μM FITC-insulin for 2.5 hr at 37° C and then trypsinized to remove surface-bound insulin. The amount of FITC–insulin internalized was then measured by flow cytometry. For the four cell lines, the mean fluorescence per cell, corrected for autofluorescence and converted to number of molecules of FITC-insulin, was highly correlated with the relative growth rate ($r = -0.977$). No significant positive correlation with insulin requirement (negative correlation with relative growth rate) was observed for cellular autofluorescence, light scattering, volume, or binding or internalization of wheat-germ agglutinin or chick erythrocyte histone. When the FITC-insulin internalization per cell was expressed per unit surface area (calculated from cell volume measurements), the high degree of correlation with relative growth rate remained ($r = -0.945$), indicating that the differences in insulin internalization were not due to differences in cell size.

* This work was supported in part by Postdoctoral Fellowship DRG–352–F from the Damon Runyon–Walter Winchell Cancer Foundation and by Grants GM–14825, GM–27576 and CA–25066 from the National Institutes of Health.

307

The high degree of correlation between insulin requirement and insulin internalization we have observed is inconsistent with simple on–off growth control models. These models would predict two distinct classes of insulin requirement and make no prediction regarding insulin internalization. Our results indicate that these two characteristics are linked.

REFERENCES

1. PASTAN, I. H. & M. C. WILLINGHAM. 1981. Science **214:** 504.
2. MURPHY, R. F., S. POWERS, M. VERDERAME, C. R. CANTOR & R. POLLACK. 1982. Cytometry **2:** 402.

METHIONINE REQUIREMENT IN SKIN FIBROBLASTS OF HUMANS WITH POLYPOSIS OF THE COLON AND THE GARDNER SYNDROME

Yves B. Mikol and Martin Lipkin

Memorial Sloan–Kettering Cancer Center
New York, New York 10021

The Gardner syndrome (GS) is an autosomal dominant hereditary disease.[1] The phenotype of epithelial and mesodermal cells from these patients leads, with an early age of onset, to the development of neoplasm in multiple sites (polyposis in the colon, hyperplasias of the stomach, adenomas of the duodenum, desmoids in soft tissues, sebaceous and bone cysts), suggesting that all the cells carry an identical genotypic abnormality leading to the phenotype of tumor cells. Only in the presence of folic acid and vitamin B_{12} can homocysteine replace methionine as an essential nutrient in the medium of mammalian cells growing in tissue culture. Since the ability of normal cell lines to grow as well in medium containing folic acid, vitamin B_{12} and methionine or homocysteine has been demonstrated in several laboratories,[2-5] the reduced growth of various tumor and transformed cell lines in methionine-deficient, homocysteine-, folic acid- and vitamin B_{12}-supplemented medium appears to be a phenotypic manifestation of an abnormal genotype. This phenotype of "increased methionine requirement" was investigated in skin fibroblasts of patients with GS and of cancer-free individuals (CFF).

The skin fibroblasts were plated and allowed to attach for 24 hours in a complete medium whilch was replaced with an identical medium but deficient in methionine and further supplemented with 60 mg/L DL-homocysteine-thiolactone, 10 mg/L folic acid, and 4 mg/L vitamin B_{12}. Cells were counted every other day for 12 days. Cell growth constants in the presence (K_M) or absence (K_H) of methionine were taken during the exponential phase of growth and used to calculate the slope of the least mean square derived by linear regression analysis.[6] All results are expressed as the mean $\pm$ standard error. In CFF, K_M was not significantly different from K_H (0.118 ± 0.007, respectively, with 7 different volunteers). K_M from GS and from CFF were not significantly different, but in GS K_H was decreased by 72% ($K_M = 0.113 \pm 0.002$ and $K_H = 0.082 \pm 0.002$, p < 0.001, in 6 different patients (FIG. 1). Pretreatment with 5×10^{-6} M N-methyl-N'-nitronitrosoguanidine for 1 hour did not alter significantly the cell growth in either group (3 patients with GS and 4 CFF).

The current data demonstrate that unlike skin fibroblasts from CFF, skin fibroblasts from patients with GS demonstrated reduced growth when homocysteine replaced methionine in the culture medium. This phenotypic abnormality has been reported in tumor and transformed cell lines.[2-6] Increased methionine requirement could be the result of a drain of methyl groups due to increased phospholipid turnover and methylation of macromolecules.[7-9] Thus, reduced growth of skin fibroblasts from GS, tumor and

309

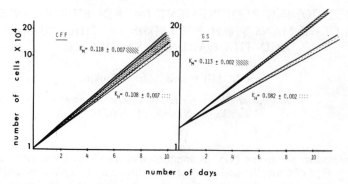

FIGURE 1. Growth curves of skin fibroblasts from CFF (*left*) and those with GS (*right*) grown in the presence (K_M) or absence (K_H) of methionine. K_M and K_H are expressed as mean ± SE ($n = 7$ CFF and 6 GS). Each shaded area delimits the curves calculated by linear regression analysis for the maximal and minimal values of K_M and K_H.

transformed cells in methionine-deficient, homocysteine-supplemented medium, appears to be a phenotypic manifestation of a genotype associated in GS patients with the development of neoplasm at multiple sites.

REFERENCES

1. GARDNER, E. J. & R. C. RICHARDS. 1953. Multiple cutaneous and subcutaneous lesions occuring simultaneously with hereditary polyposis and osteomatosis. Am. J. Human Genet. **5:** 139–147.
2. HALPERN, B. C., B. R. CLARK, D. N. HARDY, R. M. HALPERN & R. A. SMITH. 1974. The effect of replacement of methionine by homocystine on survival of malignant and normal adult mammalian cells in culture. Proc. Natl. Acad. Sci. USA. **71:** 1133–1136.
3. HOFFMAN, R. M. & R. W. ERBE. 1976. High *in vivo* rates of methionine biosynthesis in transformed human and malignant rat cells auxotrophic for methionine. Proc. Natl. Acad. Sci. USA. **73:** 1523–1527.
4. WILSON, M. J. & L. A. POIRIER. 1978. An increased requirement for methionine by transformed rat liver epithelial cells *in vitro*. Exp. Cell Res. **111:** 397–400.
5. KREIS, W., A. BAKER, V. RYAN & A. BERTASSO. 1980. Effect of nutritional and enzymatic methionine deprivation upon human normal and malignant cells in tissue culture. Cancer Res. **40:** 634–641.
6. POIRIER, L. A. & M. J. WILSON. 1980. The elevated requirement for methionine by transformed rat liver epithelial cells *in vitro*. Ann. NY Acad. Sci., **349:** 283–294.
7. BOREK, E. & P. R. SRINIVASAN. 1966. The methylation of nucleic acids. Ann. Rev. Biochem. **35:** 275–298.
8. TISDALE, M. J. 1980. Effect of methionine deprivation on methylation and synthesis of macromolecules. Br. J. Cancer **42:** 121–128.
9. KOIZUMI, K., K. TAMIYA-KOIZUMI, T. FUJII, J. OKUDA & K. KOJIMA. 1980. Comparative study of the phospholipid composition of plasma membranes isolated from rat primary hepatomas induced by 3'-methyl-4-dimethylaminoazobenzene and from normal growing rat livers. Cancer Res. **40:** 909–913.

THE RESPONSE OF EPITHELIAL CELLS OF DIFFERENT HIERARCHICAL STATUS TO CYTOTOXIC INSULT

C. S. Potten

Paterson Laboratories
Christie Hospital
Manchester M20 9BX, England

The mucosa of the small intestine is highly polarized with a functional pole, the villus, where cells become senescent, die and are discarded, and a proliferative pole in the crypts, where compensation for this cell loss occurs. This cell replacement is achieved via an hierarchical cellular organization within the crypts, that is, a cell lineage with a relatively few lineage-ancestors or stem cells. These stem cells, which are thus responsible for all the cell replacement throughout life, must be located at the origin of all the cell migration, that is, at a specific position near the base of the crypt. If cell position is carefully defined by numbering each cell along the side of a crypt, the position can be used to identify cells of differing hierarchical status within the proliferative compartment. In this way the qualitative and quantitative response of cells of differing hierarchical status to various forms of cytotoxic insult can be studied.

Various cytotoxic insults have been studied ranging from internal (^{3}H-TdR) and external irradiation to cytotoxic drugs, such as hydroxyurea (HU), vincristine (VC), cycloheximide (CH), cyclophosphamide (CP) and isopropylmethane sulphonate (IMS).

Various endpoints have been investigated, including rapid histologically identifiable cell death (recorded as apoptosis, although similar results and conclusions can be drawn if pycnosis is recorded). Apoptosis was recorded for all the agents listed above, while mitotic inhibition (G_2 delay), changes in labeling index, and thymidine incorporation (grain counts) have been studied after external irradiation.

The results are summarized in FIGURE 1 and can be stated as follows:

1. The cells that die rapidly after irradiation are few in number and are located at the crypt base (most frequently seen at cell positions 5 or 6).

2. Proliferative cells at higher cell positions rarely, if ever, die via apoptosis after any doses within the time scale considered here, that is, according to this criterion they are very radio-resistant.

3. These higher positioned proliferative cells can, however, die via apoptosis within a few hours if exposed to HU. The most frequent position for dead cells after HU treatment is cell position 10.

4. Each cytotoxic agent tends to have its own characteristic cell killing distribution, that is, it attacks a characteristic subpopulation of crypt cells. These differences are not apparently related cell kinetic parameters.

5. Some endpoints show a striking cell-position-dependence, for example, mitotic inhibition can be virtually complete at the crypt base, but unaffected at the upper crypt position.

311

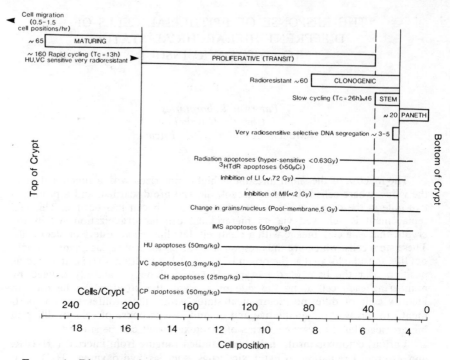

FIGURE 1. Diagrammatic representation of the crypt of the small intestine showing the cell populations and the regions of maximal change when various endpoints are studied after a range of cytotoxic agents has been administered. All data are related to the cell position within the crypt. LI = labeling index; MI = mitotic index; IMS = isopropyl methane sulphonate; HU = hydroxyurea; VC = vincristine; CH = cycloheximide; CP = cyclophosphamide. Some data are preliminary and some represent unpublished data of Ijiri and of Moore.

6. The results as a whole suggest that the qualitative and quantitative response to cytotoxic insult may vary considerably according to hierarchical position and particularly that *some* cells early in the cell lineage are very sensitive to irradiation.

CIRCADIAN RHYTHMS IN CELL PROLIFERATION IN NORMAL MICE AND IN MICE BEARING TETRAPLOID EHRLICH ASCITES CARCINOMA (EAC)

N. H. Rubin and J. A. Hokanson

University of Texas Medical Branch
Galveston, Texas 77550

Cell proliferation *in vivo* does not occur asynchronously or randomly, but rather is characterized by a circadian variation in DNA synthesis and mitosis. The uptake of tritiated thymidine and the mitotic index in normal proliferative tissues show a predictable peak (highest measured value) and trough (lowest measured value) when monitored over a 24-hour period.

An experiment was designed to use flow cytometry to explore for circadian fluctuation in cell cycle phases in two strains of normal mice (CDF_1, Swiss) and in mice bearing 7-day-old EAC (Swiss + EAC). Six animals from each group of 10-week-old, light–dark standardized (8-hr light–16-hr darkness; lights on from 0900 to 1700) male mice were killed every 3 hr for 24 hr. The epithelium of each tongue was separated from the underlying muscle, processed to a single cell suspension, and fixed in 70% ethanol. Ascitic fluid was aspirated from the tumor-bearing mice and fixed in 70% ethanol. For each sample of tongue or EAC, the DNA content of 20,000–50,000 cells was analyzed in a Coulter TPS–1 flow cytometer. From the resulting DNA histograms, the G_1, S and G_2M fractions were estimated. The data were analyzed for circadian periodicity by an innovative use of the multiple linear regression procedures found in SPSS, a commonly available computer-based statistical package. The means of the 3-hour samples were used to compute a 24-hr mean for each phase of the cell cycle in each tissue analyzed. The variation at each sample time from the overall 24-hr mean was determined.

TABLE 1

CIRCADIAN VARIATION IN DNA SYNTHESIS IN MURINE TONGUE

Time	Percent Variation from 24-hr Mean		
	CDF_1	Swiss–Control	Swiss + EAC
0900	78.4	85.5	113.4
1200	72.7	63.9	87.8
1500	53.4 (low)	—	74.4
1800	73.9	56.6 (low)	65.9 (low)
2100	101.1	75.9	81.7
2400	159.1 (high)	114.5	104.9
0300	145.5	165.1 (high)	134.2
0600	115.9	134.9	139.0 (high)
	$p < 0.001, r^2 = 0.79$	$p < 0.001, r^2 = 0.74$	$p < 0.001, r^2 = 0.53$

313

Statistically significant circadian rhythms were found in tongue in both control and tumor-bearing mice and in the tumor itself. The fluctuation from the 24-hr mean at each sample time is shown in TABLE 1 for S phase in tongue. The highest and lowest percent variation in each group are indicated.

The phasing of the 24-hr fluctuation in DNA synthesis in tongue was nearly identical when quantified by flow cytometry and by tritiated thymidine incorporation (CDF_1 mice). Statistically significant rhythms in G_1, S and G_2M were found in the tumor itself ($p < 0.02$). Analysis by light microscopy of the mitotic index of the tumor samples verified the circadian rhythm in mitosis.

It is emphasized that the only systematic variable in these experiments was the time in the 24-hr period when the animals were killed. These results show how analysis of cell proliferation *in vivo* can be more precise when the circadian system is considered and furthermore suggest that circadian rhythms in cell division should not be ignored when investigating relationships between tumor cell and normal cell kinetics and cancer therapy.

DNA LIGASE ACTIVITY IN EXTRACTS OF
MOUSE ERYTHROLEUKEMIA (MEL)
CELLS DURING DIFFERENTIATION *

Barbara M. Scher,†‡ William Scher,‡ and Samuel Waxman ‡

† Department of Microbiology and
‡ Cancer Chemotherapy Foundation Laboratory
Department of Medicine
Mount Sinai School of Medicine of the
City University of New York
New York, New York 10029

Treatment with dimethyl sulfoxide (DMSO) induces some stages of erythroid differentiation in MEL cells. The differentiating cells produce hemoglobin (Hb) and become limited in their proliferative capacity. Nuclear condensation occurs (see Reuben et al.[1] for review).

After 4 days in culture in the absence and in the presence of 1.8% (vol/vol) DMSO, DNA ligase levels were shown to be lower in DMSO-treated MEL cells than in untreated MEL cells.[2] To further characterize this effect, DNA ligase and DNAase activities were determined in cell-free extracts prepared from MEL cells grown from 1 to 5 days in the absence and in the presence of DMSO. Hb-containing cells were detectable after 67 hr of growth in the presence of DMSO and by 113 hr the percentage of such cells in the DMSO-treated cultures had risen to over 85%. In contrast, the percentage of Hb-containing cells in untreated cultures remained at less than 1%.

DNA ligase activity was measured under conditions that inhibited all major competing DNAase activities in the extracts. The specific activity of DNA ligase in extracts from DMSO-treated cells was 167, 95, 22, 12, and <4% of the activity in extracts from untreated cells after 19, 43, 67, 95, and 113 hr of DMSO treatment, respectively. When extracts from untreated and DMSO-treated cells were mixed, DNA ligase activities in the mixtures were additive and no evidence of inhibitors in the extracts from the DMSO-treated cells was noted.

DNAase activity was determined in extracts that were first dialyzed to eliminate ATP and therefore DNA ligase activity. The major DNAase activity in MEL cell extracts was inhibited by G-actin and was, therefore, presumed to be DNAase I-like. Unlike the results seen with DNA ligase, the specific activity of this DNAase did not decrease during 95 hr of DMSO treatment, but rather increased slightly.

In cell line DR–10, a variant cell line that is resistant to DMSO induction of differentiation, these DMSO-induced changes were not seen. In addition,

* This work was supported by Grants AM 16690–06 and CA 24402–03 from the United States Public Health Service, Grant CH–144 from the American Cancer Society, and by grants from the Chemotherapy Foundation and the Charles E. Merrill Trust.

315

the changes were not correlated with growth rate. These results suggest that the changes in DNA ligase activity may be related to differentiation, possibly to the limitation in cell multiplication observed in DMSO-treated MEL cells.

REFERENCES

1. REUBEN, R. C., R. A. RIFKIND & P. A. MARKS. 1980. Biochim. Biophys. Acta 605: 325.
2. SCHER, B. M., W. SCHER, A. ROBINSON & S. WAXMAN. 1982. Cancer Res. 42: 1300.

ANTIPROMOTION OF DIMETHYLHYDRAZINE-INDUCED MURINE COLONIC CARCINOMA BY DEHYDROEPIANDROSTERONE *

Jonathan W. Nyce, Peter N. Magee, and Arthur G. Schwartz

*Fels Research Institute and
Departments of Pathology and Microbiology
Temple University School of Medicine
Philadelphia, Pennsylvania 19140, and the
Department of Biology
Temple University
Philadelphia, Pennsylvania 19122*

Twenty-six of 153 BALB/c female mice given 21 mg/kg 1,2-dimethylhydrazine (DMH) subcutaneously weekly for 26 weeks developed tumors visible at the anus. None of 141 matched animals, in whom an identical regimen of DMH was administered along with 0.6% dehydroepiandrosterone (DHEA) in the diet, developed such tumors. Autopsy of 10 animals from each group at 20 weeks revealed a 16-fold reduction in colonic tumor yield per animal in DMH + DHEA-treated animals compared with those treated with DMH alone (TABLE 1). Twenty-sixth-week autopsies showed over a five-fold reduction in colonic tumor yield in the DHEA-treated animals. No tumors were visible in animals receiving control diet or DHEA alone. This tumor inhibition by DHEA appears to be antipromoting in nature since preliminary experiments indicate that levels of alkylated bases 12 hours after administration of DMH are similar at week 20 in each group (TABLE 2). This finding is surprising in view of evidence that DHEA may reduce available pools of NADPH, a required cofactor in DMH metabolism. It should be noted, however, that under conditions different from those used to produce colonic tumors (8 weeks of 0.6% DHEA in the absence of long-term DMH induction), DHEA did exert an inhibitory effect upon metabolism of a single dose of DMH (approximately 35% inhibition of 7-methylguanine/mol guanine; data not shown). DHEA appears to exert cytostatic effects upon various NADPH-dependent steps in deoxynucleotide synthesis, however. For example, uridine diphosphate levels are elevated more than four-fold in nuclei of colonic epithelial cells from DHEA-treated animals as compared with control values. Further evidence in favor of DHEA-induced depletion of NADPH comes from an apparent interference with folate metabolism suggested by the more than two-fold increase in C1 incorporation from DMH into guanine.

A reduced proliferative zone in colonic epithelial crypts in DHEA-treated animals is indicated by (1) inhibition of DNA synthesis through nucleotide depletion at NADPH-dependent steps, and (2) increased ratios of 5-methylcytosine/cytosine. Since enzymatic methylation at the 5 position of cytosine is

* This work was supported by Grants CA–14661, CA–23451 and CA–09214 from the National Institutes of Health.

TABLE 1

REDUCTIONS IN TUMOR * YIELD INDUCED BY DHEA †

	Average Number of Tumors/Animal	
	20 weeks	26 weeks
DMH ‡ plus DHEA	0.5 ± 0.71	2.5 ± 1.3
DMH only	8.3 ± 6.2	13.2 ± 6.4
Control diet	0.0	0.0
DHEA only	0.0	0.0

† 0.6% DHEA was administered in the diet.

‡ DMH was administered subcutaneously 21 mg/kg once weekly for 26 weeks.

* Tumors consist mostly of adenocarcinomas, but are unclassified as of this writing.

a postreplicational modification, the presence of fewer newly replicated, unmethylated cells in DHEA-treated epithelium is implied.

Because proliferative changes in colonic epithelium in human populations at high risk of developing colonic carcinoma resemble those observed in DMH-treated mice,[1] DHEA may have tumor-prophylactic properties in man as well. Such groups at high risk for colonic adenocarcinoma, and thus good candidates for DHEA therapy, include those with ulcerative colitis, familial polyposis coli, cancer family syndrome, and patients previously treated for colonic cancer.

In summary, DHEA is an effective prophylactic agent in DMH-induced murine colonic adenocarcinoma. NADPH-dependent deoxyribonucleotide synthesis pathways are altered following daily administration of DHEA to female BALB/c mice.

TABLE 2

COLONIC EPITHELIAL CELL DNA ALKYLATION AND C1 INCORPORATION 12 HOURS AFTER A REGULARLY SCHEDULED ADMINISTRATION OF DMH AT WEEK 20 *

	DMH at 20 Weeks	DMH + 0.6% DHEA at 20 Weeks
7-Methylguanine/mol guanine $\times 10^6$	13,546 ± 1,289	14,553 ± 1,353
0^6-Methylguanine/mol guanine $\times 10^6$	2,014 ± 191	3,936 ± 334
C1 pool-labeled guanine/mol guanine $\times 10^6$	10,353 ± 1,109	23,191 ± 1,600
(7-Methylguanine/mol guanine)/ C1 pool-labeled guanine/mol guanine)	1.32	0.628

* 21 mg/kg DMH subcutaneously, 2.13 mCi/mmol final specific activity, was substituted for normal weekly nonradioactive dose at week 20.

REFERENCE AND BIBLIOGRAPHY

1. LIPKIN, M. 1974. Phase I and phase II proliferative lesions of colonic epithelial cells in diseases leading to colonic cancer. Cancer **34:** 878–888.
2. PASHKO, L. L., A. G. SCHWARTZ, M. ABOU-GHARBIA & D. SWERN. 1981. Inhibition of DNA synthesis in mouse epidermis and breast epithelium by dehydroepiandrosterone and related steroids. Carcinogenesis **2:** 717–721.
3. DWORKIN, C. R., S. D. GORMON, L. L. PASHKO, V. J. CRISTOFALO & A. G. SCHWARTZ. Inhibition of growth of HeLa and WI-38 cells by dehydroepiandrosterone and its reversal by ribo- and deoxyribonucleosides. Exp. Cell Res. Submitted for publication.

THE CLONING OF A SPECIFIC SEGMENT
OF THE HAMSTER GENOME
REQUIRED FOR CELL PROLIFERATION *

Kenneth J. Soprano,† Shirley M. Tilghman,‡
and Renato Baserga §

*Departments of Microbiology † and Pathology §
Temple University School of Medicine
Philadelphia, Pennsylvania 19140*

*‡ Institute for Cancer Research
Philadelphia, Pennsylvania 19111*

We are interested in studying the control of cell proliferation in mammalian cells. Since different steps of the cell cycle are known to be controlled by different genes,[1] one approach to the study of this problem involves the use of mammalian cell cycle mutants. Several temperature-sensitive mutants of the cell cycle have been derived from the Syrian hamster cell line BHK-21;[2-5] ts13 is one such mutant. When shifted to the nonpermissive temperature of 39.6°C these cells arrest in the G_1 stage, 3.5 hours prior to S.[6] These cells, therefore, provide a suitable system to study at least one cellular process in G_1 which is required for passage of cells through G_1 into S.

Thus far, conventional biochemical methods have provided little information concerning the identity or function of the cellular component which would permit the proliferation of ts13 cells at the nonpermissive temperature. Such information would greatly enhance the understanding of how this gene and its product(s) might influence cell proliferation during G_1. Thus, we thought it would be very desirable to develop a system to isolate and identify genes which influence cell proliferation. With this goal in mind, we have performed experiments (1) to determine biologic complementation assays for the ts gene in ts13 cells using the ability of naked DNA derived from wild-type BHK cells to successfully transfect ts13 cells; and (2) to use these assays to select and isolate segments of the BHK genomic DNA contained in a bacteriophage Charon 4A gene library which are capable of complementing the ts defect in ts13 cells.

We constructed the BHK gene library according to the procedures of Maniatis et al.[7] using Alu I/Hae III-cleaved DNA inserted into the EcoRI-generated outer arms of Charon 4A. After *in vitro* packaging, the number of members in the library was determined by plaque assay to be 750,000. Each of these was amplified and then fractionated into 25 subpopulations, each containing 30,000 members.

These subpopulations were then screened for complementation of the ts13 defect by two methods: a colony assay and an autoradiographic assay. In the colony assay, ts13 cells were plated at 34° (0.5×10^5) in a 60-mm dish. After 24 hours these cells were transfected with phage subpopulations and then incubated for 14 days at 39.6°, the nonpermissive temperature. At the end of this

* This work was supported by Research Grant CA 12923 from the United States Public Health Service.

period of time the number of colonies present was determined (transfection frequency).

Each subpopulation was also screened by the autoradiographic assay. In this assay ts13 cells were plated at 34° in low serum on coverslips such that they entered the quiescent or G_0 state after 7 days. At this time, they were transfected with phage and, incubated at 39.6° in 10% serum and ^{3}H-labeled thymidine. After 24 hours the coverslips were harvested for autoradiography. The rationale of this assay is that upon addition of 10% serum at 39.6°, G_0 cells go to the ts point and stop unless the phage subpopulation contains an insert capable of complementing the ts block. If it does, these cells pass through G_1 and enter S, where they become labeled and thus can be detected by autoradiography.

Those subpopulations that were positive by both assays were further fractionated. After five such fractionations, a single population of phage theoretically consisting of one member was obtained. This population was "plaqued" and 10 isolated plaques were further assayed. A single plaque-purified phage (named clone #8) containing a hamster insert capable of complementing the ts13 temperature sensitive defect was isolated. DNA prepared from this phage successfully permitted growth of ts13 at its nonpermissive temperature when introduced into cells by either direct manual microinjection or by transfection.

These results suggest that genes required for cell proliferation in mammalian cells can be isolated and identified using this approach with other temperature-sensitive mutants of the cell cycle.

REFERENCES

1. BASERGA, R. 1976. Multiplication and Division in Mammalian Cells. Marcel Dekker. New York, NY.
2. MEISS, H. K. & C. BASILICO. 1972. Nature New Biol. **239:** 66.
3. BURSTIN, S. J., H. K. MEISS & C. BASILICO. 1974. J. Cell Physiol. **84:** 397.
4. NAHA, P., A. L. MEYER & K. HEWITT. 1975. Nature **258:** 49.
5. TALAVERA, A. & C. BASILICO. 1977. J. Cell Physiol. **92:** 425.
6. FLOROS, J., T. ASHIHARA & R. BASERGA. 1978. Cell Biol. Int. Rep. **2:** 259.
7. MANIATIS, T. 1978. Cell **15:** 687.

CLONAL AND BIOCHEMICAL ANALYSIS OF COMMITMENT OF HL-60 CELLS TO TERMINAL DIFFERENTIATION

Asterios S. Tsiftsoglou, Willie Wong, Mark Minden,* and Stephen H. Robinson

*Charles A. Dana Research Institute and the
Harvard-Thorndike Laboratory of the
Beth Israel Hospital, and the Department of Medicine
Beth Israel Hospital and
Harvard Medical School, Boston, Massachusetts 02115; and
* Center for Cancer Research
Massachusetts Institute of Technology,
Cambridge, Massachusetts 02139*

HL-60 cells were originally isolated from the peripheral blood of a patient with acute promyelocytic leukemia.[1] HL-60 cells grown in culture and induced to differentiate into mature granulocytes [1,2] or macrophage-like cells [3] by a variety of chemical agents (such as DMSO, retinoic acid, 6-thioguanine, the phorbol ester TPA) [1-5] serve as a model system with which to study mechanisms related to neoplasia and hematopoietic cell differentiation. Previous studies of the differentiation of HL-60 cells have been carried out with suspension cultures. We have developed a method of clonal cell culture that allows us to study the proliferative capacity of individual HL-60 cells as they respond to inducing agents. The major objectives of this report are: (1) to describe culture conditions for cloning individual HL-60 cells with high efficiency; (2) to determine the kinetics of HL-60 cell differentiation at the level of individual cells; (3) to investigate whether commitment of HL-60 cells to terminal differentiation is reversible or irreversible and is associated with major alterations in transcription and replication of DNA; and (4) to investigate whether two structurally unrelated chemical inducers of granulocytic differentiation, DMSO and retinoic acid (RA), induce the expression of the same or different phenotypes.

Clonal growth of HL-60 cells was accomplished using a modified plasma clot assay system employing the standard reagents described by McLeod et al.[6] in 1974 and L-glutamine (200 μg/ml) in DME medium supplemented with 13% FCS. Cells in primary suspension culture were treated with 1.5% DMSO, 2 μM retinoic acid (RA), or no drug, and at various times during incubation were removed from culture, washed and plated in plasma clots (400 cells/0.1 ml). Plasma clots were cultured for 10 days and stained with nitrobluetetrazolium (NBT),[7] fixed, counterstained with 1% safranin and examined microscopically (10X). Parallel biochemical and morphologic studies were carried out with the cells in primary suspension culture to determine the degree of cell maturation by morphologic criteria, the expression of NBT activity, changes in cell size, and the rates of RNA and DNA synthesis.

The major findings are summarized as follows: (1) HL-60 cells can be cloned in plasma clots with a plating efficiency of 40–60%. (2) Cells exposed to DMSO or RA in suspension culture undergo a decrease in cell size and an increase in nuclear maturation. When subcultured in plasma clots, the induced cells form colonies composed either of all NBT-positive cells or both NBT-positive and NBT-negative cells; in both types of colonies the cells are widely dispersed. With increasing time of exposure to DMSO or RA in primary culture, both colony number and size decline progressively until colony formation finally ceases to occur. Undifferentiated HL-60 cells give rise to compact NBT-negative colonies of variable size without much cell migration. (3) Commitment of HL-60 cells to terminal maturation and loss of proliferative capacity is irreversible and begins to occur within the first few hours following treatment of cells with inducing agents. (4) In contrast to DMSO, which produces cells resembling metamyelocytes, RA leads to the accumulation of further differentiated polymorphonuclear leukocytes. (5) HL-60 cell differentiation induced by either DMSO or RA is associated with a dramatic decline in both RNA (nuclear and cytoplasmic) and DNA synthesis as measured by the incorporation of [^{3}H]uridine and [^{3}H]thymidine into TCA-insoluble material, respectively. Recently, using a cloned fragment (6.6 kb) of mouse ribosomal DNA sequences,[8] which cross-hybridizes with human ribosomal DNA sequences, we found that the decline in nuclear RNA synthesis observed in RA-induced HL-60 cells involves cessation of transcription of ribosomal DNA sequences.

REFERENCES

1. COLLINS, S. J., R. C. GALLO & R. E. GALLAGHER. 1977. Nature (London) **270:** 347–349.
2. COLLINS, S. J., F. W. RUSCETTI, R. E. GALLAGHER & R. C. GALLO. 1978. Proc. Natl. Acad. Sci. USA **75:** 2458–2462.
3. ROVERA, G., D. SANTOLI & C. DAMBLEY. 1979. Proc. Natl. Acad. Sci. USA **76:** 2779–2783.
4. BREITMAN, T. R., S. E. SELONICK & S. J. COLLINS. 1980. Proc. Natl. Acad. Sci. USA **77:** 2936–2940.
5. PAPAC, R., A. E. BROWN, E. SCHWARTZ & A. C. SARTORELLI. 1980. Cancer Lett. **10:** 33–38.
6. McLEOD, D. L., M. M. SHREEVE & A. A. AXELRAD. 1974. Blood **44:** 514–534.
7. BAEHNER, R. L., L. A. BOXER & J. DAVIS. 1976. Blood **48:** 309–313.
8. TSIFTSOGLOU, A. S., V. VOLLOCH, J. F. GUSELLA, W. WONG & D. HOUSMAN. 1982. Submitted for publication.

PLASMIN-ACTIVATED ANTICANCER PRODRUGS

Michael J. Weber, Prasun K. Chakravarty,
Margaret R. Bruesch, Gail L. Johnson,
John A. Katzenellenbogen, and Philip L. Carl *

*University of Illinois
Urbana, Illinois 61801; and
* University of North Carolina
Chapel Hill, North Carolina 27514*

Many types of malignant cells and human tumors display an elevated activity of plasminogen activator, the protease responsible for converting plasminogen to the active protease, plasmin. We therefore expect that high levels of plasmin should occur in the milieu of tumors producing plasminogen activator. We have exploited this tumor-associated fibrinolytic activity in an attempt to increase the selectivity of cancer chemotherapy, by synthesizing plasmin-activatable prodrug derivatives of a number of antineoplastic drugs. We anticipate that these prodrugs will be preferentially activated at the site of the tumor.

Our strategy for preparing the prodrugs has involved coupling a specific tripeptide to an essential NH_2- of the parent drug, through an amide linkage. Since the NH_2- of the parent drug is essential for biological activity, the peptidyl drugs are biologically inactive but can be reactivated when plasmin cleaves the peptide from the drug. The peptide (D-valine-L-leucine-L-lysine) has been chosen to be an excellent substrate for plasmin on the basis of direct studies of plasmin specificity as well as analysis of the sites of plasmin cleavage during fibrinogenolysis.

We have synthesized peptidyl derivatives of acivicin, adriamycin, melphalan, and phenylenediamine mustard, and all have been shown to be substrates for plasmin. The cytotoxicity of the prodrugs and the parent drugs was tested in culture against normal chicken embryo cells, which produce little plasminogen activator, and against Rous sarcoma-virus-transformed cells, which produce high levels of plasminogen activator. In every case, the prodrugs displayed a 7–20-fold improvement in selective toxicity for the malignant cells compared with that of the parent drugs.

As a prelude to testing these drugs *in vivo,* we have examined several transplantable murine tumors for plasminogen activator activity. Of the tumors tested, B16 melanoma displayed the highest activity, which was 3 to 5 times higher than the activity of the most active of the normal organs tested (brain, lung, and kidney). Moreover, mice carrying the B16 tumor displayed a 10–30-fold elevation in the levels of fibrin degradation products in their serum. This indicates that the plasminogen activator produced by this tumor is causing markedly increased fibrinolysis *in vivo.* Thus, the B16 tumor appears to be a suitable system for *in vivo* testing of plasmin-activated prodrugs.

THE REGULATION OF EPIDERMAL GROWTH FACTOR RECEPTORS BY PLATELET-DERIVED GROWTH FACTOR

Walker Wharton,*† Edward Leof,†
W. J. Pledger,† and Edward O'Keefe †

*Experimental Pathology Group
Los Alamos National Laboratory
Los Alamos, New Mexico 87545

† Cell Biology Program
Cancer Research Center
University of North Carolina
Chapel Hill, North Carolina 27514

The traverse of G_0/G_0 in BALB/c-3T3 cells is controlled by two functionally distinct sets of peptide factors.[1] Platelet-derived growth factor (PDGF) controls the initiation of cell cycle traverse by making cells competent to respond to the progression factors in platelet-poor plasma (PPP). Although the specific plasma-derived factors that act to allow competent 3T3 cells to traverse G_0/G_1 are not known, medium supplemented with a combination of epidermal growth factor (EGF) and somatomedin C contains all the progression activity found in medium supplemented with 5% PPP.

The biochemical mechanism by which PDGF renders cells sensitive to EGF and somatomedin C is of interest. Peptide factors might act in a concerted manner if one was able to modulate either the number or affinity of the receptors for another peptide. Clemmons et al.[2] reported that PDGF caused no change in somatomedin C binding, although the treatment of competent cells with plasma-supplemented medium brought about a two-fold increase in the number of somatomedin C receptors. Here we report data concerning the relationship between PDGF treatment and the number of EGF receptors.

When quiescent 3T3 cells were exposed to PDGF, there was a concentration-dependent decrease in ^{125}I-labeled EGF binding, which was maximal after 2 hr and which persisted for at least 6 hr after PDGF addition. The effects of the partially purified PDGF preparation could not be attributed to contamination by EGF, since both by radioreceptor assay and by radioimmunoassay the undiluted PDGF did not contain detectable amounts of EGF. At PDGF concentrations that rendered 100% of the cells competent, there was an approximately 50% reduction in ^{125}I-labeled EGF binding with no further increases observed even at PDGF concentrations 10-fold higher than maximally effective levels. The effects of PDGF on EGF binding could apparently be accounted for by a decrease in the number of EGF receptors with no change in receptor affinity. Cholera toxin, which potentiates the ability of PDGF to render cells competent,[3] also potentiated the PDGF-mediated down-regulation of EGF receptors, even though it had no effect on ^{125}I-EGF binding when added alone. When PDGF and cholera toxin were added together to quiescent 3T3 cells, there was a reduction between 85 and 95% in EGF binding. The ability of PDGF and cholera toxin to decrease EGF binding was substantially inhibited by cycloheximide. Coincidental with the dramatic loss in binding was

325

an abrogated growth requirement for EGF; that is, cells treated with PDGF and cholera toxin required only somatomedin C to traverse G_0/G_1 and initiate DNA synthesis.

REFERENCES

1. PLEDGER, W. J., C. D. STILES, H. N. ANTONIADES & C. D. SCHER. 1977. Proc. Natl. Acad. Sci. USA **74:** 4481.
2. CLEMMONS, D. R., J. J. VAN WYK & W. J. PLEDGER. 1980. Proc. Natl. Acad. Sci. USA **77:** 6644.
3. WHARTON, W., E. B. LEOF, N. OLASHAW, H. S. EARP & W. J. PLEDGER. J. Cell. Physiol. In press.

Index of Contributors